Cardiac Diseases - Novel Aspects of Cardiac Risk, Cardiorenal Pathology and Cardiac Interventions

Edited by David C. Gaze and Aleksandar Kibel

Published in London, United Kingdom

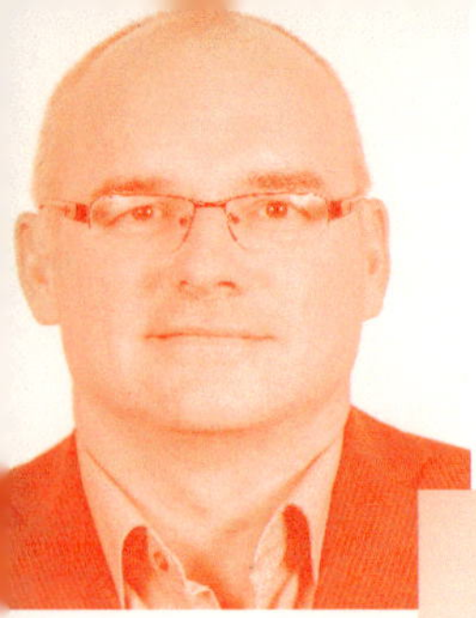
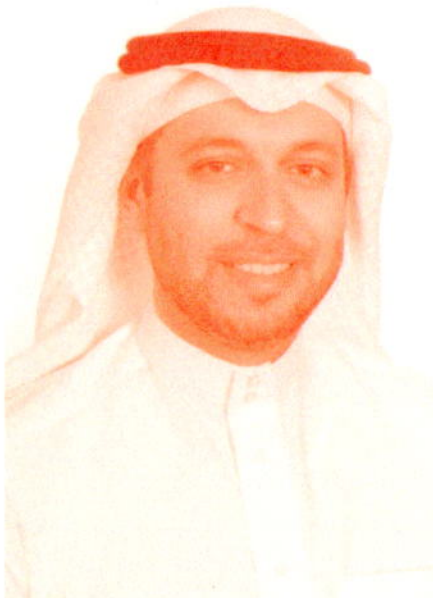
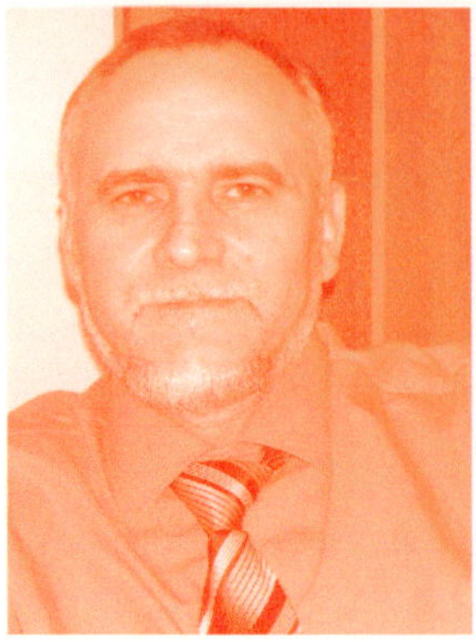
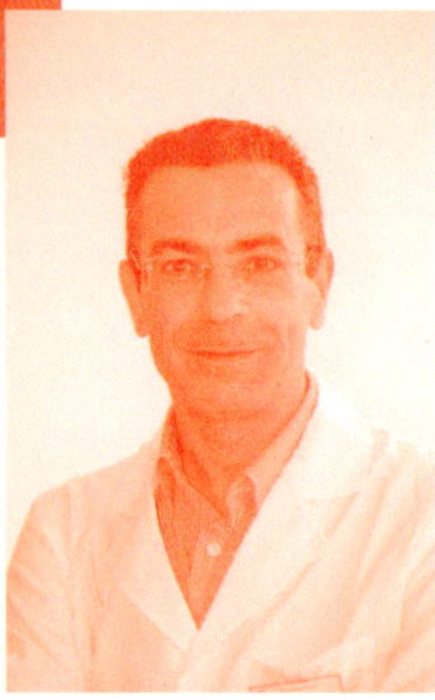
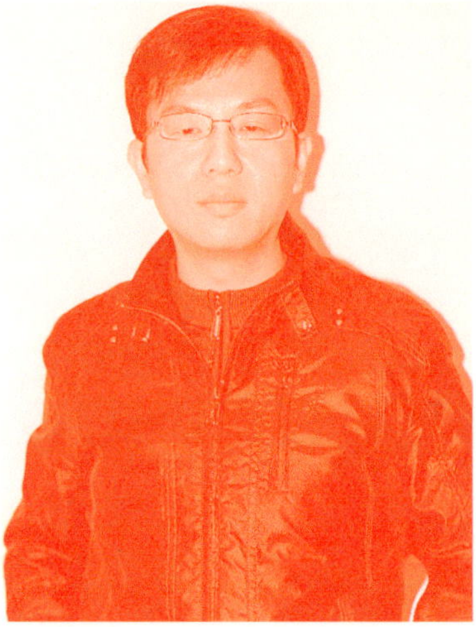
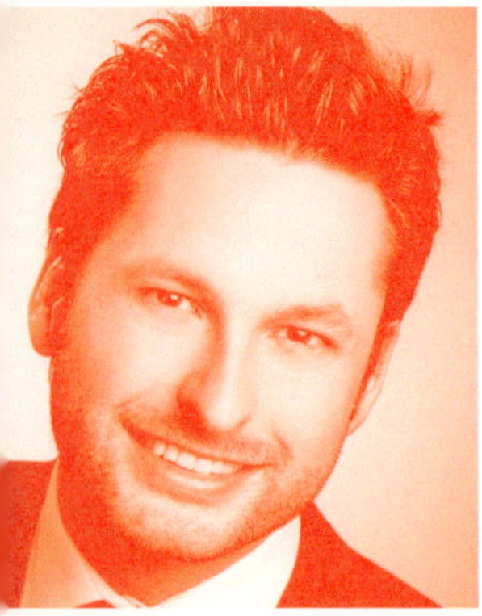
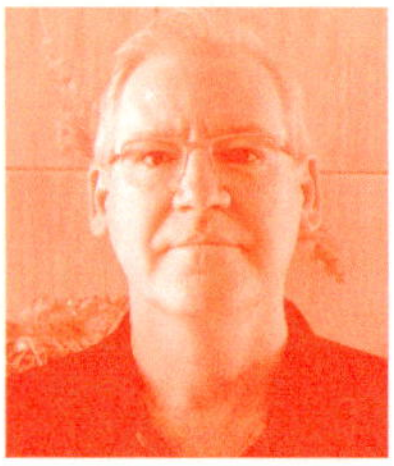

IntechOpen

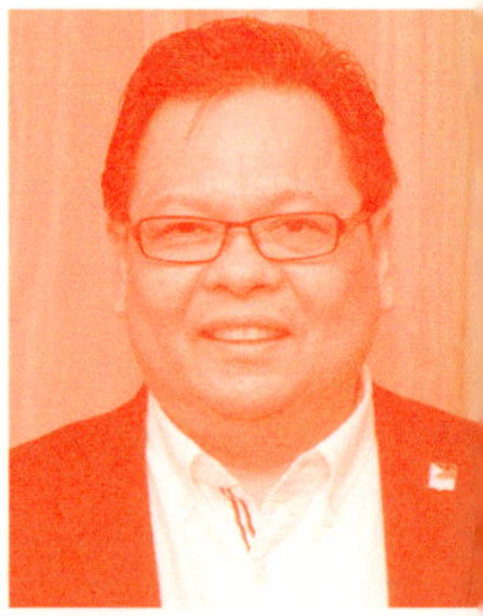
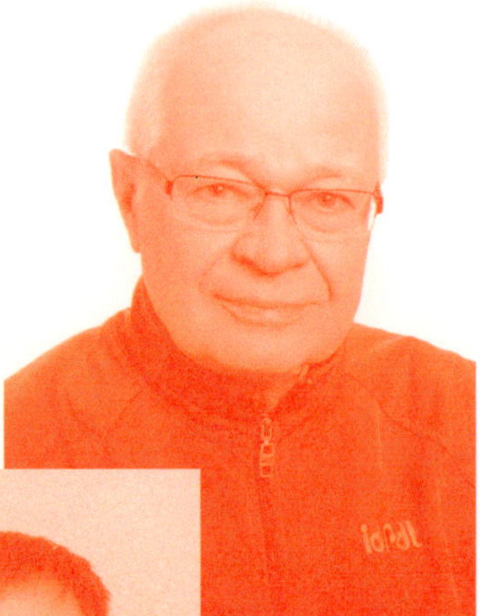
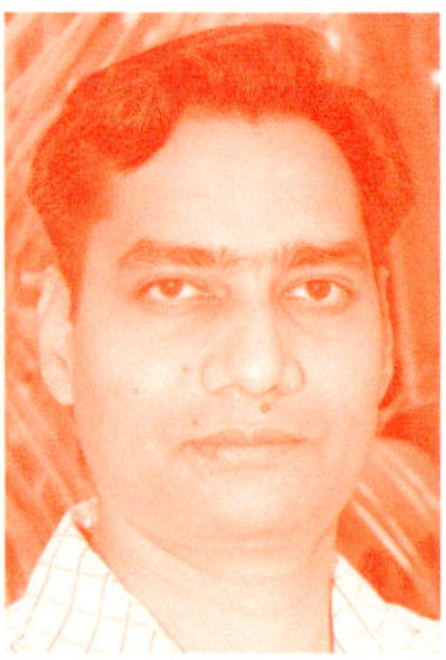
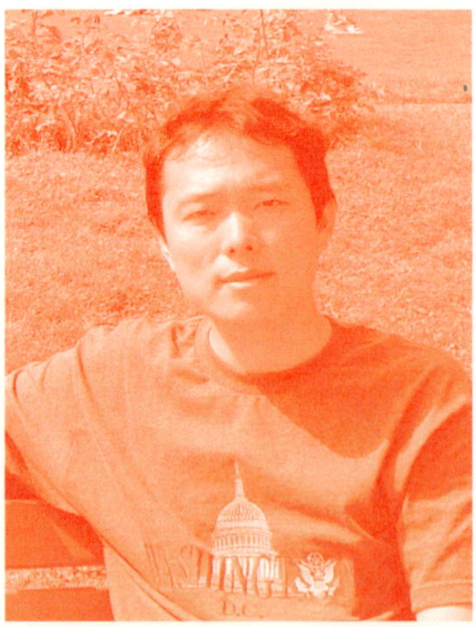
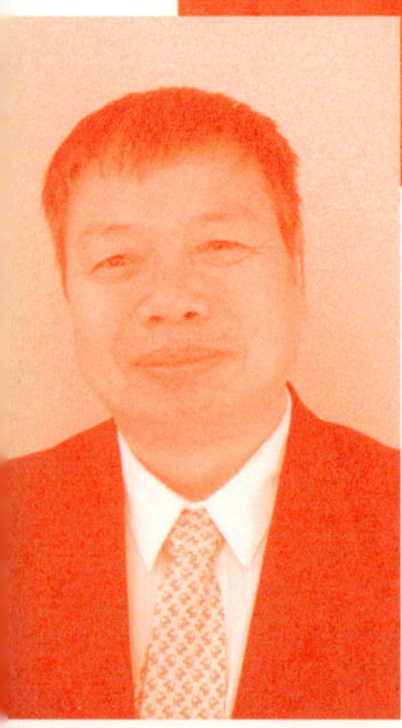
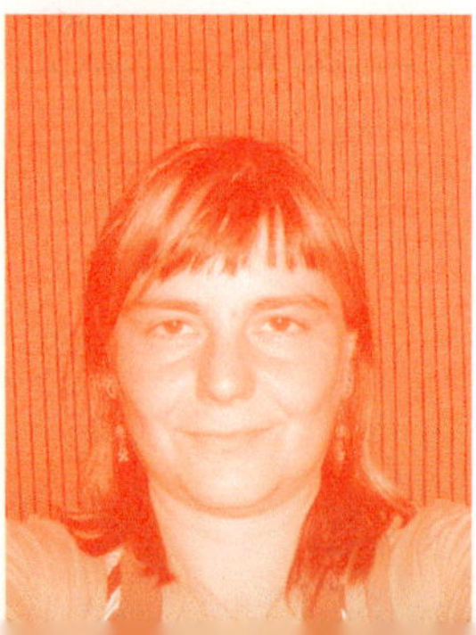

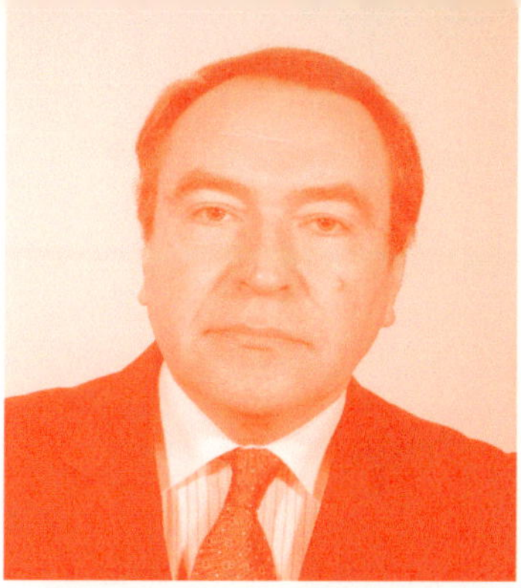

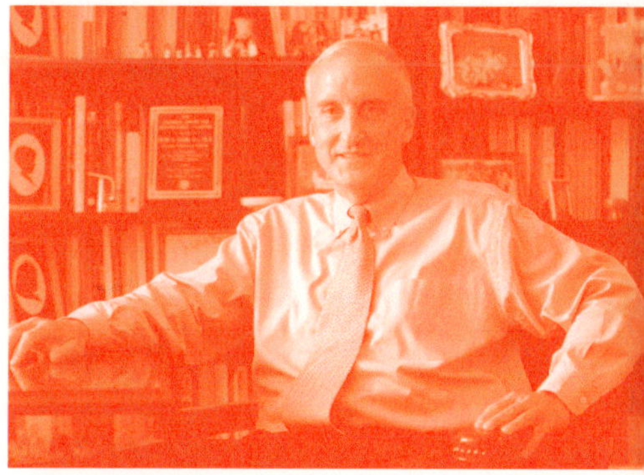

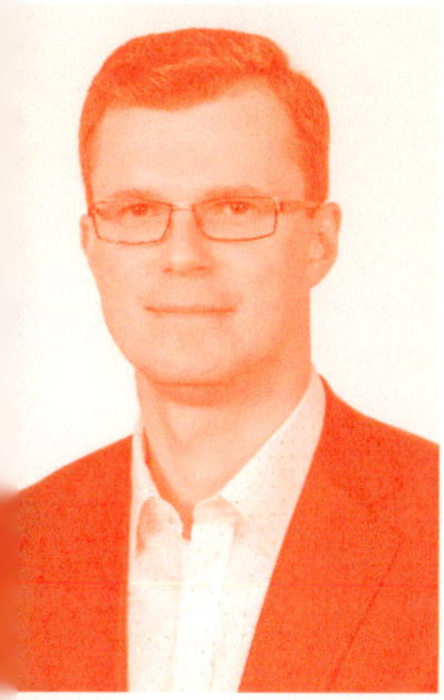

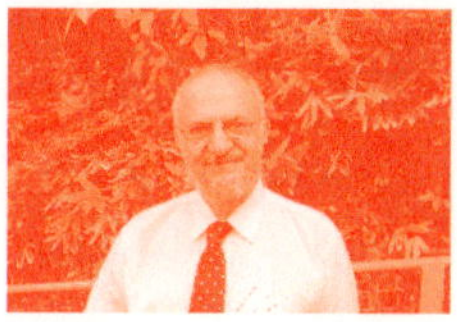

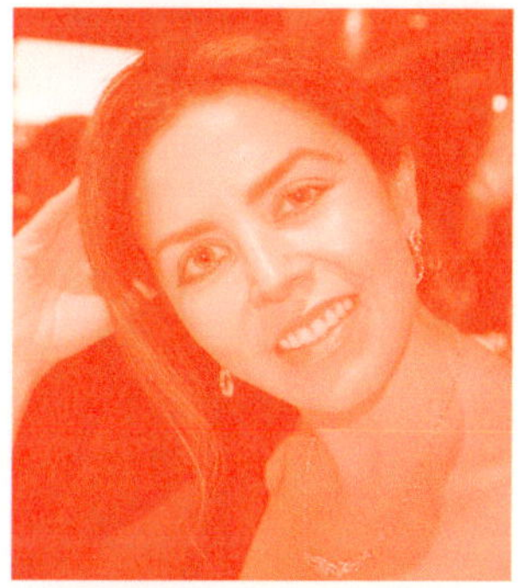

Supporting open minds since 2005

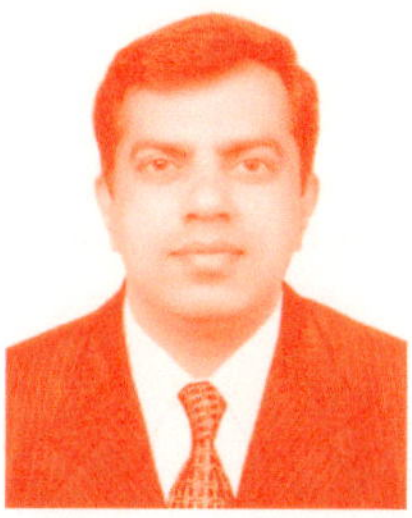

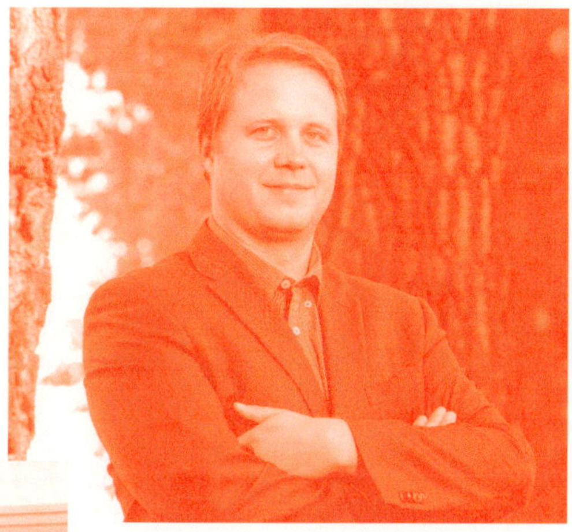

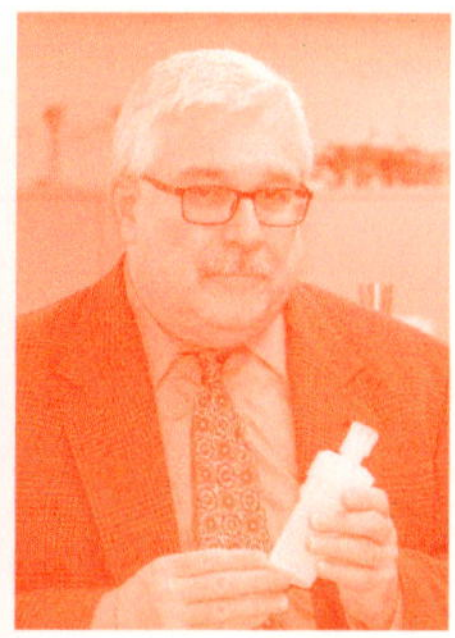

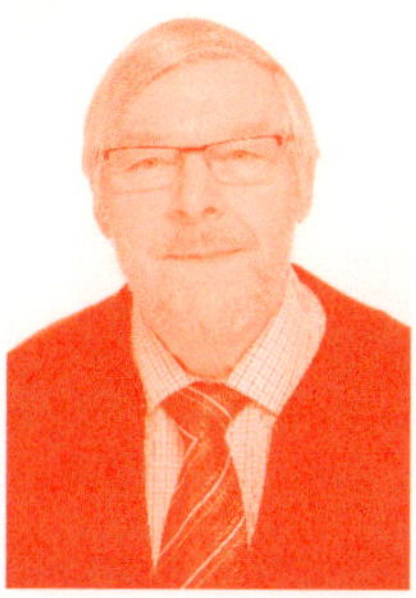

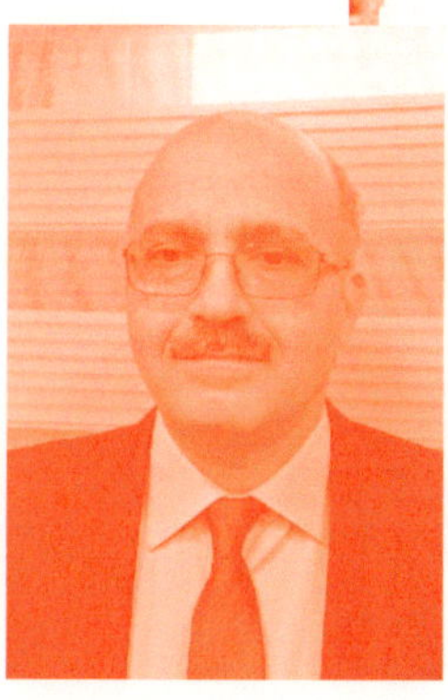

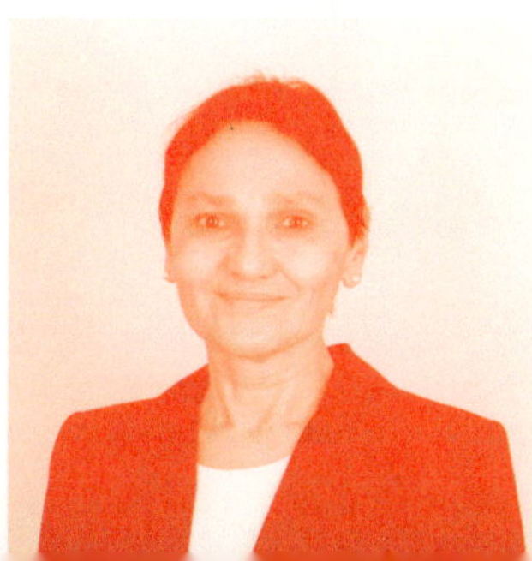

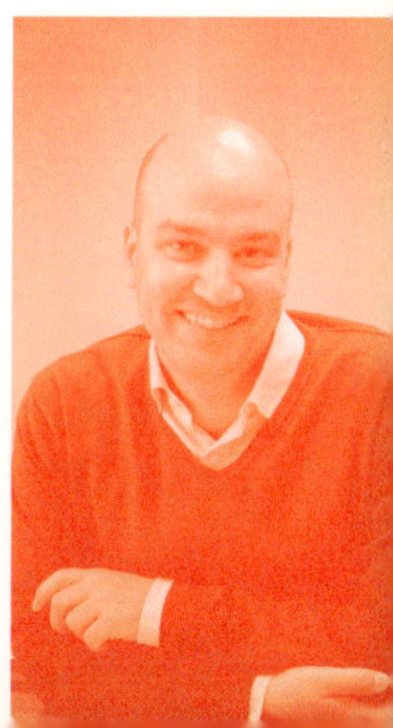

Cardiac Diseases - Novel Aspects of Cardiac Risk, Cardiorenal Pathology and Cardiac Interventions
http://dx.doi.org/10.5772/intechopen.87374
Edited by David C. Gaze and Aleksandar Kibel

Contributors
Mark Alekseevich Soborov, Ivana Škrlec, Catrin Rutland, Valentina Kubale, Ewelina Prozorowska, Kristýna Glocová, Lucy Slater, Wang Zhilu, Guo Yaya, Gao Yan, Wang Chenxia, YanPing Bai, Chuan Wang, Yang Yu, Chengxiong Gu, Jingxing Li, Iris Bararu Bojan, Oana-Viola Badulescu, Maria Vladeanu, Andrei Bojan, Manuela Ciocoiu, Miguel Alejandro Farah, Franco Farah, Miguel Angel Farah, Imran Khalil, Shogade Taiwo, Akpabio Akpabio, Pedro Ponce, ana Mateus, Hemant J. Mehta, Ketrell L. McWhorter, Yong-He Ding, Jing Zhong, Li-Ping Li, Jian-Feng Zhou, John G. Kingma, Valsalayam Raghavapanicker Sanal Kumar, Pradeep Kumar Radhakrishnan, Gayathri Ananyajyothi Ambat, Nihas Nazer, Nazer Yoosuf Abdul, David C. Gaze, Sobhi Mleyhi, Rim Miri, Raouf Denguir, Shiv Kumar Choudhary, Pradeep Kumar Radhakrishnan, Rajaghatta Sundararam Bharath, Nichith Chandrasekaran, Vigneshwaran Sankar, Ajith Sukumaran, Charlie Oommen

First published in London, United Kingdom, 2021 by IntechOpen
IntechOpen is the global imprint of INTECHOPEN LIMITED, registered in England and Wales, registration number: 11086078, 5 Princes Gate Court, London, SW7 2QJ, United Kingdom
Printed in Croatia

British Library Cataloguing-in-Publication Data
A catalogue record for this book is available from the British Library

Additional hard and PDF copies can be obtained from orders@intechopen.com

Cardiac Diseases - Novel Aspects of Cardiac Risk, Cardiorenal Pathology and Cardiac Interventions
Edited by David C. Gaze and Aleksandar Kibel
p. cm.
Print ISBN 978-1-83968-161-5
Online ISBN 978-1-83968-162-2
eBook (PDF) ISBN 978-1-83968-163-9

For EU product safety concerns:
IN TECH d.o.o., Prolaz Marije Krucifikse Kozulić 3, 51000 Rijeka, Croatia, info@intechopen.com or visit our website at intechopen.com.

Meet the editors

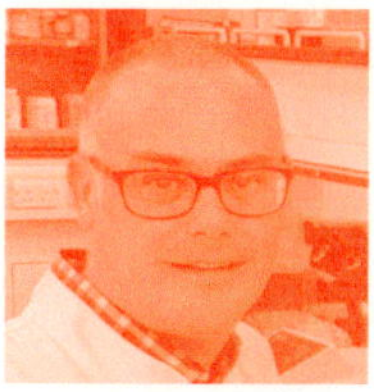

Dr. David Gaze is currently a lecturer in Clinical Biochemistry at the University of Westminster. His academic research interests are in the development and clinical utility of cardiac biomarkers for the detection of cardiovascular disease with a special interest in the cardiorenal population. He has authored and co-authored more than 150 peer-reviewed papers and 200 abstracts. He has contributed five book chapters to cardiovascular-related textbooks as well as is writing a textbook on cardiac troponin. He is a peer reviewer for 25 medical journals. He is the commissioning editor for review articles for the *Annals of Clinical Biochemistry & Laboratory Medicin*e and is Co-editor-in-chief of Practical Laboratory Medicine.

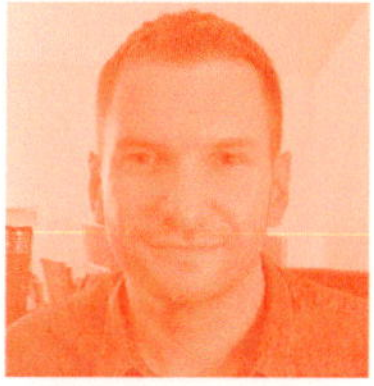

Aleksandar Kibel is an assistant professor at the Department of Physiology and Immunology at the Faculty of Medicine, University of Osijek, as well as an internal medicine specialist and cardiology subspecialist at the Department for Heart and Vascular Diseases, Osijek University Hospital Centre, Croatia. He graduated with a maximum possible grade average from the Faculty of Medicine, University of Osijek, with an MD degree in 2009, conducting experimental research activities during almost all study years and receiving awards that include the country's top scholarship ("Top Scholarship for Top Students"). Research activities included laboratory practicums and research visits at a number of foreign institutions including the University Clinic Hamburg-Eppendorf (Germany), the Medical College of Wisconsin (USA), Chulalongkorn University in Bangkok (Thailand), etc. He obtained his Ph.D. degree at the Department of Physiology and Immunology with a focus on vascular physiology and pathophysiology and teaches at the medical high school, university, and postgraduate doctoral levels. He served as a mentor on several diploma works. Prior work experience also includes work at the Emergency Medicine Department and an internship at the University Hospital Zagreb, as well as volunteer work at the Red Cross. He has published a number of scientific papers and three book chapters and has actively participated in many international scientific conferences, in research projects at the pre-clinical and clinical levels, and in pharmacological clinical trials as a sub-investigator. He is a guest editor of several special issues and an editorial board member of several international scientific journals.

Contents

Preface

This is the latest book in a series of cardiovascular-related texts from IntechOpen Publishing. The present volume considers general aspects of cardiac disease and is partitioned into three distinct sections.

1. Cardiac Risk

This section is comprised of chapters discussing the developmental risk of cardiac disease. Chapter 1 discusses the role of inflammation in the development of cardiovascular pathology, in particular the role of inflammation in the formation of thrombosis and the contribution to risk of myocardial infarction. Chapter 2 stays with myocardial infarction, offering perspectives on the pathophysiology of myocardial injury with insight into cardioprotective mechanisms. Chapter 3 examines the fascinating area of circadian rhythm disruption via an epigenetic approach to the development of cardiovascular disease. Chapter 4 specifically focuses on the global prevalence and diagnostic criteria in Takotsubo syndrome, indicating that universal acceptance of definition and diagnostic criteria is required. Chapter 5 examines the disproportionate differences in prognosis of patients according to gender following percutaneous coronary intervention with primary and secondary prevention recommendations. Chapter 6 investigates body image and obesity acceptance in relation to clinical cardiac risk factors. Study in this area suggests that the efficacy of classical risk reduction regimens (such as weight management, exercise, hypertensive and hyperglycaemic control, etc.) can be improved by the maintenance of a self-perception of 'normal' weight in reducing the risk of cardiovascular disease. Chapter 7 specialises in discussing the genetic determinants of familial dilated cardiomyopathy with a focus on genotype-targeted therapeutic strategies. Chapter 8 discusses the impact of coronavirus disease and the implication of the cardiovascular system in severe cases. The final chapter in section 1, chapter 9, the authors consider the role of the G-protein-coupled, seven-transmembrane receptors (7TMRs) and their role in the cardiovascular system and development of cardiomyopathy with attention to the role of autoimmunity and autoantibodies in cardiomyopathy.

2. Cardiorenal Pathology

Section 2 specifically examines the specialised area of cardiorenal pathology. Chapter 10 discusses the perils and opportunities of vascular access in renal patients being assessed for central venous diseases, while Chapter 11 focuses on early detection and endovascular intervention to correct dialysis vascular access failure.

3. Cardiovascular Interventions

The final section relates to surgical interventions as part of the armamentarium of medical therapies aimed to alleviate cardiovascular diseases. The section starts with Chapter 12 offering an overview of basic to advanced specialised techniques available to the interventional cardiologist to open occluded arteries in the hope of salvaging myocardial tissue. Chapter 13 focuses on the primary angioplasty in a geographic arrangement from artery to the myocardium with particular emphasis on novel treatments offering continuous myocardial protection, again to preserve tissue and improve overall prognosis. Chapter 14 turns attention to coronary artery bypass grafting (CABG) and the management of ascending aorta calcification which is an independent risk factor for cerebrovascular events post-off-pump CABG procedures. Chapter 15 deals with the surgical methodologies available for reconstructing distal aortic dissection. Chapter 16 identifies the complexities of mitral valve repair and focuses on a novel non-resectional repair technique. The penultimate chapter, chapter 17 discusses the complications of minimally invasive left ventricular assistance devices in patients with advanced cardiac failure. Last but by no means least, Chapter 18 discusses the radical approach of Sanal flow choking and its risk association to asymptomatic cardiovascular disease as demonstrated through a review of *In Vitro* and *In Silico* studies.

The eighteen chapters above offer insight into the current state of the art with respect to risk of developing cardiovascular diseases, maintenance of patent vascular access in patients with cardiorenal syndrome, and a plethora of novel interventional technologies all aimed at salvaging damaged tissue and improving prognosis and reducing mortality.

At the inception of this book, the World was a very different place. With the rapid emergence of coronavirus diseases, the value of the content of this book is now more important than ever; especially through the open-access platform allowing such knowledge to be freely available to those in less fortunate situations.

The editors wish to thank the authors of each chapter for providing their expert insight into the chapter content and responding rapidly to our revision requests. Our gratitude is also extended most humbly to those authors and co-authors who have turned any clinical responsibilities to the fight against COVID-19.

We also wish to extend our thanks to the publishing management team at IntechOpen Publishing, notably to Sandra Maljavac and Dolores Kuzelj.

Dr. David C. Gaze
University of Westminster,
London, United Kingdom

Dr. Aleksandar Kibel
Osijek University Hospital,
Osijek, Croatia

Dedication

Mr Charles Benjamin Flint

20th March 1936 – 17th April 2020

One of the many victims of the COVID-19 Pandemic DCG

Section 1

Cardiac Risk

Chapter 1

Correlations between Inflammation and Thrombosis in the Pathogeny of Myocardial Infarction

Iris Bararu Bojan, Oana-Viola Badulescu, Maria Vladeanu, Andrei Bojan and Manuela Ciocoiu

Abstract

Atherosclerosis is the main cause of myocardial infarction. This process involves a complex interplay between metabolic pathways governing lipid deposition, inflammatory and immune responses to oxidized lipids, and endothelial dysfunction. Myocardial infarction appears when these processes culminate with a thrombotic event. Markers of inflammation, such as C-reactive protein (CRP), myeloperoxidase (MPO) and leukocyte levels are strong predictors of cardiovascular death, myocardial infarction, and stroke. This process involves a complex interplay between metabolic pathways governing lipid deposition, inflammatory and immune responses to oxidized lipids, and endothelial dysfunction. Myocardial infarction appears when these processes culminate with a thrombotic event. Markers of inflammation, such as C-reactive protein (CRP), myeloperoxidase (MPO) and leukocyte levels are strong predictors of cardiovascular death, myocardial infarction, and stroke. This review will summarize the molecular and cellular links between inflammation and thrombosis in the context of myocardial infarction, which support the concept of a thrombo inflammatory state leading to the vessel obstruction and to the subsequent myocardial necrosis.

Keywords: thrombosis, inflammation, atherosclerosis

1. Introduction

Myocardial infarction is a form of coronary artery disease, in which the occlusion of the coronary artery induces ischemia of the subsequent territory and eventually leads to the destruction of up to a billion myocardic cells.

Atherosclerosis is the main cause of myocardial infarction. This process involves a complex interplay between metabolic pathways governing lipid deposition, inflammatory and immune responses to oxidized lipids, and endothelial dysfunction.

Myocardial infarction appears when these processes culminate with a thrombotic event. Markers of inflammation, such as C-reactive protein (CRP), myeloperoxidase (MPO) and leukocyte levels are strong predictors of cardiovascular death, myocardial infarction, and stroke [1].

IntechOpen

As the human heart cannot regenerate, the acute myocardial infarction is associated with the destruction of large proportion of myocardium that will lead to the development of a collagen scar. This process is associated with an evident inflammatory reaction. This inflammatory reaction will lead to the chemotaxis of leukocytes that will be preferentially localized at the border of the necrotic myocardium. These leukocytes may lead to cytotoxic reactions that can increase the injured zone [2].

2. The role of inflammation in myocardial infarction

The acute pro-inflammatory process triggered by the onset of myocardial infarction consists in multiple processes such as the production of reactive oxygen species and DAMPs (damage associated molecular patterns) which are in fact the substrate for PRRs (pattern recognition receptors). These processes will eventually lead to the formation of cytokines and chemokines that will mediate the attraction of thee inflammatory cells to the border zone of the myocardial infarction.

After the onset of a myocardial infarction the healing process involves three important phases: the inflammatory response, the proliferation and in the end the maturation.

During the inflammatory response the necrotic cardiomyocytes release danger signals, called alarmins that will signalize some particular types of receptors called TLRs (toll-like receptors) and RAGE (receptor for advanced glycation end products), thus stimulating the immune cells, the endothelial ones and the fibroblasts to secrete chemokines and cytokines. The inflammatory phase is also characterized by the activation of the complement cascade. The complement cascade can be activated in three different manners: the classic pathway, the lectin and the alternate way [1–3]. These pathways all lead to the common pathway that results in opsonization, subsequent inflammation attracting others phagocytes, or activation of thee cell killing membrane attack complex – **Figure 1**.

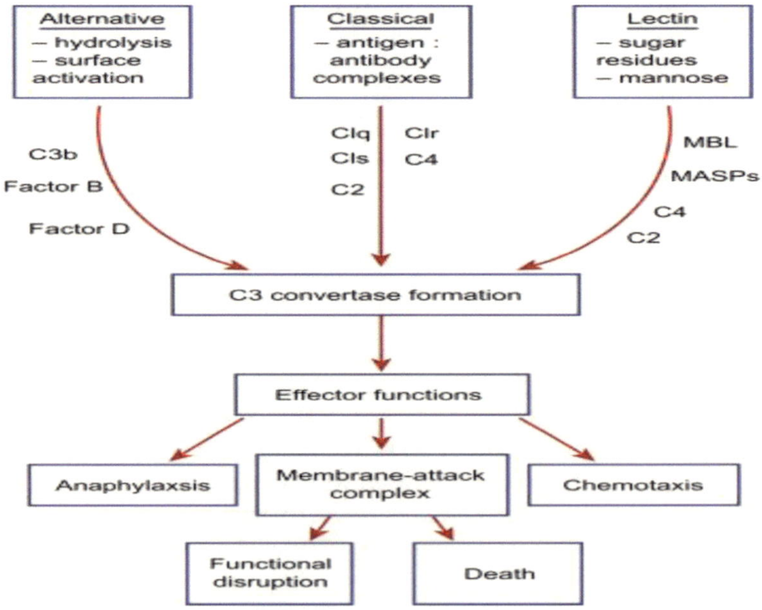

Figure 1.
The complement cascade – https://www.sciencedirect.com/topics/medicine-and-dentistry/complement-system.

The inflammatory process and the activation of the complement cascade determine the release of pro-inflammatory cytokines, such as Tumor Necrosis Factor (TNF)-α, IL-1β and IL-6.

A key role in the activation of the inflammatory reaction is played by the IL-1 signaling pathway. This pathway stimulates the production of chemokines by fibroblasts and leukocytes, but inhibits the conversion of fibroblasts in myofibroblasts. Damaged myocardial cells release IL-1α, while IL-1β is upregulated after infarction. An important key for this mechanism is represented by the inflammasome, which triggers the activation of caspase-1 and thus transforms active pro-IL-1β into IL-1β. It was shown that the inflammasome can be found both in myocardial and in interstitial cells in the ischemic myocardium. The pharmacological blockage of IL-1 or the genetic inhibition proved to reduce left ventricle remodelation after myocardial infarction [4, 5].

IL-6 is associated with both pro and anti-inflammatory effects. Myocardial infarction is associated with increased circulating IL-6. Some studies showed that the genetic polymorphisms of the IL-6 receptor signaling pathway may lead to a diminished plasma level of high-sensitivity C-reactive protein (hs-CRP) and thus may lead to the decrease of cardiovascular risk [6].

The post-infarction inflammatory response determines a chemokine upregulation, which are responsible for the recruitment of other leukocytes in the infarcted area.

The neutrophils are activated by CXC chemokines containing the Glu-Leu-Arg sequence (the ELR motif), such as CXCL8/IL-8, while the CC chemokines, such as monocyte chemo attractant protein-(MCP)-1/CCL2 and CCL7 attract monocytes. The phagocytosis is activated and the necrotic detritus is eliminated, so that the healing process may start. When the infiltrated neutrophils enter the apoptotic process, the inflammatory phase comes to an end [7].

From this moment on the apoptotic cells are scavenged by professional phagocytes, thus leading to a process called efferocytosis. This phase consists in the release of cytokines with anti-inflammatory effect such as IL-10 and TGF-β. These mediators induce an endogenous intracellular signal, such as Interleukin-receptor associated kinase-M that inhibits the pro-inflammatory process in the healing areas of the myocardium. The inhibition of inflammatory signaling and the removal of the inflammatory infiltrate is determined by the presence of inhibitory leukocyte, such as anti-inflammatory monocyte subpopulations and regulatory T cells [8].

The remaining cardiomyocytes in the infarct border zone secrete mediators with anti-inflammatory properties that lead to the diminishment of the affected area. If the inflammatory response is unrestrained or is very expansive, the result will consist in rapid left ventricle remodeling, which can be implicated in inducing heart failure in patients surviving an acute myocardial infarction.

When the proliferative phase of myocardial infarction has begun, the diminishment of pro-inflammatory molecules such as IL-1β and Interferon-γ-inducible Protein (IP)-10 causes the transformation of fibroblasts in myofibroblasts. These compounds have an extensive endoplasmic reticulum and possess a contractile protein that is called α-smooth muscle actin (α-SMA) and are capable of inducing an increased synthesis of matrix protein [7–9].

When the proliferative phase comes to an end, the mature scar starts to form. The myofibroblasts enter apoptosis and matrix cross-linking occurs. This mechanism seems to be mediated by the removal of growth factors, the inhibition of TGF-β mediated response and the modification of the composition of the matrix.

In the remaining healthy myocardium the fibroblasts may rest chronically active as s result of a pressure overload. This will induce the fibrosis of the myocardium and will lead to diastolic dysfunction.

As inflammation plays a key-role in the pathogenesis of myocardial infarction, some authors thought that giving anti-inflammatory therapy to patients with acute coronary syndrome would be beneficial, but the results proved that treatment with corticosteroids or with NSAIDs is associated with a worsened outcome. Due to the non-selective inhibition of the inflammatory cascade, these drugs have potentially catastrophic consequences. Therefore the current guidelines are against the use of broad range anti-inflammatory therapy in patients with acute coronary syndrome [10, 11].

A better understanding of the process of inflammation in myocardial infarction leads to the conclusion that targeted inhibition of selected inflammatory routes may add up to the protection of the vulnerable myocardium without harming the reparative response. There are studies that showed that a targeted neutralization of specific inflammatory mediators such as chemokines and cytokines can reduce the size of the infarction.

3. The role of thrombosis in myocardial infarction

Inflammation is responsible for inducing an active atheroclerotic plaque, but this plaque is not sufficient to induce a myocardial. After the plaque has ruptured, the hemostatic balance is impaired, thus leading to coronary thrombosis. The alterations of the hemostatic balance consist in increased platelet adhesion, coagulation cascade activation and subsequent. Over-activated procoagulation determines a thrombophillic status that can be acquired from complex patterns of inheritance or environmental risk factors.

The thrombotic events may be caused by an increase of different coagulation factors. Plasmatic fibrinogen is an important cardiovascular risk factor. It was proven that increased levels of Interleukin 6, may lead to an increased hepatic synthesis of fibrinogen, thus representing an important link between inflammation and thrombophilic status.

Thrombin or FIIa is a serin protease which has an important clotting effect. The importance of thrombin in the clotting anomalies is rather disputed. Some studies have shown that the concentration of thrombin in patients with coronary artery disease is normal and that it does not represent a predicting factor for vascular complications, while other researchers have stipulated that thrombin is one of the most important factors responsible for the thrombotic complications. Nevertheless, increased levels of thrombin are associated with the presence of denser thrombus structures, with a diminished permeability, which is resistant to fibrinolysis [12–14].

Clotting factor XIII is involved in hemostasis, fibrinolysis, vascular remodeling and tissue repair. It is important to do the genotyping of factor XIII in order to assess the prothrombotic status because the existing data in the literature rest unclear. Clotting factor XIII is a pro-transglutaminase with tetrameric structure consisting of two active subunits A and two inhibitory/protective subunits B. The clotting factor XIII genotyping has shown that mixed FXIII heterozygous mutants (formed from a wild allele and a mutant one) were associated with increased levels of total and LDL-cholesterol and with elevated concentrations of CRP, while the other genotypes of clotting factor XIII have not been correlated with these changes [15–18].

From our personal experience, from a clinical study including 60 patients with myocardial infarction, we found out that 25% of patients had heterozygous mutants of factor XIII (wild type + mutant type), the majority of them being elderly men. Almost one third of the patients with PAI-1 4G/4G genotype and a quarter of those with genotype 5G/5G were associated with heterozygous mutants of FXIII

(WT + MT); the combined 4G/5G genotype was associated only with wild-type FXIII. The clotting factor XIII genotyping realized during the current research has shown that mixed FXIII heterozygous mutants (formed from a wild allele and a mutant one) were associated with increased levels of total and LDL cholesterol and with elevated concentrations of C-reactive protein, while the other genotypes of clotting factor XIII have not been correlated with these changes – **Figure 2**.

These genomic changes appear to be responsible for the decreased permeability of the formed thrombus and for the inhibition of the fibrinolysis process, which explains the higher incidence of acute coronary syndromes and complex coronary artery lesions in type 2 diabetic patients [19, 20].

The atherothrombotic complications may be caused also by a modification in fibrinolysis. The fibrinolysis is initiated by the conversion of plasminogen in plasmin, a process which is mediated mainly by the tisular plasminogen activator (tPA).

The plasminogen activator inhibitor type 1 (PAI-1) is the primary inhibitor of the fibrinolysis, which acts by forming a complex with tPA. PAI-1 gene is situated on the 7th chromosome and contains 8 introns and 9 exons. The effect of PAI-1 is the down-regulation of the fibrinolytic process as it inhibits the transformation of plasminogen to plasmin regulated by tissue-plasminogen activator and urokinase [21–23].

PAI-1 levels are proportional with the degree of the inflammatory process, induce atherosclerosis and are linked to the presence of metabolic syndrome. Obesity and diabetes mellitus type 2 are pathological conditions associated with increased PAI-1 levels that may lead to extensive atherosclerosis. Human CD 34+ cells exert high levels of PAI-1 especially in patients with diabetes and micro vascular complications. High levels of PAI-1 are associated with visceral adiposity because this molecule is produced by ectopic fat depots. The inflammatory state conferred by the high PAI-1 levels cause a dysfunctional activity of the cytokines (IL-8, leukotriene B4) and can determine impaired monocyte migration [24].

There are 5 polymorphisms of the PAI-1 gene: 675 4G/5G, 844 A > G, Ala15Thr, Val17Ile and Asn195Ile. The 4G/5G polymorphism (the deletion/insertion of guanosine in the 675 position of the PAI-1 gene promoter) is a major genetic determinant of PAI-1 levels. Some authors have suggested that the 4G allele association with other thrombophilic defects (factor V Leiden, prothrombin mutation, hyperhomocysteinemia, and decreased activity of protein C or S) increases the risk of thrombosis. In patients with coronary artery disease the presence of PAI-1 4G/4G genotype was associated with an increased risk of sudden death. When PAI-1 has an increased activity, the high circulating levels of PAI-1 may induce the persistence of microthrombi, therefore leading to a prothrombotic state in an early myocardial infarction please, which will affect the short-term outcome of patients with acute coronary syndrome. Even more PAI-1 levels are linked to the degree of myocardial fibrosis that can lead to detrimental left ventricle remodeling and poor long-term prognosis [25–28].

From our personal experience from a research involving 60 patients with acute coronary syndrome, we found out that the majority of patients had the 4G/4G

Figure 2.
Identification of factor XIII Val34Leu polymorphism.

genotype, which was associated with elevated levels of glycated hemoglobin and with a high concentration of LDL cholesterol and fibrinogen and with multivessel atherosclerosis, while the other genotypes of PAI-1 were not correlated with these changes – **Figures 3** and **4**.

In our studied group, 65% of patients had the PAI-1 4G/4G genotype, while 15% of patients had a heterozygote 4G/5G genotype. Not only did PAI-1 4G/4G genotype associate more frequently with atherogenic dyslipidemia, but it also showed a slight direct correlation with the inflammatory parameters – **Figure 5**.

As a consequence we can assume that the prothrombotic status found in patients with myocardial infarction seems to be modulated by the genomic polymorphism of clotting factor XIII, which is responsible for the formation of a more stable cruoric thrombus which is more resistant to fibrinolysis. Even more, these patients show a deficiency of the endogenous fibrinolysis, which predisposes the development of a thrombophilic status. This decrease in the thrombolytic process seems to derive from the genomic polymorphism of plasminogen activator inhibitor type 1. The most common genotype of PAI-1 associated with an increased cardiovascular risk is PAI-1 4G genotype. These polymorphisms are correlated with the presence of metabolic disorders and an abnormal inflammatory process in patients with acute coronary syndrome, thereby inducing an increased cardiovascular risk in these patients.

Fibrinogen and PAI polimorphism

Genotype	N	Mean	Std. Deviation	Std. Error	CI 95%		Min	Max	Test t-Student p
					-95%CI	+95%CI			
PAI-1									
4G	39	5.43	0.92	0.18	5.06	5.80	3.81	7.32	0.037
5G	12	5.59	0.46	0.16	5.20	5.97	5..00	6.21	
4G/5G	9	6.42	0.58	0.24	5.81	7.02	5.90	7.20	

Figure 3.
The relationship between PAI-1 polymorphism and the plasmatic level of fibrinogen.

LDL Cholesterol and the genomic polimorphism

Genotype	N	Mean	Std. Deviation	Std. Error	CI 95%		Min	Max	Test t-Student p
					-95%CI	+95%CI			
PAI-1									
4G	39	199.00	29.72	5.83	187.00	211.00	136	240	0.037
5G	12	200.38	42.91	15.17	164.51	236.24	150	265	
4G/5G	9	161.67	20.48	8.36	140.17	183.16	131	180	

Figure 4.
The relationship between PAI-1 polymorphism and the plasmatic level of LDL-cholesterol.

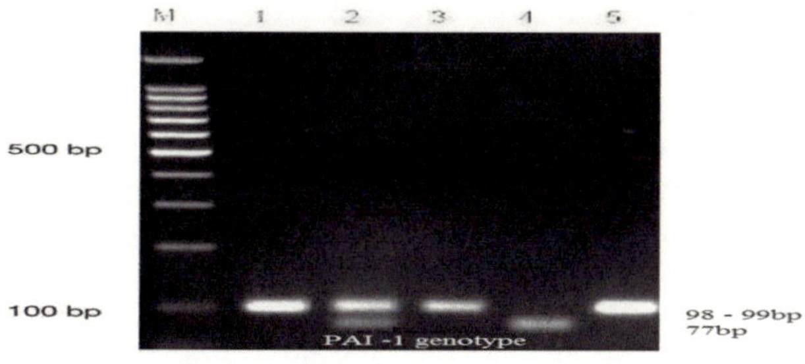

Figure 5.
Identification of PAI-1 polymorphism.

In conclusion, a better understanding of the inflammatory and thrombotic processes that lead to myocardial infarction can help improve the manner of treatment for this patients, thus increasing their quality of life and their prognostic.

Author details

Iris Bararu Bojan, Oana-Viola Badulescu*, Maria Vladeanu, Andrei Bojan and Manuela Ciocoiu
University of Medicine and Pharmacy Gr. T. Popa, Iași, Romania

*Address all correspondence to: violabadulescu@yahoo.com

References

[1] Saxena A, Russo I, Frangogiannis NG. Inflammation as a therapeutic target in myocardial infarction: Learning from past failures to meet future challenges. Translational Research. 2016;**167**(1):152-166. DOI: 10.1016/j.trsl.2015.07.002

[2] Frangogiannis NG. The immune system and the remodeling infarcted heart: Cell biological insights and therapeutic opportunities. Journal of Cardiovascular Pharmacology. 2014;**63**:185-195

[3] Entman ML, Youker K, Shoji T, et al. Neutrophil induced oxidative injury of cardiac myocytes. A compartmented system requiring CD11b/CD18-ICAM-1 adherence. The Journal of Clinical Investigation. 1992;**90**:1335-1345

[4] Chen C, Feng Y, Zou L, et al. Role of extracellular RNA and TLR3-Trif signaling in myocardial ischemia-reperfusion injury. Journal of the American Heart Association. 2014;**3**:e000683

[5] Zhang W, Lavine KJ, Epelman S, et al. Necrotic myocardial cells release damage-associated molecular patterns that provoke fibroblast activation in vitro and trigger myocardial inflammation and fibrosis in vivo. Journal of the American Heart Association. 2015;**4**

[6] Harrison SC, Smith AJ, Jones GT, et al. Interleukin-6 receptor pathways in abdominal aortic aneurysm. European Heart Journal. 2013;**34**(48):3707-3716. DOI: 10.1093/eurheartj/ehs354

[7] Ong SB, Hernández-Reséndiz S, Crespo-Avilan GE, et al. Inflammation following acute myocardial infarction: Multiple players, dynamic roles, and novel therapeutic opportunities. Pharmacology & Therapeutics. 2018;**186**:73-87. DOI: 10.1016/j.pharmthera.2018.01.001

[8] Empana JP, Jouven X, Canoui-Poitrine F, Luc G, Tafflet M, Haas B. C-reactive protein, interleukin 6, fibrinogen and risk of sudden death in European middle-aged men: The PRIME study. Arteriosclerosis, Thrombosis, and Vascular Biology. 2010;**30**:2047-2052

[9] Swerdlow DI, Holmes MV, Kuchenbaecker KB, Engmann JE, Shah T, Sofat R. The interleukin-6 receptor as a target for prevention of coronary heart disease: A Mendelian randomisation analysis. Lancet. 2012;**379**:1214-1224

[10] Serhan CN, Chiang N, Van Dyke TE. Resolving inflammation: Dual anti-inflammatory and pro-resolution lipid mediators. Nature Reviews. Immunology. 2008;**8**:349-361

[11] Shinde AV, Frangogiannis NG. Fibroblasts in myocardial infarction: A role in inflammation and repair. Journal of Molecular and Cellular Cardiology. 2014;**70**:74-82

[12] Li C, Ren H, Chen H, et al. Prothrombin G20210A (rs1799963) polymorphism increases myocardial infarction risk in an age-related manner: A systematic review and meta-analysis. Scientific Reports. 2017;**7**(1):13550. DOI: 10.1038/s41598-017-13623-6

[13] Ridker PM, Hennekens CH, Miletich JP. G20210A mutation in prothrombin gene and risk of myocardial infarction, stroke, and venous thrombosis in a large cohort of US men. Circulation. 1999;**99**:999-1004

[14] Sode BF, Allin KH, Dahl M, Gyntelberg F, Nordestgaard BG. Risk of venous thromboembolism and myocardial infarction associated with factor V Leiden and prothrombin mutations and blood type. CMAJ. 2013;**185**:E229-E237. DOI: 10.1503/cmaj.121636

[15] Rosendaal FR. Clotting and myocardial infarction: A cycle of insights. Journal of Thrombosis and Haemostasis. 2003;**1**:640-642. DOI: 10.1046/j.1538-7836.2003.00233.x

[16] Wu W, Liu R, Chen L, Chen H, Zhang S. Disequilibrium of blood coagulation and fibrinolytic system in patients with coronary artery ectasia. Medicine (Baltimore). 2016;**95**:e2779. DOI: 10.1097/MD.0000000000002779

[17] Silvain J, Pena A, Vignalou JB, Hulot JS, Galier S, Cayla G, et al. FXIII-A Leu34 genetic variant in premature coronary artery disease: A genotype–phenotype case control study. Thrombosis and Haemostasis. 2011;**106**:511-520

[18] Board PG. Genetic polymorphism of the B subunit of human coagulation factor XIII. American Journal of Human Genetics. 1980;**32**:348-353

[19] Leifheit HJ, Cleve H. Analysis of the genetic polymorphism of coagulation factor XIIIB (FXIIIB) by isoelectric focusing. Electrophoresis. 1988;**9**:426-429. DOI: 10.1002/elps.1150090814

[20] Komanasin N, Catto AJ, Futers TS, van HylckamaVlieg A, Rosendaal FR, Ariens RA. A novel polymorphism in the factor XIII B-subunit (His95Arg): Relationship to subunit dissociation and venous thrombosis. Journal of Thrombosis and Haemostasis. 2005;**3**:2487-2496

[21] Nordt TK, Lohrmann J, Bode C. Regulation of PAI-1 expression by genetic polymorphism. Impact on atherogenesis. Thrombosis Research. 2001;**103**(Suppl. 1):S1-S5

[22] Dai Y, Gao RL, Ye Y, Wu YJ, Chen JL, et al. The 4G/5G genetic polymorphism of the plasminogen activator inhibitor-1 (PAI-1) gene is not associated with plasma PAI-1 antigen level and the risk of coronary artery disease in Chinese. Chinese Circulation Journal. 2001;**16**:275-278

[23] Li XS, Xian SX, Huang HQ. Relationship between plasminogen activator inhibitor-1 gene and coronary heart disease with blood-stagnation syndrome. Journal of Guangzhou University of Traditional Chinese Medicine. 2002;**19**:261-264

[24] Fu Y, Wang XD, Zhai YL, Fan Z, Yang L, et al. The 4G/5G polymorphism of the plasminogen activator inhibitor-1 gene in patients with coronary heart disease. Journal of Capital University of Medical Sciences. 2001;**22**:119-122

[25] Xu K, Liu X, Yang F, et al. PAI-1 -675 4G/5G polymorphism in association with diabetes and diabetic complications susceptibility: A meta-analysis study. PLoS One. 2013;**8**(11):e79150. DOI: 10.1371/journal.pone.0079150

[26] Thomas WJ, Ansgar JP, Gunnar P, Frank-Chris S. Hemostatic risk factors in patients with coronary artery disease and type 2 diabetes - a two year follow-up of 243 patients. Cardiovascular Diabetology. 2009;**8**:48-52

[27] Tengyue Z, Chong P, Ningdong L, Elaine Z, Kanxing Z. Plasminogen activator inhibitor-1 4G/5G polymorphism and retinopathy risk in type 2 diabetes: A meta-analysis. BMC Medicine. 2013;**11, 1**:120-124

[28] Lopes C, Dina C, Durand E, Froguel P. PAI-1 polymorphisms modulate phenotypes associated with the metabolic syndrome in obese and diabetic Caucasian population. Diabetologia. 2003;**46**:1284-1290

Chapter 2

Acute Myocardial Infarction: Perspectives on Physiopathology of Myocardial Injury and Protective Interventions

John G. Kingma

Abstract

Diffuse coronary artery injury produces a host of physiopathological, structural and metabolic changes in cardiocytes that, if not rectified, result in significant loss of functional myocardium to cause cardiac contractile dysfunction. Restoration of blood perfusion to the infarct-related artery helps to limit the acute effects of myocardial infarction; however, cardiocyte injury may be exacerbated because of the restoration of blood perfusion to the ischemic zone (i.e. reperfusion injury). Various manifestations of reperfusion injury include no-reflow, myocardial stunning or hibernation and ventricular arrhythmias. Consequently, reperfusion of an infarct related artery is often viewed in the context of being a "double-edged sword." Pharmacologic and non-pharmacologic interventions have been investigated in pre-clinical and clinical studies in the hunt to develop strategies to protect cardiomyocytes against the long-term effects of ischemia, or delay development of necrosis (resulting from ischemia or reperfusion). This book chapter will update current thinking on cardioprotective strategies to improve clinical outcomes in patients with coronary artery disease.

Keywords: acute myocardial infarction, cardioprotection, ischemic conditioning, myocardial ischemia, reperfusion injury

1. Introduction

Physiopathological mechanisms responsible for myocardial cell death (necrosis, apoptosis, autophagy, etc.) caused by coronary artery disease have been abundantly discussed over the past several decades. Acute myocardial infarction is a leading cause of sudden cardiac death among urban dwellers in North America and Europe. Clinical treatment of patients with coronary artery disease is focused on limiting the deleterious consequences that follow coronary artery occlusion; however, to do so it is fundamental to understand the mechanisms, at the molecular and cellular level, that are involved in cell death and survival. Existing knowledge has progressed massively over the years and useful clinical interventions, both pharmacologic and non-pharmacologic, are currently available to limit, but not abrogate, effects of ischemia. An important question that remains concerns the existence of "reperfusion-induced injury"; many adhere to the notion that significant cellular death can occur once blood flow is restored to an infarct-related artery. While definitive proof is lacking myocardial stunning, vascular no-reflow (perfusion deficit) and ventricular arrhythmias are often attributed to this form of cardiomyocyte loss after ischemia. The objective of the present chapter is to update current thinking on the question of lethal reperfusion injury and to summarize current treatments used to limit overall effects.

1.1 Acute myocardial infarction

Myocardial ischemia is defined as *the condition where coronary blood flow across the ventricular wall is insufficient to conserve steady-state metabolism*. Acute disruption of the blood supply to any region of the heart causes cardiomyocyte injury and eventually cellular death depending on the duration of perfusion deficit. Cardiac cell injury is characterized to be either *reversible* (if reperfusion of the infarct-related artery can be instituted rapidly, ≤15 minutes), or *irreversible* (poor, or no, cellular survival even if blood flow is restored). Cardiomyocyte necrosis progresses as a transmural gradient across the ventricular wall, from endocardium to epicardium, in most animal models studied [1, 2]. Early development of necrosis in the subendocardium is probably related to higher oxygen requirements (due to greater contribution to myocardial contraction) of that layer compared to the subepicardium [3–5]; myocardial perfusion is coupled to myocardial oxygen consumption. Although we agree that progression of coronary heart disease and symptom phenotypes may differ in relation to sex this subject is beyond the scope of this review.

Myocardial ischemia initiates multiple changes in cardiomyocyte structure including marked swelling, development of contraction bands, mitochondrial calcification and membrane disruption; the pathobiology of cellular changes produced by ischemia have been characterized in earlier studies [6–8]. Different modes (apoptosis, autophagy, oncosis, and necrosis) of cellular injury have been described [9] and are discussed elsewhere [10]. The cardiomyocyte cytoskeleton (i.e. structure needed to maintain cellular morphology and physiology) is markedly altered by biochemical changes caused by disruption of oxygen and nutrient supply [11]. Cardiomyocyte death occurs with disruption of the cellular membrane and subsequent leakage of intracellular components into the extracellular fluid [12–14]. Irreversibly injured cardiomyocytes display small breaks in the plasmalemma along with cellular swelling and sarcolemmal blebbing [1]. Necrosis in non-cardiac cells is not well described but it is clear that other cell types within the myocardium (i.e. vascular endothelial and smooth muscle cells, nervous system cells, etc.) are affected by ischemia.

Restoration of blood flow to the perfusion bed of the infarct-related artery can limit damage to cardiomyocyte as long as reperfusion is instituted within a reasonable period. Indeed, this is the basis for widespread use of percutaneous coronary interventions for relief of symptoms in patients with coronary artery disease and is responsible for manifest reduction in mortality. Thousands of studies have examined the physiopathology of ischemia-reperfusion injury over the past half-century with the aim to elucidate pathways leading to cellular necrosis; increased knowledge gained from these studies has led to the realization that this is a complex and multifaceted scenario.

1.2 Lethal reperfusion injury

It is clear that restoration of blood flow to ischemic myocardium is the most effective treatment against myocyte necrosis [15, 16]. Timely opening of an infarct-related artery is essential as the amount of myocardium salvaged rapidly decreases when reperfusion interventions are delayed. Furthermore, reperfusion may itself cause further cellular damage; thus it is often viewed in the context of being a "double-edged sword" [17]. Studies have confirmed that reperfusion triggers abrupt metabolic, electrophysiologic, morphologic and functional changes. The term "lethal reperfusion injury" designates damage to viable cardiomyocytes caused after successful restoration of blood flow to the ischemic perfusion bed. Several possible forms of reperfusion injury such as coronary artery no-reflow, myocardial hibernation, myocardial stunning, ventricular arrhythmias, etc. have been advanced [18, 19]; however, definitive proof that reperfusion injury exists remains to be established. With that in mind, we believe that reperfusion might accelerate expression of injury produced by ischemia but does not itself cause *de novo* cardiomyocyte injury.

Physiopathological mechanisms that produce reperfusion injury are complex and multifactorial; no specific mechanism has been shown to take precedence over others. In experimental animal models, the release of an acute coronary occlusion produces a prolonged hyperemic response particularly in the deeper myocardial layers (subendocardium > subepicardium); hyperemic responses vary depending on the duration of ischemia [20–22]. Reperfusion of the ischemic myocardium depends on arterial driving pressure and extravascular compressive forces; this is particularly important for the function of coronary collateral vessels that supply much needed oxygen and nutrients to surviving cardiomyocytes post-ischemia. As such, restoration of coronary blood flow in the infarct-related artery does not guarantee homogeneous perfusion of blood across the ventricular wall. Indeed, areas where blood flow is less than normal (i.e. no-reflow) are mostly associated with myocardial regions where injury is irreversible.

1.2.1 No-reflow

No-reflow is caused by injury at the structural level (i.e. cell swelling, membrane gaps, etc.) [23, 24]; microvessels might be more resistant to short periods of ischemia compared to cardiomyocytes because their endothelial oxygen requirements are modest and they are in close proximity to oxygen supply. No-reflow does not precede tissue damage but follows it; furthermore, it does not expand myocardial infarct size (role in pathogenesis of tissue damage is considered to be minor) [25, 26]. However, it has been suggested to contribute to infarct expansion, ventricular dilatation and remodeling by limiting access of inflammatory cells to the ischemic zone to initiate cardiac repair [27, 28]. Microvessel damage is also manifest as hemorrhage due to abnormalities in vessel permeability [29].

No-reflow occurs in patients with cardiovascular disease [30, 31]; pharmacotherapy appears to normalize ischemic zone perfusion and reduce mortality.

1.2.2 Myocardial stunning and hibernation

Reperfusion injury is associated with depletion of high-energy phosphate stores, cellular swelling, increases in capillary permeability and reduced microvessel reactivity [32–34]. Restoration of blood flow to the ischemic myocardium mitigates myocardial injury; however, restoration of contractile function is not necessarily immediate. When blood supply to the heart is limited, myocardial contraction is restricted as described for the "smart heart theory" [35]. In normal myocardium, increases in metabolic demand due to intensification of myocardial work are met by regional increases in blood flow as well as increases in oxygen extraction [36]. Post-ischemic myocardial stunning and myocardial hibernation have been described in animals [37, 38] and patients [35, 39] and designate viable but chronically dysfunctional states [40]. Myocardial stunning refers to persistent (but reversible) contractile dysfunction [41, 42] produced by a relatively brief ischemic period [43]. Myocardial hibernation, on the other hand, refers to viable but chronically dysfunctional myocardium that may be related to poor resting perfusion [35], or general absence of perfusion abnormalities [44, 45] but the latter has not been clearly established [46, 47]. Recent findings suggest that repetitive ischemia, chronic stunning and hibernation are linked as a continuum [40]; in other words, stunned myocardium can progressively transform into hibernating myocardium. For both dysfunctional myocardial states, downregulation of contractile function might be a cellular adaptive mechanism to facilitate preservation of myocardial integrity and viability [35]. Perfusion-contraction matching may be key to myocardial hibernation but this may not be so for myocardial stunning; a number of review articles on this subject are available [48–50]. Whether contractile dysfunction can be reversed by improved revascularization in stunned or hibernating myocardium is moot after the formation of scar [40].

1.2.3 Ventricular arrhythmias

Development of life threatening ventricular arrhythmias, which range from ventricular premature beats with long coupling intervals to ventricular fibrillation early after onset of reperfusion, also represent a form of reperfusion injury [51, 52]. Although the physiopathology causing ventricular arrhythmias during reperfusion is ill understood they are known to be initiated by complex cellular changes with regard to electrophysiological, metabolic and structural properties [53]; potential chemical mediators of arrhythmogenesis have been presented [54, 55]. In rat hearts subject to brief coronary artery occlusion (~5 minutes) followed by reperfusion severe ventricular arrhythmias occur [56]. However, in larger animal species, incidence of lethal ventricular arrhythmias increases when reperfusion is instituted within 30 minutes after coronary occlusion [57]. The overall incidence of ventricular arrhythmias decreases significantly when reperfusion follows longer durations of ischemia [58, 59].

2. Cardioprotection strategies

Strategies designed to protect against myocardial injury caused by ischemia, or reperfusion have been extensively studied. In animal models reduction of infarct size is reported with the use of single, or multiple pharmacologicals; however, translation of cardioprotection to patients remains disappointing. Efficacy of interventions is dependent on a host of factors that include time of administration of treatment (i.e. during ischemia, at reperfusion, late reperfusion), duration of occlusion, reperfusion status, species, cell types and end targets (i.e. molecular, biochemical, etc.). In patients, cellular protection is more difficult; however, multi-target studies continue to attempt to limit cardiomyocyte injury. The presence of comorbidities also affects the cardioprotective capability of different treatments. Development of reliable interventions (i.e. pharmacologic, non-pharmacologic) remains an ongoing challenge; findings from basic science and clinical studies on understanding of mechanisms involved in cellular injury and death have been significant but more work is necessary.

2.1 Pharmacologic strategies

For more than 50 years a host of pharmacologic interventions have been employed to limit the extent of myocardial necrosis in animal models and clinical studies. Some cardioprotection has been reported for different manifestations of ischemic injury but no long-lasting protection has yet been afforded by any drug. Many different exogenously administered compounds, which act at different levels (i.e. cell membrane receptors, intracellular signaling pathways, platelet aggregation pathways, inflammation, etc.), have been tested, but results are highly variable. In patients with coronary artery disease/acute myocardial infarction, a "golden window of opportunity" may exist after onset of symptoms to attenuate ischemic injury [60]; however, to date most pharmacologic strategies to delay progression of ischemic injury have not shown great promise with regard to clinical outcomes. Potential reasons include problems regarding timing of drug administration and drug dosage as well as the heterogeneity of comorbidities within patient populations [61]. Recent studies have focused on use of pharmaceuticals that target molecular mechanisms and signal transduction at different cellular levels (i.e. cell membrane, mitochondria, etc.); however, translation of protection with pharmaceuticals that act by stimulating intracellular signaling pathways remains a challenge [62, 63]. While numerous pharmacologic compounds have been tested in animal models and humans to date, none offers protection greater than that afforded by ischemic conditioning (cf. below).

Current pharmacologic interventions targeting ischemia-reperfusion injury include use of beta-blockers; these drugs were among the first reported to delay progression of ischemic injury more than 40 years ago [64–67]. Infarct limiting properties were mostly attributed to reductions in myocardial energy and oxygen consumption. More recently, the selective β1-adrenergic receptor antagonist, metoprolol, administered before reperfusion has been shown to inhibit neutrophil-platelet interactions and protect ischemic myocardium in patients [68]; other elements (i.e. neutrophil trafficking, formation of neutrophil-platelet co-aggregates, etc.) associated with neutrophil dynamics might also be involved [69, 70]. The role of neutrophils in ischemia-reperfusion injury is well established. Protection by metoprolol could be due to reduced microvessel plugging, or microvascular obstruction, by neutrophil-platelet plugs, or other inflammatory cell aggregates. Additionally, metoprolol could directly affect platelet aggregation but this remains to be proven.

Platelet aggregation is a crucial factor for post-ischemic vessel re-occlusion in patients with coronary artery disease even after successful percutaneous coronary interventions. Activated platelets release potent chemotactic factors that stimulate formation of thrombus and microaggregates, which can cause microvascular obstruction underperfusion of the ischemic myocardium [71–73]. Anti-platelet and anti-thrombotic interventions provide significant protection against ischemic injury; though poorly understood, protection is probably mediated through pathways that are similar to those activated by ischemic conditioning [74, 75]. In animal studies, platelet aggregation inhibitors such as ticagrelor ($P2Y_{12}$ receptor blocker) markedly reduce myocardial infarct size that effectively translates to improved cardiac contractile function [76–78]. However, this is not necessarily true for drugs such as clopidogrel (thienopyridine—class of platelet aggregation blockers) which efficiently limits platelet aggregation but does not influence ischemic myocardial injury [75, 79]. Protection probably occurs through adenosine-related mechanisms more than anti-platelet aggregation actions [80, 81]. Other classes of platelet activation blockers (i.e. glycoprotein 2b/3a blockers, etc.) have also reported significant anti-necrosis and anti-arrhythmic effects [82, 83]; however, cardioprotective efficacy of these agents may be limited with extended ischemic durations [84].

Mitochondria are considered an important target for reduction of ischemia-reperfusion injury [85]; mitochondria are responsible for generation of high-energy phosphates and contribute to ion homeostasis, formation of reactive oxygen species and Ca^{2+} handling. Myocardial ischemia-reperfusion markedly alters mitochondrial function that can ultimately lead to cell death. Recent studies have focused on a large conductance pore of the mitochondrial membrane—mitochondrial transition pore (mPTP) located in the inner mitochondrial membrane, which opens at onset of reperfusion leading to osmotic swelling and a decrease in oxidative phosphorylation. In the heart, mPTP inhibitors have been studied in animal models of ischemia-reperfusion injury; several have been reported to be cardioprotective [86–88]. In clinical studies, pharmacologicals that target mitochondrial function have not had positive results with respect to limiting ischemic injury [89–92].

To date, no single pharmacologic compound has achieved a level of cardioprotection greater than that obtained by ischemic conditioning. In an attempt to enhance protection, new initiatives have begun to examine the efficacy of combined treatments (i.e. drug plus ischemic conditioning) that target different cellular mechanisms (i.e. insulin signaling, energy metabolism, etc.) affected by ischemia and reperfusion. For instance, combined glucose-insulin-potassium-exenatide with remote conditioning reduced infarct size in a large animal model [93]. In a combined basic science and clinical study from Hauerslev's laboratory, it was shown that treatment with glyceryl trinitrate (nitric oxide donor) in combination with remote conditioning abolished the individual protective effects obtained with either intervention alone [94]. Similar results have been reported in patients [95] but not all data are consistent [96]. In a canine study from our laboratory, we reported that ischemic conditioning (classic and delayed) significantly reduced ischemic injury; however, combined treatment with EMD 87580 (NHE1 blocker) and ischemic conditioning did not affect the level of cardioprotection [97]. These findings suggest that the level of protection possible with any intervention is limited (i.e. not additive). Underlying explanations for these controversial findings need to be resolved with further investigation.

2.2 Non-pharmacologic strategies

In the clinical setting, percutaneous coronary interventions (PCI) remain the benchmark to restore perfusion in the infarct related artery; however, efficacy of these interventions is variable. An unfortunate aspect of PCI that is often underestimated is the release of micro particulate debris and platelet micro-aggregates that can cause additional myocardial injury downstream at the level of the microvasculature [98–100]. As a result, mechanical thrombectomy (i.e. passive aspiration, active mechanical catheters, etc.) is being developed to limit untoward effects of distal embolization by atherothrombotic debris [101–103].

Keeping in mind that "time is muscle" it is clear that any delay in onset of treatment considerably influences overall success. Combined pharmacotherapy with mechanical reperfusion (i.e. facilitated PCI) is being tested to improve clinical outcomes [104, 105].

Cardiac regeneration therapies (i.e. cardiomyocyte transplantation, biocompatible matrices, etc.) to repair damaged myocardium is another promising intervention to restore post-ischemic cardiac dysfunction (cf. recent review from Kingma [106]). Basic studies designed to better understand underlying mechanisms are ongoing; however, many limitations (i.e. rejection of transplanted cells, presence of scar, poor vascularization, tumor formation, myocardial location, etc.) underscore initial optimism afforded to these interventions for improvement of ventricular function.

Cardiac conditioning (also organ conditioning) is a promising intervention that may eventually prove to be useful for protection of ischemic myocardium (or other organs) in patients; this intervention was first described as ischemic preconditioning more than 30 years ago [107]. Since then, more than 8000 studies have consistently reported protection against necrosis, ventricular dysrhythmias and myocardial contractile dysfunction in experimental animal and in clinical studies [108–111]. At the moment, the clinical usefulness of ischemic conditioning as a preventive strategy for tissue protection remains controversial; the presence of multiple comorbidities may be important [112, 113] but their effect may be overcome depending on the scale of stimulus that is used to trigger cytoprotective pathways [114].

In the original ischemic preconditioning study by Murry and colleagues, dog hearts were exposed *in situ* to brief, repetitive non-lethal cycles of ischemia-reperfusion prior to a prolonged ischemic event [107]. Development of myocardial necrosis was initially delayed and protection was transient depending on the duration of coronary occlusion. An essential requirement for protection against ischemic injury by this intervention is reperfusion of the ischemic region [18]. Publication of this landmark paper paved the way for numerous studies not only with respect to the heart on potential contributory endogenous cellular protection pathways. To date, anesthetic drugs, other pharmacologic or remote interventions, have all demonstrated ischemic conditioning (pre-, per-, post-conditioning) mediated protection. A cross-tolerance phenomenon could also be involved since many triggers for intracellular signaling pathway-mediated protection are similar [115–117]. Prospective contributory mechanisms to conditioning mediated protection have been reviewed elsewhere [109, 118–120].

The principal difficulty with ischemic conditioning strategies is the inability to translate success in animal models to the clinical setting to improve overall outcomes. A major liability is the requirement to physically apply an ischemic conditioning intervention prior to onset of acute ischemia (incapacity to determine its occurrence). The observation that remote ischemic conditioning could provide robust protection against ischemic injury is promising [121]. In their initial canine cardiac ischemia-reperfusion injury study, Przyklenk and coworkers pretreated a region of the heart with brief non-lethal cycles of repetitive ischemia and reperfusion and showed marked protection (i.e. reduced infarct size) of a distant adjacent region in the same heart. Since the publication of this study, others have reported significant limitation of different manifestations of ischemic injury in various experimental models [122]. A crucial question concerns the mechanism(s) by which cytoprotective signals are transported from conditioned tissue to the distant target tissue. Blood or perfusate-borne humoral factors, neuronal stimulation and transmission as well as systemic alteration of circulating immune cells have all been proposed [123–125]. Findings, in animal models, from our laboratory tend to favor the humoral hypothesis; in dogs subject to acute ischemia-reperfusion injury, protection was not reversed after either pharmacologic or surgical decentralization of the intrinsic cardiac nervous system [126]. On this basis we hypothesized that inter-organ crosstalk did not require an intact autonomic nervous system. Stimulation of the nervous system, either locally or within cardiac ganglia could potentially stimulate release of cardioprotective substances (chemokines, leukotrienes, microRNA, etc.) into the bloodstream to initiate downstream effects [109, 127–129]. Interestingly, activation of the sympathetic nervous system is not required for classical ischemic conditioning, however, it is essential for second-window, or delayed, conditioning [130, 131].

A key element for protection by remote conditioning is restoration of blood flow to affected tissues [111, 132]; without it transfer of triggering mediators would be constrained. In humans, it is not clear that conditioning strategies afford significant protection (against endothelial dysfunction, increased permeability, structural alterations, etc.) at the level of the microcirculation in the deeper myocardial tissue layers [115, 133, 134]. Nonetheless, improved myocardial perfusion with remote conditioning may occur based on findings of higher TIMI (thrombosis in myocardial infarction) scores, myocardial blush grade and coronary reserve in cardiac patients. Restoration of blood flow to the deeper layers of the myocardial wall is a crucial risk factor for ventricular remodeling and major adverse cardiac events [135–137].

In the clinical setting, results with this intervention (i.e. repeated arm or leg ischemia-reperfusion) are mixed; studies report either manifest cardioprotection [138, 139], no benefit [18, 140, 141] or exacerbation of injury [112, 142]. Failure to provide protection by remote conditioning in patients may be associated with the use of anesthetics such as propofol that abrogates protection [18]; volatile anesthetics are mostly recommended for at-risk cardiac patients [143, 144]. In proof-of-concept studies, other forms of remote conditioning, such as remote ischemic perconditioning (intervention performed during evolving myocardial infarction) have reported protection against tissue injury, ST-segment resolution and biomarker release in animal models and patients [145–147].

3. Concluding comments

Pathogenesis of lethal reperfusion injury remains to be established; the principle that reperfusion injury contributes to post-ischemic myocardial dysfunction is generally accepted but definitive evidence for its existence is lacking. While evaluation of the nature of cellular changes produced by ischemia and subsequent reperfusion has produced significant novel insights it is unclear that cardiomyocytes are the only cell types (within the myocardium) that are at risk of further injury. Of principle importance is that interventions to limit myocardial injury be instituted at the time of, or in conjunction with other reperfusion strategies. Pharmacologic compounds currently being used in the clinical setting delay, at best, short-term progression of cellular injury; long-term effects of these treatments in large animal ischemia-reperfusion injury models have not been properly investigated. The concept of a "magic bullet" intervention remains utopic, at present, considering the complexity of physiopathological mechanisms involved in cell death and myocardial remodeling. Utilization of exogenous interventions such as ischemic conditioning in combination with pharmacologic treatments remains a significant challenge. Further investigations into combination therapy, particularly in longer-term studies should be envisaged; consideration should also be paid to the existence of comorbidities within the patient population since overall efficacy of any treatment option will be affected.

Author details

John G. Kingma
Faculty of Medicine, Department of Medicine, Université Laval, Québec, Canada

*Address all correspondence to: john.kingma@fmed.ulaval.ca

References

[1] Jennings RB. Historical perspective on the pathology of myocardial ischemia/reperfusion injury. Circulation Research. 2013;**113**(4):428-438. DOI: 10.1161/CIRCRESAHA.113.300987

[2] Reimer KA, Jennings RB. The "wavefront phenomenon" of myocardial ischemic cell death. II. Transmural progression of necrosis within the framework of ischemic bed size (myocardium at risk) and collateral flow. Laboratory Investigation. 1979;**40**(6):633-644

[3] Vinten-Johansen J, Weiss HR. Oxygen consumption in subepicardial and subendocardial regions of the canine left ventricle. The effect of experimental acute valvular aortic stenosis. Circulation Research. 1980;**46**(1): 139-145. DOI: 10.1161/01.res.46.1.139

[4] Hoffman JI, Buckberg GD. The myocardial oxygen supply: Demand index revisited. Journal of the American Heart Association. 2014;**3**(1):e000285. DOI: 10.1161/JAHA.113.000285

[5] Hoffman JI. Determinants and prediction of transmural myocardial perfusion. Circulation. 1978;**58**(3 Pt 1): 381-391. DOI: 10.1161/01.cir.58.3.381

[6] Ganote CE. Contraction band necrosis and irreversible myocardial injury. Journal of Molecular and Cellular Cardiology. 1983;**15**:67-73

[7] Reimer KA, Jennings RB, Tatum AH. Pathobiology of acute myocardial ischemia: Metabolic, functional and ultrastructural studies. The American Journal of Cardiology. 1983;**52**:72A-81A

[8] Kloner RA, Darsee JR, DeBoer LWV, Carlson N. Early pathologic detection of acute myocardial infarction. Archives of Pathology & Laboratory Medicine. 1981;**105**:403-406

[9] Galluzzi L, Bravo-San Pedro JM, Vitale I, Aaronson SA, Abrams JM, Adam D, et al. Essential versus accessory aspects of cell death: Recommendations of the NCCD 2015. Cell Death and Differentiation. 2015;**22**(1):58-73. DOI: 10.1038/cdd.2014.137

[10] JG K. Acute myocardial injury: A perspective on lethal reperfusion injury. Cardiovascular Pharmacology: Open Access. 2017;**6**:8. DOI: 10.4172/2329-6607.1000216

[11] Ganote C, Armstrong S. Ischaemia and the myocyte cytoskeleton: Review and speculation. Cardiovascular Research. 1993;**27**:1387-1403

[12] Steenbergen C, Hill ML, Jennings RB. Cytoskeletal damage during myocardial ischemia: Changes in vinculin immunofluorescence staining during total in vitro ischemia in canine heart. Circulation Research. 1987;**60**(4):478-486

[13] Jennings RB, Hawkins HK, Lowe JE, Hill ML, Klotman S, Reimer KA. Relation between high energy phosphate and lethal injury in myocardial ischemia in the dog. The American Journal of Pathology. 1978;**92**(1):187-214

[14] Jennings RB, Reimer KA, Steenbergen C. Myocardial ischemia revisited. The osmolar load, membrane damage, and reperfusion. Journal of Molecular and Cellular Cardiology. 1986;**18**:769-780

[15] Downey JM, Cohen MV. Reducing infarct size in the setting of acute myocardial infarction. Progress in Cardiovascular Diseases. 2006;**48**(5):363-371. DOI: 10.1016/j.pcad.2006.02.005

[16] Goel K, Pinto DS, Gibson CM. Association of time to reperfusion with

left ventricular function and heart failure in patients with acute myocardial infarction treated with primary percutaneous coronary intervention: A systematic review. American Heart Journal. 2013;**165**(4):451-467. DOI: 10.1016/j.ahj.2012.11.014

[17] Braunwald E, Kloner RA. Myocardial reperfusion: A double-edged sword? The Journal of Clinical Investigation. 1985;**76**:1713-1719

[18] Heusch G. Cardioprotection: Chances and challenges of its translation to the clinic. Lancet. 2013;**381**(9861):166-175. DOI: 10.1016/S0140-6736(12)60916-7

[19] Bernink FJ, Timmers L, Beek AM, Diamant M, Roos ST, Van Rossum AC, et al. Progression in attenuating myocardial reperfusion injury: An overview. International Journal of Cardiology. 2014;**170**(3):261-269. DOI: 10.1016/j.ijcard.2013.11.007

[20] Kloner RA, Ganote CE, Jennings RB. The "no-reflow" phenomenon after temporary coronary occlusion in the dog. The Journal of Clinical Investigation. 1974;**54**(6):1496-1508. DOI: 10.1172/JCI107898

[21] Willerson JT, Powell WJ Jr, Guiney TE, Stark JJ, Sanders CA, Leaf A. Improvement in myocardial function and coronary blood flow in ischemic myocardium after mannitol. The Journal of Clinical Investigation. 1972;**51**(12):2989-2998. DOI: 10.1172/JCI107126

[22] Camilleri JP, Joseph D, Fabiani JN, Deloche A, Schlumberger M, Relland J, et al. Microcirculatory changes following early reperfusion in experimental myocardial infarction. Virchows Archiv. A, Pathological Anatomy and Histology. 1976;**369**(4):315-333. DOI: 10.1007/bf00432452

[23] Ambrosio G, Weisman HF, Mannisi JA, Becker LC. Progressive impairment of regional myocardial perfusion after initial restoration of postischemic blood flow. Circulation. 1989;**80**(6):1846-1861

[24] Jeremy RW, Links JM, Becker LC. Progressive failure of coronary flow during reperfusion of myocardial infarction: Documentation of the no reflow phenomenon with positron emission tomography. Journal of the American College of Cardiology. 1990;**16**(3):695-704

[25] Kloner RA, Rude RE, Carlson N, Maroko PR, DeBoer LWV, Braunwald E. Ultrastructural evidence of microvascular damage and myocardial cell injury after coronary artery occlusion: Which comes first? Circulation. 1980;**62**:945-952

[26] Cobb FR, Bache RJ, Rivas F, Greenfield JC Jr. Local effects of acute cellular injury on regional myocardial blood flow. The Journal of Clinical Investigation. 1976;**57**:1359-1368

[27] Kloner RA. No-reflow phenomenon: Maintaining vascular integrity. Journal of Cardiovascular Pharmacology and Therapeutics. 2011;**16**(3-4):244-250. DOI: 10.1177/1074248411405990

[28] Vinten-Johansen J. Involvement of neutrophils in the pathogenesis of lethal myocardial reperfusion injury. Cardiovascular Research. 2004;**61**(3):481-497. DOI: 10.1016/j.cardiores.2003.10.011

[29] Bresnahan GF, Roberts R, Shell WE, Ross J Jr, Sobel BE. Deleterious effects due to hemorrhage after myocardial reperfusion. The American Journal of Cardiology. 1974;**33**(1):82-86. DOI: 10.1016/0002-9149(74)90742-5

[30] Rezkalla SH, Dharmashankar KC, Abdalrahman IB, Kloner RA. No-reflow phenomenon following percutaneous coronary intervention for acute myocardial infarction: Incidence,

outcome, and effect of pharmacologic therapy. Journal of Interventional Cardiology. 2010;**23**(5):429-436. DOI: 10.1111/j.1540-8183.2010.00561.x

[31] Rezkalla SH, Kloner RA. Coronary no-reflow phenomenon: From the experimental laboratory to the cardiac catheterization laboratory. Catheterization and Cardiovascular Interventions. 2008;**72**(7):950-957. DOI: 10.1002/ccd.21715

[32] Becker LC, Ambrosio G. Myocardial consequences of reperfusion. Progress in Cardiovascular Diseases. 1987;**30**:23-44

[33] Reimer KA, Hill ML, Jennings RB. Prolonged depletion of ATP and of the adenine nucleotide pool due to delayed resynthesis of adenine nucleotides following reversible myocardial ischemic injury in dogs. Journal of Molecular and Cellular Cardiology. 1981;**13**(2):229-239. DOI: 10.1016/0022-2828(81)90219-4

[34] Kloner RA, DeBoer LW, Darsee JR, Ingwall JS, Hale S, Tumas J, et al. Prolonged abnormalities of myocardium salvaged by reperfusion. The American Journal of Physiology. 1981;**241**(4):H591-H599. DOI: 10.1152/ajpheart.1981.241.4.H591

[35] Rahimtoola SH. The hibernating myocardium. American Heart Journal. 1989;**117**(1):211-221

[36] Feigl EO. Coronary physiology. Physiological Reviews. 1983;**63**:1-205

[37] Heyndrickx GR, Baig H, Nellens P, Leusen I, Fishbein MC, Vatner SF. Depression of regional blood flow and wall thickening after brief coronary occlusions. American Journal of Physiology. Heart and Circulatory Physiology. 1978;**234**:H653-H6H9

[38] Heyndrickx GR, Millard RW, McRitchie RJ, Maroko PR, Vatner SF. Regional myocardial functional and electrophysiological alterations after brief coronary artery occlusion in conscious dogs. The Journal of Clinical Investigation. 1975;**56**:978-985

[39] Chatterjee K, Swan HJ, Parmley WW, Sustaita H, Marcus HS, Matloff J. Influence of direct myocardial revascularization on left ventricular asynergy and function in patients with coronary heart disease. With and without previous myocardial infarction. Circulation. 1973;**47**(2):276-286. DOI: 10.1161/01.cir.47.2.276

[40] Benz DC, von Dahlen AP, Huang W, Messerli M, von Felten E, Benetos G, et al. No differences in rest myocardial blood flow in stunned and hibernating myocardium: Insights into the pathophysiology of ischemic cardiomyopathy. European Journal of Nuclear Medicine and Molecular Imaging. 2019;**46**(11):2322-2328. DOI: 10.1007/s00259-019-04440-2

[41] Bolli R. Postischemic myocardial stunning: Pathogenesis, pathophysiology, and clinical relevance. In: Yellon DM, Jennings RB, editors. Myocardial Protection: The Pathophysiology of Reperfusion and Reperfusion Injury. 1st ed. New York: Raven Press; 1992. pp. 105-149

[42] Bolli R. Myocardial 'stunning' in man. Circulation. 1992;**86**(6):1671-1691

[43] Benz DC, Gaemperli O. The right timing for post-ischemic stunning. Journal of Nuclear Cardiology. 2017;**24**(4):1302-1304. DOI: 10.1007/s12350-016-0473-8

[44] Canty JM Jr, Fallavollita JA. Hibernating myocardium. Journal of Nuclear Cardiology. 2005;**12**(1):104-119. DOI: 10.1016/j.nuclcard.2004.11.003

[45] Heusch G, Schulz R, Rahimtoola SH. Myocardial hibernation:

A delicate balance. American Journal of Physiology. Heart and Circulatory Physiology. 2005;**288**(3):H984-HH99. DOI: 10.1152/ajpheart.01109.2004

[46] Camici PG, Rimoldi OE. Myocardial blood flow in patients with hibernating myocardium. Cardiovascular Research. 2003;**57**(2):302-311

[47] Camici PG, Wijns W, Borgers M, De Silva R, Ferrari R, Knuuti J, et al. Pathophysiological mechanisms of chronic reversible left ventricular dysfunction due to coronary artery disease (hibernating myocardium). Circulation. 1997;**96**(9):3205-3214. DOI: 10.1161/01.cir.96.9.3205

[48] Heusch G, Schulz R. Perfusion-contraction match and mismatch. Basic Research in Cardiology. 2001;**96**(1): 1-10. DOI: 10.1007/s003950170072

[49] Heusch G. Hibernating myocardium. Physiological Reviews. 1998;**78**(4):1055-1085

[50] Ross JJ. Myocardial perfusion-contraction matching. Implications for coronary heart disease and hibernation. Circulation. 1991;**83**(3):1076-1083

[51] Manning AS, Hearse DJ. Reperfusion-induced arrhythmias: Mechanisms and prevention. Journal of Molecular and Cellular Cardiology. 1984;**16**:497-518

[52] Majidi M, Kosinski AS, Al-Khatib SM, Lemmert ME, Smolders L, van Weert A, et al. Reperfusion ventricular arrhythmia 'bursts' in TIMI 3 flow restoration with primary angioplasty for anterior ST-elevation myocardial infarction: A more precise definition of reperfusion arrhythmias. Europace. 2008;**10**(8):988-997. DOI: 10.1093/europace/eun123

[53] Akar JG, Akar FG. Regulation of ion channels and arrhythmias in the ischemic heart. Journal of Electrocardiology. 2007;**40**(6 Suppl):S37-S41. DOI: 10.1016/j.jelectrocard.2007.05.020

[54] Curtis MJ, Pugsley MK, Walker MJ. Endogenous chemical mediators of ventricular arrhythmias in ischaemic heart disease. Cardiovascular Research. 1993;**27**(5):703-719. DOI: 10.1093/cvr/27.5.703

[55] van der Weg K, Prinzen FW, Gorgels AP. Editor's choice-reperfusion cardiac arrhythmias and their relation to reperfusion-induced cell death. European Heart Journal Acute Cardiovascular Care. 2019;**8**(2):142-152. DOI: 10.1177/2048872618812148

[56] Bernier M, Hearse DJ, Manning AS. Reperfusion-induced arrhythmias and oxygen-derived free radicals: Studies with "anti-free radical" interventions and a free radical-generating system in the isolated perfused rat heart. Circulation Research. 1986;**58**:331-340

[57] Balke CW, Kaplinsky E, Mickelson EL, Naito N, Dreifus LS. Reperfusion ventricular tachyarrhythmias: Correlation with antecedent coronary artery occlusion, tachyarrhythmias and duration of myocardial ischemia. American Heart Journal. 1981;**101**:449-456

[58] Sommers HM, Jennings RB. Ventricular fibrillation and myocardial necrosis after transient ischemia. Effect of treatment with oxygen, procainamide, reserpine, and propranolol. Archives of Internal Medicine. 1972;**129**(5):780-789

[59] Tanaka K, Hearse DJ. Reperfusion-induced arrhythmias in the isolated rabbit heart: Characterization of the influence of the duration of regional ischemia and the extracellular potassium concentration. Journal of Molecular and Cellular Cardiology. 1988;**20**(3):201-211. DOI: 10.1016/s0022-2828(88)80053-1

[60] Gersh BJ, Stone GW, White HD, Holmes DR Jr. Pharmacological facilitation of primary percutaneous coronary intervention for acute myocardial infarction: Is the slope of the curve the shape of the future? Journal of the American Medical Association. 2005;**293**(8):979-986. DOI: 10.1001/jama.293.8.979

[61] Sharma V, Bell RM, Yellon DM. Targeting reperfusion injury in acute myocardial infarction: A review of reperfusion injury pharmacotherapy. Expert Opinion on Pharmacotherapy. 2012;**13**(8):1153-1175. DOI: 10.1517/14656566.2012.685163

[62] Kloner RA. Current state of clinical translation of cardioprotective agents for acute myocardial infarction. Circulation Research. 2013;**113, 4**:451-463. DOI: 10.1161/CIRCRESAHA.112.300627

[63] Bulluck H, Yellon DM, Hausenloy DJ. Reducing myocardial infarct size: Challenges and future opportunities. Heart. 2016;**102**(5):341-348. DOI: 10.1136/heartjnl-2015-307855

[64] Ibanez B, Heusch G, Ovize M, Van de Werf F. Evolving therapies for myocardial ischemia/reperfusion injury. Journal of the American College of Cardiology. 2015;**65**(14):1454-1471. DOI: 10.1016/j.jacc.2015.02.032

[65] Boyle DM, Barber JM, McIlmoyle EL, Salathia KS, Evans AE, Cran G, et al. Effect of very early intervention with metoprolol on myocardial infarct size. British Heart Journal. 1983;**49**(3):229-233. DOI: 10.1136/hrt.49.3.229

[66] Kudoh Y, Maxwell MP, Hearse DJ, Downey JM, Yellon DM. Inability of metoprolol to achieve a sustained limitation of infarct size 24 h after coronary artery embolization in the closed chest dog. Journal of Cardiovascular Pharmacology. 1984;**6**(6):1201-1209

[67] Ibanez B, Cimmino G, Prat-Gonzalez S, Vilahur G, Hutter R, Garcia MJ, et al. The cardioprotection granted by metoprolol is restricted to its administration prior to coronary reperfusion. International Journal of Cardiology. 2011;**147**(3):428-432. DOI: 10.1016/j.ijcard.2009.09.551

[68] Garcia-Prieto J, Villena-Gutierrez R, Gomez M, Bernardo E, Pun-Garcia A, Garcia-Lunar I, et al. Neutrophil stunning by metoprolol reduces infarct size. Nature Communications. 2017;**8**:14780. DOI: 10.1038/ncomms14780

[69] Antoniucci D. Block the ischemia and reperfusion damage: An old adjunctive drug for a new reperfusion strategy. Journal of the American College of Cardiology. 2014;**63**(22):2363-2364. DOI: 10.1016/j.jacc.2014.03.015

[70] Kim MH, Gorouhi F, Ramirez S, Granick JL, Byrne BA, Soulika AM, et al. Catecholamine stress alters neutrophil trafficking and impairs wound healing by beta2-adrenergic receptor-mediated upregulation of IL-6. The Journal of Investigative Dermatology. 2014;**134**(3):809-817. DOI: 10.1038/jid.2013.415

[71] Shen YT, Wiedmann RT, Lynch JJ Jr, Gould RJ. Platelet glycoprotein IIb/IIIa receptor inhibitor preserves coronary flow reserve during progressive coronary arteriostenosis in swine. Arteriosclerosis, Thrombosis, and Vascular Biology. 2000;**20**(10):2309-2315

[72] Rendu F, Brohard-Bohn B. The platelet release reaction: Granules' constituents, secretion and functions. Platelets. 2001;**12**(5):261-273. DOI: 10.1080/09537100120068170

[73] Yuan X, Xiang Y, Zhu N, Zhao X, Ye S, Zhong P, et al. Salvianolic acid a protects against myocardial ischemia/reperfusion injury by reducing platelet activation and inflammation. Experimental and Therapeutic Medicine. 2017;**14**(2):961-966. DOI: 10.3892/etm.2017.4619

[74] Yang XM, Cui L, Alhammouri A, Downey JM, Cohen MV. Triple therapy greatly increases myocardial salvage during ischemia/reperfusion in the in situ rat heart. Cardiovascular Drugs and Therapy. 2013;**27**(5):403-412. DOI: 10.1007/s10557-013-6474-9

[75] Yang XM, Liu Y, Cui L, Yang X, Liu Y, Tandon N, et al. Platelet P2Y(1)(2) blockers confer direct postconditioning-like protection in reperfused rabbit hearts. Journal of Cardiovascular Pharmacology and Therapeutics. 2013;**18**(3):251-262. DOI: 10.1177/1074248412467692

[76] Nanhwan MK, Ling S, Kodakandla M, Nylander S, Ye Y, Birnbaum Y. Chronic treatment with ticagrelor limits myocardial infarct size: An adenosine and cyclooxygenase-2-dependent effect. Arteriosclerosis, Thrombosis, and Vascular Biology. 2014;**34**(9):2078-2085. DOI: 10.1161/ATVBAHA.114.304002

[77] Ye Y, Birnbaum GD, Perez-Polo JR, Nanhwan MK, Nylander S, Birnbaum Y. Ticagrelor protects the heart against reperfusion injury and improves remodeling after myocardial infarction. Arteriosclerosis, Thrombosis, and Vascular Biology. 2015;**35**(8):1805-1814. DOI: 10.1161/ATVBAHA.115.305655

[78] Vilahur G, Gutierrez M, Casani L, Varela L, Capdevila A, Pons-Llado G, et al. Protective effects of Ticagrelor on myocardial injury after infarction. Circulation. 2016;**134**(22):1708-1719. DOI: 10.1161/CIRCULATIONAHA.116.024014

[79] Wang K, Zhou X, Huang Y, Khalil M, Wiktor D, van Giezen JJ, et al. Adjunctive treatment with ticagrelor, but not clopidogrel, added to tPA enables sustained coronary artery recanalisation with recovery of myocardium perfusion in a canine coronary thrombosis model. Thrombosis and Haemostasis. 2010;**104**(3):609-617. DOI: 10.1160/TH09-12-0823

[80] Armstrong D, Summers C, Ewart L, Nylander S, Sidaway JE, van Giezen JJ. Characterization of the adenosine pharmacology of ticagrelor reveals therapeutically relevant inhibition of equilibrative nucleoside transporter 1. Journal of Cardiovascular Pharmacology and Therapeutics. 2014;**19**(2):209-219. DOI: 10.1177/1074248413511693

[81] van Giezen JJ, Sidaway J, Glaves P, Kirk I, Bjorkman JA. Ticagrelor inhibits adenosine uptake in vitro and enhances adenosine-mediated hyperemia responses in a canine model. Journal of Cardiovascular Pharmacology and Therapeutics. 2012;**17**(2):164-172. DOI: 10.1177/1074248411410883

[82] Willerson JT, Golino P, McNatt J, Eidt J, Yao S-K, Buja LM. Role of new antiplatelet agents as adjunctive therapies in thrombolysis. The American Journal of Cardiology. 1991;**67**:12A-18A

[83] Kingma JG Jr, Plante S, Bogaty P. Platelet GPIIb/IIIa receptor blockade reduces infarct size in a canine model of ischemia-reperfusion. Journal of the American College of Cardiology. 2000;**36**(7):2317-2324

[84] Kingma JG. Effect of platelet GPIIb/IIIa receptor blockade with MK383 on infarct size and myocardial blood flow in a canine reocclusion model. Journal of Cardiovascular Pharmacology and Therapeutics. 2018;**24**(2):182-192. DOI: 10.1177/1074248418808389

[85] Boengler K, Lochnit G, Schulz R. Mitochondria "THE" target of myocardial conditioning. American Journal of Physiology. Heart and Circulatory Physiology. 2018;**315**(5):H1215-H1H31. DOI: 10.1152/ajpheart.00124.2018

[86] Argaud L, Gateau-Roesch O, Raisky O, Loufouat J, Robert D, Ovize M. Postconditioning inhibits mitochondrial permeability transition. Circulation. 2005;**111**(2):194-197. DOI: 10.1161/01.CIR.0000151290.04952

[87] Argaud L, Gomez L, Gateau-Roesch O, Couture-Lepetit E, Loufouat J, Robert D, et al. Trimetazidine inhibits mitochondrial permeability transition pore opening and prevents lethal ischemia-reperfusion injury. Journal of Molecular and Cellular Cardiology. 2005;**39**(6):893-899. DOI: 10.1016/j.yjmcc.2005.09.012

[88] Gomez L, Thibault H, Gharib A, Dumont JM, Vuagniaux G, Scalfaro P, et al. Inhibition of mitochondrial permeability transition improves functional recovery and reduces mortality following acute myocardial infarction in mice. American Journal of Physiology. Heart and Circulatory Physiology. 2007;**293**(3):H1654-H1661. DOI: 10.1152/ajpheart.01378.2006

[89] Gibson CM, Giugliano RP, Kloner RA, Bode C, Tendera M, Janosi A, et al. EMBRACE STEMI study: A phase 2a trial to evaluate the safety, tolerability, and efficacy of intravenous MTP-131 on reperfusion injury in patients undergoing primary percutaneous coronary intervention. European Heart Journal. 2016;**37**(16):1296-1303. DOI: 10.1093/eurheartj/ehv597

[90] Lincoff AM, Roe M, Aylward P, Galla J, Rynkiewicz A, Guetta V, et al. Inhibition of delta-protein kinase C by delcasertib as an adjunct to primary percutaneous coronary intervention for acute anterior ST-segment elevation myocardial infarction: Results of the PROTECTION AMI randomized controlled trial. European Heart Journal. 2014;**35**(37):2516-2523. DOI: 10.1093/eurheartj/ehu177

[91] Ottani F, Latini R, Staszewsky L, La Vecchia L, Locuratolo N, Sicuro M, et al. Cyclosporine a in reperfused myocardial infarction: The multicenter, controlled, open-label CYCLE trial. Journal of the American College of Cardiology. 2016;**67**(4):365-374. DOI: 10.1016/j.jacc.2015.10.081

[92] Piot C, Croisille P, Staat P, Thibault H, Rioufol G, Mewton N, et al. Effect of cyclosporine on reperfusion injury in acute myocardial infarction. The New England Journal of Medicine. 2008;**359**(5):473-481. DOI: 10.1056/NEJMoa071142

[93] Alburquerque-Bejar JJ, Barba I, Inserte J, Miro-Casas E, Ruiz-Meana M, Poncelas M, et al. Combination therapy with remote ischaemic conditioning and insulin or exenatide enhances infarct size limitation in pigs. Cardiovascular Research. 2015;**107**(2):246-254. DOI: 10.1093/cvr/cvv171

[94] Hauerslev M, Mork SR, Pryds K, Contractor H, Hansen J, Jespersen NR, et al. Influence of long-term treatment with glyceryl trinitrate on remote ischemic conditioning. American Journal of Physiology. Heart and Circulatory Physiology. 2018;**315**(1):H150-H1H8. DOI: 10.1152/ajpheart.00114.2018

[95] Candilio L, Malik A, Ariti C, Barnard M, Di Salvo C, Lawrence D, et al. Effect of remote ischaemic preconditioning on clinical outcomes in patients undergoing cardiac bypass surgery: A randomised controlled clinical trial. Heart. 2015;**101**(3):185-192. DOI: 10.1136/heartjnl-2014-306178

[96] Kleinbongard P, Thielmann M, Jakob H, Peters J, Heusch G, Kottenberg E. Nitroglycerin does not interfere with protection by remote ischemic preconditioning in patients with surgical coronary revascularization under isoflurane anesthesia. Cardiovascular Drugs and Therapy. 2013;**27**(4):359-361. DOI: 10.1007/s10557-013-6451-3

[97] Kingma JG. Inhibition of Na(+)/H(+) exchanger with EMD 87580 does not confer greater cardioprotection beyond preconditioning on ischemia-reperfusion injury in Normal dogs. Journal of Cardiovascular Pharmacology and Therapeutics. 2018;**23**(3):254-269. DOI: 10.1177/1074248418755120

[98] Heusch G, Kleinbongard P, Skyschally A, Levkau B, Schulz R, Erbel R. The coronary circulation in cardioprotection: More than just one confounder. Cardiovascular Research. 2012;**94**(2):237-245. DOI: 10.1093/cvr/cvr271

[99] Babu GG, Walker JM, Yellon DM, Hausenloy DJ. Peri-procedural myocardial injury during percutaneous coronary intervention: An important target for cardioprotection. European Heart Journal. 2011;**32**(1): 23-31. DOI: 10.1093/eurheartj/ehq393

[100] Skyschally A, Walter B, Heusch G. Coronary microembolization during early reperfusion: Infarct extension, but protection by ischaemic postconditioning. European Heart Journal. 2013;**34**(42):3314-3321. DOI: 10.1093/eurheartj/ehs434

[101] Heusch G, Kleinbongard P, Bose D, Levkau B, Haude M, Schulz R, et al. Coronary microembolization: From bedside to bench and back to bedside. Circulation. 2009;120(18):1822-1836. DOI: 10.1161/CIRCULATIONAHA.109.888784

[102] Giglioli C, Cecchi E, Sciagra R, Baldereschi GJ, Meucci F, Valente S, et al. COmparison between COronary THrombus aspiration with Angiojet(R) or export(R) catheter in patients with ST-elevation myocardial infarction submitted to primary angioplasty: The COCOTH study. International Journal of Cardiology. 2016;**203**:757-762. DOI: 10.1016/j.ijcard.2015.03.158

[103] Svilaas T, Vlaar PJ, van der Horst IC, Diercks GF, de Smet BJ, van den Heuvel AF, et al. Thrombus aspiration during primary percutaneous coronary intervention. The New England Journal of Medicine. 2008;**358**(6):557-567. DOI: 10.1056/NEJMoa0706416

[104] Brodie BR. Facilitated percutaneous coronary intervention. Heart. 2005;**91**(12):1527-1529. DOI: 10.1136/hrt.2005.064618

[105] Brodie BR, Stuckey TD, Hansen C, Muncy D. Benefit of coronary reperfusion before intervention on outcomes after primary angioplasty for acute myocardial infarction. The American Journal of Cardiology. 2000;**85**(1):13-18

[106] Kingma JG. Myocardial infarction: Perspectives on cardiac regeneration and cardiac remote conditioning interventions to limit cellular injury. World Journal of Cardiovascular Diseases. 2020;**10**:188-207. DOI: 10.4236/wjcd.2020.104019

[107] Murry CE, Jennings RB, Reimer KA. Preconditioning with ischemia: A delay of lethal cell injury in ischemic myocardium. Circulation. 1986;**74**:1124-1136

[108] Rosenberg JH, Werner JH, Moulton MJ, Agrawal DK. Current modalities and mechanisms underlying cardioprotection by ischemic conditioning. Journal of Cardiovascular Translational Research.

2018;**11**(4):292-307. DOI: 10.1007/s12265-018-9813-1

[109] Hausenloy DJ, Barrabes JA, Botker HE, Davidson SM, Di Lisa F, Downey J, et al. Ischaemic conditioning and targeting reperfusion injury: A 30 year voyage of discovery. Basic Research in Cardiology. 2016;**111**(6):70. DOI: 10.1007/s00395-016-0588-8

[110] Przyklenk K. Ischaemic conditioning: Pitfalls on the path to clinical translation. British Journal of Pharmacology. 2015;**172**(8):1961-1973. DOI: 10.1111/bph.13064

[111] Kingma JG. Conditioning strategies limit cellular injury? World Journal of Cardiovascular Diseases. 2014;**4**:539-547

[112] Ovize M, Thibault H, Przyklenk K. Myocardial conditioning: Opportunities for clinical translation. Circulation Research. 2013;**113**(4):439-450. DOI: 10.1161/CIRCRESAHA.113.300764

[113] Vander Heide RS, Steenbergen C. Cardioprotection and myocardial reperfusion: Pitfalls to clinical application. Circulation Research. 2013;**113**(4):464-477. DOI: 10.1161/CIRCRESAHA.113.300765

[114] Tsang A, Hausenloy DJ, Mocanu MM, Carr RD, Yellon DM. Preconditioning the diabetic heart: The importance of Akt phosphorylation. Diabetes. 2005;**54**(8):2360-2364. DOI: 10.2337/diabetes.54/8/2360

[115] Kingma JG. The myocardial microcirculation: A key target for salvaging ischemic myocardium? World Journal of Cardiovascular Diseases. 2013;**3**:8-16. DOI: 10.4236/wjcd.2013.35A002

[116] Yellon DM, Downey JM. Preconditioning the myocardium: From cellular physiology to clinical cardiology. Physiological Reviews. 2003;**83**(4):1113-1151

[117] Downey JM, Davis AM, Cohen MV. Signaling pathways in ischemic preconditioning. Heart Failure Reviews. 2007;**12**(3-4):181-188. DOI: 10.1007/s10741-007-9025-2

[118] Hausenloy DJ, Yellon DM. Preconditioning and postconditioning: Underlying mechanisms and clinical application. Atherosclerosis. 2009;**204**(2):334-341. DOI: 10.1016/j.atherosclerosis.2008.10.029

[119] Dawn B, Bolli R. Role of nitric oxide in myocardial preconditioning. Annals of the New York Academy of Sciences. 2002;**962**:18-41

[120] Hausenloy DJ. Signalling pathways in ischaemic postconditioning. Thrombosis and Haemostasis. 2009;**101**(4):626-634

[121] Przyklenk K, Bauer B, Ovize M, Kloner RA, Whittaker P. Regional ischemic preconditioning protects remote virgin myocardium from subsequent coronary occlusion. Circulation. 1993;**87**:893-899

[122] Bromage DI, Pickard JM, Rossello X, Ziff OJ, Burke N, Yellon DM, et al. Remote ischaemic conditioning reduces infarct size in animal in vivo models of ischaemia-reperfusion injury: A systematic review and meta-analysis. Cardiovascular Research. 2017;**113**(3):288-297. DOI: 10.1093/cvr/cvw219

[123] Weber C. Far from the heart: Receptor cross-talk in remote conditioning. Nature Medicine. 2010;**16**(7):760-762. DOI: 10.1038/nm0710-760

[124] Dickson EW, Tubbs RJ, Porcaro WA, Lee WJ, Blehar DJ,

Carraway RE, et al. Myocardial preconditioning factors evoke mesenteric ischemic tolerance via opioid receptors and K(ATP) channels. American Journal of Physiology. Heart and Circulatory Physiology. 2002;**283**(1):H22-HH8

[125] Przyklenk K, Darling CE, Dickson EW, Whittaker P. Cardioprotection 'outside the box'—The evolving paradigm of remote preconditioning. Basic Research in Cardiology. 2003;**98**(3):149-157

[126] Kingma JG, Simard D, Voisine P, Rouleau JR. Role of the autonomic nervous system in cardioprotection by remote preconditioning in isoflurane-anaesthetized dogs. Cardiovascular Research. 2011;**89**(2):384-391. DOI: 10.1093/cvr/cvq306

[127] Jensen RV, Stottrup NB, Kristiansen SB, Botker HE. Release of a humoral circulating cardioprotective factor by remote ischemic preconditioning is dependent on preserved neural pathways in diabetic patients. Basic Research in Cardiology. 2012;**107**(5):285. DOI: 10.1007/s00395-012-0285-1

[128] Li J, Rohailla S, Gelber N, Rutka J, Sabah N, Gladstone RA, et al. MicroRNA-144 is a circulating effector of remote ischemic preconditioning. Basic Research in Cardiology. 2014;**109**(5):423. DOI: 10.1007/s00395-014-0423-z

[129] Davidson SM, Selvaraj P, He D, Boi-Doku C, Yellon RL, Vicencio JM, et al. Remote ischaemic preconditioning involves signalling through the SDF-1alpha/CXCR4 signalling axis. Basic Research in Cardiology. 2013;**108**(5):377. DOI: 10.1007/s00395-013-0377-6

[130] Kudej RK, Shen YT, Peppas AP, Huang CH, Chen W, Yan L, et al. Obligatory role of cardiac nerves and alpha1-adrenergic receptors for the second window of ischemic preconditioning in conscious pigs. Circulation Research. 2006;**99**(11):1270-1276

[131] Haessler R, Wolff RA, Chien GL, Davis RF, Van Winkle DM. High spinal anesthesia does not alter experimental myocardial infarction size or ischemic preconditioning. Journal of Cardiothoracic and Vascular Anesthesia 1997;11(1):72-79. DOI: 10.1016S1053-0770(97)90257-3

[132] Dickson EW, Lorbar M, Porcaro WA, Fenton RA, Reinhardt CP, Gysembergh A, et al. Rabbit heart can be "preconditioned" via transfer of coronary effluent. American Journal of Physiology. Heart and Circulatory Physiology. 1999;**277**(6):H2451-H24H7

[133] Ma XJ, Zhang XH, Li CM, Luo M. Effect of postconditioning on coronary blood flow velocity and endothelial function in patients with acute myocardial infarction. Scandinavian Cardiovascular Journal. 2006;**40**(6):327-333. DOI: 10.1080/14017430601047864

[134] Laskey WK, Yoon S, Calzada N, Ricciardi MJ. Concordant improvements in coronary flow reserve and ST-segment resolution during percutaneous coronary intervention for acute myocardial infarction: A benefit of postconditioning. Catheterization and Cardiovascular Interventions. 2008;**72**(2):212-220. DOI: 10.1002/ccd.21583

[135] Bolognese L, Carrabba N, Parodi G, Santoro GM, Buonamici P, Cerisano G, et al. Impact of microvascular dysfunction on left ventricular remodeling and long-term clinical outcome after primary coronary angioplasty for acute

myocardial infarction. Circulation. 2004;**109**(9):1121-1126. DOI: 10.1161/01.CIR.0000118496.44135.A7

[136] Dwivedi G, Janardhanan R, Hayat SA, Lim TK, Greaves K, Senior R. Relationship between myocardial perfusion with myocardial contrast echocardiography and function early after acute myocardial infarction for the prediction of late recovery of function. International Journal of Cardiology. 2010;**140**(2):169-174. DOI: 10.1016/j.ijcard.2008.11.052

[137] Dwivedi G, Janardhanan R, Hayat SA, Swinburn JM, Senior R. Prognostic value of myocardial viability detected by myocardial contrast echocardiography early after acute myocardial infarction. Journal of the American College of Cardiology. 2007;**50**(4):327-334. DOI: 10.1016/j.jacc.2007.03.036

[138] Przyklenk K. Reduction of myocardial infarct size with ischemic "conditioning": Physiologic and technical considerations. Anesthesia and Analgesia. 2013;**117**(4):891-901. DOI: 10.1213/ANE.0b013e318294fc63

[139] Loukogeorgakis SP, Panagiotidou AT, Broadhead MW, Donald A, Deanfield JE, MacAllister RJ. Remote ischemic preconditioning provides early and late protection against endothelial ischemia-reperfusion injury in humans: Role of the autonomic nervous system. Journal of the American College of Cardiology. 2005;**46**(3):450-456

[140] Hausenloy DJ, Candilio L, Evans R, Ariti C, Jenkins DP, Kolvekar S, et al. Remote ischemic preconditioning and outcomes of cardiac surgery. The New England Journal of Medicine. 2015;**373**(15):1408-1417. DOI: 10.1056/NEJMoa1413534

[141] Meybohm P, Bein B, Brosteanu O, Cremer J, Gruenewald M, Stoppe C, et al. A multicenter trial of remote ischemic preconditioning for heart surgery. The New England Journal of Medicine. 2015;**373**(15):1397-1407. DOI: 10.1056/NEJMoa1413579

[142] Ghaemian A, Nouraei SM, Abdollahian F, Naghshvar F, Giussani DA, Nouraei SA. Remote ischemic preconditioning in percutaneous coronary revascularization: A double-blind randomized controlled clinical trial. Asian Cardiovascular & Thoracic Annals. 2012;**20**(5):548-554. DOI: 10.1177/0218492312439999

[143] Zaugg M, Lucchinetti E, Behmanesh S, Clanachan AS. Anesthetic cardioprotection in clinical practice from proof-of-concept to clinical applications. Current Pharmaceutical Design. 2014;**20**(36):5706-5726. DOI: 10.2174/1381612820666140204120829

[144] Landoni G, Greco T, Biondi-Zoccai G, Nigro Neto C, Febres D, Pintaudi M, et al. Anaesthetic drugs and survival: A Bayesian network meta-analysis of randomized trials in cardiac surgery. British Journal of Anaesthesia. 2013;**111**(6):886-896. DOI: 10.1093/bja/aet231

[145] Schmidt MR, Smerup M, Konstantinov IE, Shimizu M, Li J, Cheung M, et al. Intermittent peripheral tissue ischemia during coronary ischemia reduces myocardial infarction through a KATP-dependent mechanism: First demonstration of remote ischemic perconditioning. American Journal of Physiology. Heart and Circulatory Physiology. 2007;**292**(4):H1883-H1890. DOI: 10.1152/ajpheart.00617.

[146] Yellon DM, Ackbarkhan AK, Balgobin V, Bulluck H, Deelchand A, Dhuny MR, et al. Remote ischemic conditioning reduces myocardial infarct size in STEMI patients treated by thrombolysis. Journal of the American College of Cardiology.

2015;**65**(25):2764-2765. DOI: 10.1016/j.jacc.2015.02.082

[147] Rentoukas I, Giannopoulos G, Kaoukis A, Kossyvakis C, Raisakis K, Driva M, et al. Cardioprotective role of remote ischemic perconditioning in primary percutaneous coronary intervention: Enhancement by opioid action. JACC. Cardiovascular Interventions. 2010;**3**(1):49-55. DOI: 10.1016/j.jcin.2009.10.015

Chapter 3

Epigenetics of Circadian Rhythm Disruption in Cardiovascular Diseases

Ivana Škrlec

Abstract

Circadian rhythm influences the regulation of homeostasis and physiological processes, and its disruption could lead to metabolic disorders and cardiovascular diseases (CVD). CVDs are still the dominant cause of death worldwide, which are related to numerous environmental and hereditary risk factors. Environmental and hereditary factors can clarify a small fraction of the CVD risk discrepancy. Epigenomics is a very bright strategy that will complement the knowledge of the genetic basis of CVDs. Epigenetic mechanisms allow cells to reply promptly to environmental changes and include DNA methylation, histone modification, and noncoding RNA alterations. According to research data, the circadian rhythm regulates many epigenetic regulators. The challenge is to understand how epigenetic events happen rhythmically in tissues that are involved in the development of CVDs. Epigenetic events are possibly reversible through their interface with environmental and nutritional factors, allowing innovative preventive and therapeutic strategies in cardiovascular diseases.

Keywords: circadian rhythm, cardiovascular disease, epigenetics, DNA methylation, histone modification, microRNA

1. Introduction

The word epigenetics comes from the Greek word 'epi' that means above; that is, hereditary variations in phenotype that do exclude alterations in the nucleotide sequence in DNA [1]. Epigenetic mechanisms involve DNA methylation, post-translational histone modifications, and noncoding RNAs (ncRNAs) [1]. Many studies focus on the epigenetic mechanisms of various diseases. Epigenetic processes are essential for the healthy growth and development of an organism [1]. Epigenetic mechanisms are implicated in the expression of circadian genes in the suprachiasmatic nucleus (SCN) neurons and peripheral tissues [2]. The accumulation of lifestyle and age-related epigenetic changes could result in the development of metabolic disorders and atherosclerosis [2].

The influence of epigenetic changes on the cardiovascular system is an essential link between genotype to phenotype diversity [3]. Epigenetic changes are potentially reversible and may be affected by environmental factors, nutrition, as well as gene-environment interactions. Identifying and understanding epigenetic factors represent a new insight into our knowledge of the risks of cardiovascular disease (CVD) [1].

1.1 Circadian rhythm

The circadian clock is a preserved system that allows organisms to adapt to frequent daily variations, such as the day and night and food availability [4]. This center clock receives signals from the environment and coordinates the daily activity of peripheral clocks found in almost all tissues [4]. The molecular clock is vital in maintaining metabolic and physiological homeostasis [5]. The circadian clock is linked to cellular metabolism so that dysregulation of the circadian rhythm can contribute to various pathological conditions such as diabetes, obesity, metabolic syndrome, inflammation, sleep disorders, and CVDs [5–8].

Genome-wide studies show that 10–15% of all transcripts have a circadian pattern in different tissues involved in the control of metabolism, such as the cardiovascular function [4, 6, 8, 9]. The onset of ischemic cardiopathy is irregularly distributed during the day [1, 10, 11]. A chronobiological strategy to heart disease may present new possibilities to enhance drug development to improve therapeutic outcomes [1]. Genetic evidence supports the function of circadian rhythm in the adjustment of metabolism.

1.2 Cardiovascular diseases

Cardiovascular diseases are complex and diverse. They include hypertension, coronary artery disease, heart failure, and stroke and are a main worldwide reason for morbidity and death in advanced economies and carry a substantial economic burden [1, 3, 12–15]. CVDs are associated with a variety of hereditary and variable risk factors, but environmental and genetic impacts may explain a smaller fraction of CVD risk variability [1, 12]. Studies showed that there is a wide range between 40 and 80% of the genetic contribution to the onset of cardiovascular disease [16].

The complex pathogenesis of CVD is due to the abundance of genetic and environmental factors, of which epigenetic changes are a significant factor [3]. Several risk factors of CVD, like diet, smoking, stress, circadian rhythm, and pollution, are related to epigenetic modifications [1]. Disorders such as hypertension, diabetes, and obesity are often utilized to recognize and cure people at increased CVDs risk [1]. Epigenetic modifications are associated with the processes involved in the CVD in humans or directly affect the gene expression involved in a major cardiac complication, myocardial infarction (MI). Hypertension is one of the leading causes of CVDs [3], while insulin resistance is one of the most significant precursors of type 2 diabetes and associated cardiometabolic conditions [17].

Changes in the style of living and diet could decrease the risk of CVDs [14]. Epigenetic factors indicate there is interindividual variability from birth. It can be stable over the life span and is considered to be an initiator of early programming for adult-onset diseases [12, 18]. The understanding of epigenetics in the onset of CVDs may provide a new perspective on diseases [14].

1.3 Epigenetics

Epigenetics studies heritable variations in gene expression that exclude any change in the DNA sequence [16, 19]. Epigenetic changes include modifications of the DNA base, post-translational histone modifications, and ncRNA mechanisms that run in the nucleus [16, 20]. The epigenome moves the genome from a transcriptionally active to a transcriptionally inactive state [4, 21]. Epimutation transmissions occur throughout the life of the individual [2]. The rate of epigenetic variation is higher than that of genetic mutations because the formation of new inherited changes allows adjustment to a new environment [14, 16].

The most studied epigenetic change is cytosine methylation. It is also a method for suppressing gene expression [22]. DNA methyltransferase (DNMT) enzymes perform DNA methylation. DNMTs bind the methyl group to the 5-site cytosine [16]. The methyl group most commonly binds to the cytosine at a CpG site. It is the fundamental and ubiquitous epigenetic mechanism [14]. The DNMT enzyme family, consisting of DNMT1, DNMT3a, and DNMT3b, methylates cytosine into 5-methylcytosine [14]. Promoter methylation is usually connected with inhibition of transcription [14]. DNMT1 controls the mitotic inheritance of methylated DNA, while DNMT3a and DNMT3b are mainly in charge of *de novo* methylation [14]. The different epigenetic modification is DNA hydroxymethylation, including 5-hydroxymethylated cytosines [14]. Different nutritional and lifestyle factors can affect the methylation of particular CpG sites in gene promoters and into adulthood [22].

Nucleosomes are composed of histone proteins around which DNA is wound into chromatin [16]. Nucleosomes consist of eight histone proteins: two dimers of H2A/H2B and two dimers of H3/H4. Each histone has an adjustable amino-acid tail [16]. Histones can change at more than 30 amino acid residues within amino-terminal tails [4]. Histone modifications include various processes such as acetylation, methylation, phosphorylation, sumoylation, and ubiquitination. It has a function in the organization of chromatin composition and gene expression by altering the intensity of chromatin condensation [1, 14, 23]. Histones are mostly acetylated on lysine (K) residues. Histone acetyltransferase (HAT) and histone deacetylase (HDAC) regulate histone acetylation [14]. Histone methyltransferase regulates histone methylation, while histone demethylase catalyzes demethylation. Transcription activation is usually associated with acetylation of lysine residues at histones 3 (H3) and 4 (H4). Depending on the location of the target lysines in the histone tail and the number of methyl groups added, methylation can either activate or inhibit gene expression [14, 24]. Histone phosphorylation is a marker of cell division and has a function in DNA repair, chromatin condensation during division, and regulation of gene expression [14, 25]. The addition of ubiquitin to lysine residues in histones is called ubiquitination and is implicated in DNA repair and control of transcription [14]. Sumoylation is a changeable post-translational adjustment using small ubiquitin-like proteins (SUMO) and has a crucial function in various mechanisms, such as transcription, and cell cycle progression [14, 26].

RNA-based epigenetic mechanisms include long noncoding RNAs (lncRNAs) and microRNAs (miRNAs) [14]. NcRNAs are functional RNAs that do not translate into proteins and play an essential part in epigenetic regulation [14, 16]. The lncRNAs are extremely tissue-specific relative to protein-coding genes [16]. The miRNAs are short (20–22 nucleotides), single-stranded, evolutionarily-conserved ncRNAs that modulate the expression at the post-transcriptional level of more than 50% of cellular genes [13, 14, 27].

Changes in the environment, including temperature, light, and nutritional habits, trigger reversible epigenomic modification that can influence numerous physiological processes [28]. Epigenome-wide association studies (EWAS) provide information about associations between epigenomic perturbations and traits associated with human diseases [29]. EWAS try to evaluate the environmental impact on genetic regulation. The epigenetic variations could explain missing parts of heritability of chronic diseases that have not yet been determined by genome-wide association studies [29].

2. Molecular background of circadian rhythm

The primary clock genes show circadian expression in the SCN, and light is one of the key drivers that can reset the rhythm phases. There are several crucial proteins in SCN. Transcription activators are aryl hydrocarbon receptor nuclear translocator-like (ARNTL or BMAL1) and circadian locomotor output cycle caps (CLOCK). Transcription inhibitors are period (PER) and cryptochrome (CRY) [30, 31]. Within 24 h, the entire process of activation and inhibition of gene expression takes place [32, 33]. The circadian system controls gene expression through various mechanisms as a basis of global gene regulation. The first is via E-boxes (promoter and enhancer regulatory elements) of oscillator proteins such as CLOCK, ARNTL, and NPAS2 (neuronal PAS domain protein 2). The second mechanism is using other oscillator proteins such as RORα (retinoic acid receptor-related orphan receptor) and REV-ERBα (or NR1D1, orphan nuclear receptor) via REV-ERB/ROR response element (RRE), which are present in the promoters of specific clock-controlled genes (CCGs) (**Figure 1**). The third mechanism is the daily chromatin remodeling [2, 19, 34, 35].

The ARNTL-CLOCK heterodimers enhance *CRY* and *PER* expression, as well as the expression of additional CCGs. Phosphorylated CRY-PER heterodimers repress the action of ARNTL-CLOCK heterodimer. As a result, *CRY* and *PER* gene transcription is decreased during the day, while ubiquitin degradation reduces the CRY and PER protein levels. The PER2 has histone deacetylase activity and modified chromatin structure, followed by transcription termination [36–39]. The new cycle begins with the termination of the ARNTL-CLOCK repression during the day. Casein kinase 1 (CK1) regulates the quantity of CRY-PER heterodimers' phosphorylation or degradation. CK1 controls protein activity via its phosphorylation [40]. An additional negative loop is REV-ERBα. It binds to the RRE of the *ARNTL* and *CLOCK* genes and inhibits their transcription. Overnight, REV-ERBα degrades, and RORα elevates the *ARNTL* gene transcription [2, 32, 41]. ARNTL-CLOCK heterodimers increase transcription of the nuclear receptors *RORα* and *REV-ERBα* and form an additional circadian rhythm loop [31, 42].

Nearly 10% of the transcripts show circadian rhythmicity [19]. Rhythmic expression of crucial metabolic genes is impaired due to clock gene mutations and lead to metabolic disorders [28]. Fasting glucose levels decrease, and insulin sensitivity

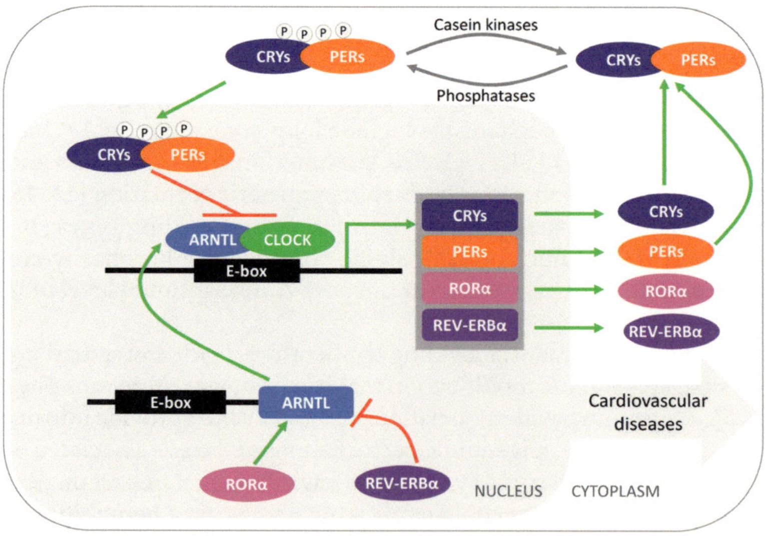

Figure 1.
Circadian rhythm gene regulation in cardiovascular diseases. ARNTL and CLOCK activate transcription of CRY *and* PER *and nuclear receptors (*REV-ERBα *and* RORα*). CRY and PER heterodimerize and phosphorylate by casein kinases and translate into the nucleus where they prevent binding of the ARNTL-CLOCK to the regulatory regions of target genes. In the second feedback loop, REV-ERBα prevents the transcription of* ARNTL*, while overnight the RORα activates transcription of* ARNTL*. ARNTL—aryl hydrocarbon receptor nuclear translocator-like, CLOCK—circadian locomotor output cycle kaput, CRY—cryptochrome, PER—period, P—phosphate, RORα—retinoic-related orphan receptor alpha, Ub—ubiquitin.*

increases in overexpression of the *CRY1* [28]. *ARNTL* deletion and *CLOCK* mutation disturb lipid metabolism [28, 43]. REV-ERBα is involved in liver circadian lipid biosynthesis, and REV-ERBα and ARNTL manage adipocyte differentiation [28]. A primary regulator of bile acid synthesis is REV-ERBα, while the *PER1* and *PER2* deletion upregulates bile acid biosynthesis and causes hepatic cholestasis [28].

Based on circadian rhythms in SCN neurons and peripheral cells, epigenetic mechanisms participate in the formation of circadian rhythms of gene expression [2]. One of the primary circadian genes, CLOCK, has the function of histone acetyltransferase. Chromatin remodeling is an essential underlying mechanism of the clock rhythm and reveals an association between cellular physiology and histone acetylation [2]. ARNTL-CLOCK heterodimer or ARNTL-NPAS2 complex mobilizes HATs and HDACs [28, 44]. To maintain metabolic homeostasis and avoid metabolic disorders, the crosstalk between circadian rhythm and metabolism is necessary [28].

3. Epigenetic changes in circadian rhythm in cardiovascular diseases

Rapid adaptation of cells to environmental changes is facilitated by epigenetic mechanisms that also offer a link between genes and the environment [1]. The phenotypic variations observed in humans are more significant than genotype variations alone, and changes in epigenetic gene modification explain them [1, 45]. CVDs, such as atherosclerosis, cardiac hypertrophy, myocardial infarction, and heart failure, are associated with epigenetic mechanisms ranging from DNA methylation, histone modification, to ncRNAs [13]. An essential way of developing CVD early in life involves epigenetic changes [12]. The underlying mechanism providing the link between the early life environment and the subsequent CVD risk is epigenetic modifications [12].

The association of methylation with specific genes may be useful in assessing the risk of a disease or in monitoring the response to a particular treatment [14]. In the process of DNA methylation, homocysteine, an amino acid that does not enter into protein composition, is essential [46]. The lack of folate in the diet leads to an increase in plasma homocysteine, which contributes to the rise of S-adenosyl homocysteine. It represses transmethylation reactions and decreases methylation all over the epigenome [1, 46]. In atherogenesis are included homocysteine-induced changes in DNA methylation in smooth muscle vascular cells [1, 47, 48]. Endothelial dysfunction and different aspects of CVD are epigenetically associated with folic acid deficiency [16]. Genomic DNA is hypomethylated in human atherosclerotic lesions [1, 2, 12]. Inflammatory processes involved in the development of atherosclerotic plaques are associated with hypermethylation [1, 49]. There are rhythmic changes in global DNA methylation in human blood, and there is an increased level at night [35]. Changes in circadian rhythm genes methylation were observed in aging mice, but are tissue-dependent [35, 50]. For example, in the stomach of older mice, the methylation of the *PER1* promoter decreased, while the methylation of the *ARNTL*, *CRY1*, and *NPAS2* promoters in the spleen was increased [35]. Sleep disorders affect circadian rhythm gene methylation, especially *ARNTL*, *CRY1*, and *PER1* [35, 51]. Temporary epigenetic changes linked with rhythmic gene expression lead to circadian epiphenotypes [2]. Based on this, it can be concluded that DNA methylation may be reversed by conventional drugs, independent of DNA replication [2].

The histone code is involved in many aspects of cardiovascular physiology, from endothelial cell responses to hypoxia to recovery from MI [16]. CLOCK has enzymatic properties of histone acetyltransferase (HAT). It performs acetylation at Lys537 of H3 histone and ARNTL, which is necessary for circadian rhythm [1, 9]. CLOCK works in collaboration with other HATs to maintain circadian rhythm in the acetylation state of histones at CCG promoters [6]. HDAC activity has an essential function in defining the intensity of myocardial ischemia, especially after MI [16]. Inhibition of HDAC can promote angiogenesis and reduce myocardial damage after MI [16], such as valproic acid (VPA), which is an HDAC inhibitor [2]. Histone deacetylases, SIRT1 (sirtuin 1), and SIRT6 participate in the histone modification, thus controlling gene expression [35] and providing a molecular connection among metabolism and circadian rhythm [6]. SIRT1 deacetylates regulatory proteins and acts as a rhythm-promoting agent in circadian oscillators [35]. SIRT1 has a unique role in central and peripheral circadian rhythms [35]. The purpose of histone phosphorylation in CVDs is minimal [14], while SUMO proteins influence the activity of several essential factors that are important for cardiac development [14]. There are connections between circadian rhythm regulators, chromatin modifications, and cellular metabolism [1, 52].

Numerous lncRNAs have essential regulatory functions in various CVDs [14]. The miRNAs regulate cholesterol metabolism, oxidative stress, and endothelial dysfunction, diverse cellular processes involved in atherosclerosis [14]. MiRNAs may be relevant regulators of circadian rhythm [1]. Circulating miRNA-145 and miRNA-126 are decreased in patients with coronary artery disease, while miRNA-1, miRNA-499, and miRNA-133b are increased during acute myocardial infarction [13]. All those miRNAs can be biomarkers of CVD.

Circadian rhythms combine metabolic and environmental signals and alter gene expression when adapting the organism to particular circumstances [6]. Many epigenetic regulators in some tissues are controlled in a circadian fashion [19, 53]. The challenge is to determine whether epigenetic variations happen in a rhythmic pattern in tissues included in the CVD development [12, 19]. Epigenetics can contribute to enhancing CVD therapies and finding new markers for CVD screening [16, 54].

4. DNA methylation and CVDs

DNA methylation is a durable, relatively constant epigenetic change. It involves the covalent attachment of a methyl group to the cytosine [3, 55]. The primary role of DNA methylation is to regulate gene expression by altering the availability of DNA to the transcription factors [3, 13].

DNA methylation links the steady genome and the changing environment. It is an instrument through which environmental changes influence metabolism [7]. Disruption of DNA methylation has been associated with different metabolic diseases such as diabetes [56], obesity, and insulin resistance [57]. Furthermore, the epigenetic mechanisms control circadian rhythm, and circadian disturbance leads to DNA methylation changes of the clock genes [7, 51, 58]. Adiposity, metabolic syndrome, and weight loss are linked to DNA methylation changes of the *ARNTL*, *CLOCK*, and *PER2* gene promoters [7]. It indicates the significance of determining the impact of DNA methylation in epigenetic studies in complex human disorders [7].

DNA methylation is cell- or tissue-specific, but epimutations are not restricted to the affected tissue and may also be observed in peripheral blood [7]. Compared to other genes, the regulatory regions of circadian rhythm genes are plentiful in CpG sites [59, 60]. Patients with coronary artery disease have altered methylation patterns relative to controls [1, 61, 62]. All mentioned supports the assumption that epigenetic variations are associated with an increased CVD risk [1].

Epigenetic alterations of circadian genes are related to obesity and metabolic disorders [17, 63]. A positive association was found between the alteration of the *ARNTL* gene methylation and weight loss, and its activity is included in the control of adipogenesis and lipid metabolism [63]. The long-term shiftwork, associated with obesity and metabolic syndrome risk, induces hypomethylation of the *CLOCK* gene promoter [22]. *CLOCK* gene SNPs are associated with a predisposition to metabolic syndrome [22, 64]. Long-term shift work, obesity, and metabolic syndrome are associated with *CRY2* hypermethylation in peripheral blood [22]. Genetic variants of the human *PER2* gene are related to abdominal obesity and CVDs [22, 65]. The methylation status of CpG sites in the *PER2* gene is associated with obesity, metabolic syndrome, and weight loss [7, 22].

Global hypomethylation of DNA is present in atherosclerotic lesions [3, 66]. The severity of atherosclerotic lesions correlates with DNA methylation [3, 14, 67, 68]. There are notable variations in DNA methylation after an MI event [69, 70]. DNA methylation status in blood samples is related to CVD [71, 72].

Environmental and behavioral factors, such as inflammation, smoking, physical activity, or stress, can alter the epigenome [63, 73]. Elevated gene expression in the inflammatory pathway is associated with decreased gene methylation [46]. DNA methylation relies on the accessibility of methyl groups obtained from methionine, and the existence of certain nutrients in the food influences epigenetic changes with possible cardiovascular outcomes [46]. Although methylation changes are related to healthy aging, they could be in the background of the development of some diseases, such as CVD [46, 74]. Reduction in global DNA methylation occurs throughout the human lifespan [46].

5. Histone modification and CVDs

Post-translational modifications occur at amino acid residues in the amino-terminal regions of histone and cover histone acetylation, methylation, phosphorylation, sumoylation, and ubiquitination. It controls chromatin remodeling and gene expression [3, 23]. Histone acetylation is a sign of transcription activation [75], while histone methylation can both stimulate and inhibit transcription [28, 75]. Post-translational histone modifications control genes coding clock proteins [46, 75]. Epigenetic irregularities are related to different disorders, including atherosclerosis [4, 76].

Histone modifications occur at the CCG promoters in a circadian fashion [4, 44, 77, 78]. The core clock protein, CLOCK, has HAT activity. It revealed the molecular association among epigenetic mechanisms and circadian rhythm [4, 19, 59, 79]. CLOCK acetylates ARNTL, which facilitates CRY-dependent repression [19, 28], and interaction of CRY1 with the ARNTL-CLOCK heterodimer [9]. CLOCK and NPAS2 attract different HATs to the promoter of the *PER1* in vascular tissues [59, 78]. The rhythmic binding of ARNTL and CLOCK transcriptional activators directly influences the acetylation of specific histone lysine residues near the DNA-binding site without the involvement of additional HAT enzymes [59]. CLOCK acetylates additional non-histone proteins that have crucial roles in the regulation of different cellular events [4].

SIRT1 is an NAD + -dependent histone deacetylase [4, 59, 80]. It is needed for rhythmic transcription of some clock genes, such as *ARNTL*, *CRY1*, and *PER2* [80, 81]. STIR1 represents the molecular connection between metabolic processes, chromatin remodeling, and circadian physiology [4]. SIRT1 plays a crucial role in metabolism. It deacetylates some proteins of the metabolic pathways and regulates gene expression by histone deacetylation [75]. *SIRT1* expression levels are nearly constant over 24 h, just like relatively constant *CLOCK* gene expression levels*** [4, 82–85]. The HAT function of CLOCK is balanced by SIRT1, which deacetylates H3 and ARNTL, and PER2 [79, 83, 86]. SIRT1 binds to ARNTL-CLOCK within a chromatin complex that, in a circadian fashion, binds to CCG promoters [4, 87]. ARNTL and PER2 are SIRT1 targets [4]. SIRT1 associates with ARNTL-CLOCK heterodimers and improves the deacetylation and degradation of PER2 [86]. SIRT1 deacetylates clock proteins in a circadian fashion [4]. HDAC3 is a deacetylase that modulates histone acetylation of circadian genes, especially those included in lipid metabolism, such as REV-ERBα [88–92]. Mutations of circadian rhythm proteins that can either modify histones (such as CLOCK) or link to histone modifiers (such as ARNTL, PER2, and REV-ERBα) are related to metabolic syndrome [75, 79]. Endogenous SIRT1 plays a crucial role in mediating cell death/survival processes and is involved in the pathogenesis of the CVDs [28, 93]. The ARNTL sumoylation plays an essential role in ARNTL accumulation and circadian rhythmicity [86].

Histone modifications, and particularly HDACs, have a significant role in the control of vascular homeostasis. Dysregulation of HDAC could lead to the formation of atherosclerotic lesions [14, 94]. In human carotid arteries, histone methylation and acetylation present recognizable patterns depending on the seriousness of the plaque [46]. Inhibition of HDACs leads to reduced inflammation and atherogenesis [46, 95]. In animal studies, HDAC inhibitors reduce the size of MI and ischemia-reperfusion injury after revascularization [46, 96]. The inhibition of HDAC may improve myocardial recovery and block post-infarction remodeling [46]. Fibrosis after MI was reduced by valproic acid, an HDAC inhibitor [14, 97].

6. MicroRNAs and CVDs

MicroRNAs (miRNAs) are small noncoding RNA molecules that repress the expression of target messenger RNAs [1, 3, 5, 98]. MicroRNA dysregulation is associated with cardiovascular diseases, lipid metabolism, endothelial function, ventricular hypertrophy, and post-infarction dysrhythmias [1, 5].

Oscillating microRNAs, based on external triggers, could affect the expression of target genes in a circadian fashion independently of clock genes [5, 99]. In plasma and serum of CVD patients are observed decreased levels of numerous miRNAs, such as miRNA-126, miRNA-17, miRNA-145, miRNA-92a, and miRNA-155 [3].

MiRNAs control the development of atherosclerosis through their action on endothelial function, plaque progression and rupture, and blood vessel development [46]. MiRNA-126 expressed by endothelial cells serves as an adverse adjuster of vascular inflammation, while miRNA-33 plays a vital role in inhibiting the critical genes implicated in cellular cholesterol export [14, 100]. Some miRNAs target DNMTs and thus regulate the level of DNA methylation in atherosclerotic lesions [14]. MiRNA-148 changes HDL and LDL cholesterol levels in murine models and thus has a vital function in lipid metabolism [46, 101, 102].

MiRNA-24, 29a, and 30a influence the circadian rhythm by regulating the stability and translation of PER1 and PER2 mRNAs [5]. The ARNTL-CLOCK heterodimer controls miRNA-142–3p and, in turn, can target ARNTL [5, 103, 104]. MiRNA-21 is a PER2-dependent miRNA and mediates PER2-obtained cardioprotection [5, 105]. Through cellular stress, PER2-dependent miRNA-21 controls cellular glycolysis. Myocardial ischemia causes activation of pathways aimed at increasing the efficiency of myocardial oxygen [5, 106]. Suppression of miRNA-21 reduces the fibrotic response and enhances cardiac activity [5].

A valuable sign of myocardial cell death is the plasma levels of miRNA-208 [3, 107]. MiRNAs have a function in remodeling after MI, a mechanism closely associated with the expansion of tissue fibrosis [14]. A more sensitive biomarker of acute non-STEM MI is miRNA-499 than cardiac troponin T [46].

MicroRNAs could potentially become new modulators of circadian rhythms and could have a positive effect on cardiovascular physiology [5]. MiRNAs regulate about 60% of all human genes [46]. Therapeutic strategies should target specific microRNAs and thus reduce their capacity to inhibit circadian rhythm components or circadian rhythm output genes [5, 108–112]. Administration of microRNAs in a circadian-dependent fashion could serve to adapt the impaired circadian system, advance metabolism by enhancing efficient oxygen pathways, and thereby promote cardioprotection from ischemia [5].

7. Conclusion

The epigenetic variations of an individual change throughout a lifetime and epigenome profiles, instead of genotypes, are reflected in phenotypes in epigenetic epidemiological studies. Therefore, epigenetic modifications are the reason or a result of a pathological condition. Understanding the epigenetic contribution to CVD pathology may help to develop new treatments and diagnostic approaches. Epigenetic biomarkers might be very useful in treatment monitoring and predicting disease outcome. Epigenetic events can potentially be reversibly altered depending on environmental and nutritional factors. Understanding epigenetic mechanisms may identify valuable, novel biomarkers for disease.

Conflict of interest

The author declares no conflict of interest.

Author details

Ivana Škrlec
Histology, Genetics, Cellular, and Molecular Biology Laboratory, Faculty of Dental Medicine and Health, Department of Biology and Chemistry, J.J. Strossmayer University of Osijek, Croatia

*Address all correspondence to: iskrlec@fdmz.hr

References

[1] Ordovás J, Smith C. Epigenetics and cardiovascular disease. Nature Reviews. Cardiology. 2011;7:510-519. DOI: 10.1038/nrcardio.2010.104.Epigenetics

[2] Gallou-Kabani C, Vigé A, Junien C. Lifelong circadian and epigenetic drifts in metabolic syndrome. Epigenetics. 2007;**2**:137-146. DOI: 10.4161/epi.2.3.4897

[3] Udali S, Guarini P, Moruzzi S, Choi S-W, Friso S. Cardiovascular epigenetics: From DNA methylation to microRNAs. Molecular Aspects of Medicine. 2013;**34**:883-901. DOI: 10.1016/j.mam.2012.08.001

[4] Bellet MM, Sassone-Corsi P. Mammalian circadian clock and metabolism—The epigenetic link. Journal of Cell Science. 2010;**123**:3837-3848. DOI: 10.1242/jcs.051649

[5] Oyama Y, Bartman CM, Gile J, Eckle T. Circadian microRNAs in cardioprotection. Current Pharmaceutical Design. 2017;**23**:3723-3730. DOI: 10.2174/1381612823666170707165319

[6] Aguilar-Arnal L, Sassone-Corsi P. Chromatin landscape and circadian dynamics: Spatial and temporal organization of clock transcription. PNAS. 2015;**112**:6863-6870. DOI: 10.1073/pnas.1411264111

[7] Peng H, Zhu Y, Goldberg J, Vaccarino V, Zhao J. DNA methylation of five core circadian genes jointly contributes to glucose metabolism: A gene-set analysis in monozygotic twins. Frontiers in Genetics. 2019;**10**:329. DOI: 10.3389/fgene.2019.00329

[8] Duez H, Staels B, Ne Duez ÉÈHL, Staels B. Circadian control of epigenetic modifications modulates metabolism. Circulation Research. 2011;**109**:353-355. DOI: 10.1161/RES.0b013e31822be420

[9] Grimaldi B, Nakahata Y, Kaluzova M, Masubuchi S, Sassone-Corsi P. Chromatin remodeling, metabolism and circadian clocks: The interplay of CLOCK and SIRT1. The International Journal of Biochemistry & Cell Biology. 2009;**41**:81-86. DOI: 10.1016/j.biocel.2008.08.035

[10] Hermida RC, Ayala DE, Fernández JR, Calvo C. Chronotherapy improves blood pressure control and reverts the nondipper pattern in patients with resistant hypertension chronotherapy in resistant hypertension. Hypertension. 2007;**51**:69-76. DOI: 10.1161/HYPERTENSIONAHA.107.096933

[11] Martino TA, Sole MJ. Molecular time: An often overlooked dimension to cardiovascular disease. Circulation Research. 2009;**105**:1047-1061. DOI: 10.1161/CIRCRESAHA.109.206201

[12] Sun C, Burgner DP, Ponsonby AL, Saffery R, Huang RC, Vuillermin PJ, et al. Effects of early-life environment and epigenetics on cardiovascular disease risk in children: Highlighting the role of twin studies. Pediatric Research. 2013;**73**:523-530. DOI: 10.1038/pr.2013.6

[13] Voelter-Mahlknecht S. Epigenetic associations in relation to cardiovascular prevention and therapeutics. Clinical Epigenetics. 2016;**8**:1-17. DOI: 10.1186/s13148-016-0170-0

[14] Prasher D, Greenway SC, Singh RB. The impact of epigenetics on cardiovascular disease. Biochemistry and Cell Biology. 2019;**98**:12-22. DOI: 10.1139/bcb-2019-0045

[15] Kearney PM, Whelton M, Reynolds K, Muntner P, Whelton PK, He J. Global burden of hypertension: Analysis of worldwide data. Lancet. 2005;**365**:217-223. DOI: 10.1016/s0140-6736(05)17741-1

[16] Webster ALH, Yan MSC, Marsden PA. Epigenetics and cardiovascular disease. The Canadian Journal of Cardiology. 2013;**29**:46-57. DOI: 10.1016/j.cjca.2012.10.023

[17] Arpón A, Milagro FI, Ramos-Lopez O, Mansego ML, Santos JL, Riezu-Boj JI, et al. Epigenome-wide association study in peripheral white blood cells involving insulin resistance. Scientific Reports. 2019;**9**:2445. DOI: 10.1038/s41598-019-38980-2

[18] Campión J, Milagro FI, Martínez JA. Individuality and epigenetics in obesity. Obesity Reviews. 2009;**10**:383-392. DOI: 10.1111/j.1467-789X.2009.00595.x

[19] Sahar S, Sassone-Corsi P. Circadian rhythms and memory formation: Regulation by chromatin remodeling. Frontiers in Molecular Neuroscience. 2012;**5**:1-4. DOI: 10.3389/fnmol.2012.00037

[20] Kim JK, Samaranayake M, Pradhan S. Epigenetic mechanisms in mammals. Cellular and Molecular Life Sciences. 2009;**66**:596-612. DOI: 10.1007/s00018-008-8432-4

[21] Borrelli E, Nestler EJ, Allis CD, Sassone-Corsi P. Decoding the epigenetic language of neuronal plasticity. Neuron. 2008;**60**:961-974. DOI: 10.1016/j.neuron.2008.10.012

[22] Milagro FI, Gómez-Abellán P, Campión J, Martínez JA, Ordovás JM, Garaulet M. CLOCK, PER2 and BMAL1 DNA methylation: Association with obesity and metabolic syndrome characteristics and monounsaturated fat intake. Chronobiology International. 2012;**29**:1180-1194. DOI: 10.3109/07420528.2012.719967

[23] Bannister AJ, Kouzarides T. Regulation of chromatin by histone modifications. Cell Research. 2011;**21**:381-395. DOI: 10.1038/cr.2011.22

[24] Ripperger JA, Schibler U. Rhythmic CLOCK-BMAL1 binding to multiple E-box motifs drives circadian Dbp transcription and chromatin transitions. Nature Genetics. 2006;**38**:369-374. DOI: 10.1038/ng1738

[25] Rossetto D, Avvakumov N, Côté J. Histone phosphorylation: A chromatin modification involved in diverse nuclear events. Epigenetics. 2012;**7**:1098-1108. DOI: 10.4161/epi.21975

[26] Wilkinson KA, Henley JM. Mechanisms, regulation and consequences of protein SUMOylation. The Biochemical Journal. 2010;**428**:133-145. DOI: 10.1042/BJ20100158

[27] Liu X, Liu S. Role of microRNAs in the pathogenesis of diabetic cardiomyopathy. Biomedical Reports. 2017;**6**:140-145. DOI: 10.3892/br.2017.841

[28] Feng D, Lazar MA. Clocks, metabolism, and the epigenome. Molecular Cell. 2012;**47**:158-167. DOI: 10.1016/j.molcel.2012.06.026

[29] Xie T, Gorenjak VG, Stathopoulou M, Dadé S, Marouli E, Masson C, et al. Epigenome-wide association study (EWAS) of blood lipids in healthy population from STANISLAS family study (SFS). International Journal of Molecular Sciences. 2019;**20**:1014. DOI: 10.3390/ijms20051014

[30] Kelleher FC, Rao A, Maguire A. Circadian molecular clocks and cancer. Cancer Letters. 2014;**342**:9-18. DOI: 10.1016/j.canlet.2013.09.040

[31] Škrlec I, Marić S, Včev A. Myocardial infarction and circadian rhythm. In: Tsipis A, editor. Visions Cardiomyocyte—Fundam. Concepts Hear. Life Dis. 1st ed. London: IntechOpen; 2019. DOI: 10.5772/INTECHOPEN.83393

[32] Škrlec I. Circadian rhythm and myocardial infarction. Medicina

Fluminensis. 2019;**55**:32-42. DOI: 10.21860/medflum2019_216321

[33] Antypa N, Mandelli L, Nearchou FA, Vaiopoulos C, Stefanis CN, Serretti A, et al. The 3111T/C polymorphism interacts with stressful life events to influence patterns of sleep in females. Chronobiology International. 2012;**29**:891-897. DOI: 10.3109/07420528.2012.699380

[34] Škrlec I, Milić J, Heffer M, Wagner J, Peterlin B. Circadian clock genes and circadian phenotypes in patients with myocardial infarction. Advances in Medical Sciences. 2019;**64**:224-229. DOI: 10.1016/j.advms.2018.12.003

[35] Hardeland R. Melatonin and chromatin. Melatonin Research. 2019;**2**:67-93. DOI: 10.32794/mr11250012

[36] Langmesser S, Tallone T, Bordon A, Rusconi S, Albrecht U. Interaction of circadian clock proteins PER2 and CRY with BMAL1 and CLOCK. BMC Molecular Biology. 2008;**9**:41. DOI: 10.1186/1471-2199-9-41

[37] Ohdo S, Koyanagi S, Matsunaga N. Chronopharmacological strategies: Intra- and inter-individual variability of molecular clock. Advanced Drug Delivery Reviews. 2010;**62**:885-897. DOI: 10.1016/j.addr.2010.04.005

[38] Partch CL, Green CB, Takahashi JS. Molecular architecture of the mammalian circadian clock. Trends in Cell Biology. 2014;**24**:90-99. DOI: 10.1016/j.tcb.2013.07.002

[39] Takeda N, Maemura K. Cardiovascular disease, chronopharmacotherapy, and the molecular clock. Advanced Drug Delivery Reviews. 2010;**62**:956-966. DOI: 10.1016/j.addr.2010.04.011

[40] Virag JAI, Lust RM. Circadian influences on myocardial infarction. Frontiers in Physiology. 2014;**5**:422. DOI: 10.3389/fphys.2014.00422

[41] Kumar J, P Challet E, Kalsbeek A. Circadian rhythms in glucose and lipid metabolism in nocturnal and diurnal mammals. Molecular and Cellular Endocrinology. 2015;**418**:74-88. DOI: 10.1016/j.mce.2015.01.024

[42] Leu H-B, Chung C-M, Lin S-J, Chiang K-M, Yang H-C, Ho H-Y, et al. Association of circadian genes with diurnal blood pressure changes and non-dipper essential hypertension: A genetic association with young-onset hypertension. Hypertension Research. 2015;**38**:155-162. DOI: 10.1038/hr.2014.152

[43] Rudic RD, McNamara P, Curtis A-M, Boston RC, Panda S, Hogenesch JB, et al. BMAL1 and CLOCK, two essential components of the circadian clock, are involved in glucose homeostasis. PLoS Biology. 2004;**2**:e377. DOI: 10.1371/journal.pbio.0020377

[44] Curtis AM, Seo SB, Westgate EJ, Rudic RD, Smyth EM, Chakravarti D, et al. Histone acetyltransferase-dependent chromatin remodeling and the vascular clock. The Journal of Biological Chemistry. 2004;**279**:7091-7097. DOI: 10.1074/jbc.M311973200

[45] Turan N, Katari S, Coutifaris C, Sapienza C. Explaining inter-individual variability in phenotype: Is epigenetics up to the challenge? Epigenetics. 2010;**5**:16-19. DOI: 10.4161/epi.5.1.10557

[46] Aslibekyan S, Claas SA, Arnett DK. Epigenetics in cardiovascular disease. Translating Epigenetics to the Clinic. 2017;**1**:135-157. DOI: 10.1016/B978-0-12-800802-7.00006-X

[47] Turunen MP, Aavik E, Ylä-Herttuala S. Epigenetics and atherosclerosis. Biochimica et Biophysica Acta. 1790;**2009**:886-891. DOI: 10.1016/j.bbagen.2009.02.008

[48] Gluckman PD, Hanson MA, Buklijas T, Low FM, Beedle AS. Epigenetic mechanisms that underpin metabolic and cardiovascular diseases. Nature Reviews. Endocrinology. 2009;**5**:401-408. DOI: 10.1038/nrendo.2009.102

[49] Libby P, Okamoto Y, Rocha VZ, Folco E. Inflammation in atherosclerosis: Transition from theory to practice. Circulation Journal. 2010;**74**:213-220. DOI: 10.1253/circj.CJ-09-0706

[50] Zhang L, Lin QL, Lu L, Yang CC, Li YL, Sun FL, et al. Tissue-specific modification of clock methylation in aging mice. European Review for Medical and Pharmacological Sciences. 2013;**17**:1874-1880

[51] Bhatti P, Zhang Y, Song X, Makar KW, Sather CL, Kelsey KT, et al. Nightshift work and genome-wide DNA methylation. Chronobiology International. 2015;**32**:103-112. DOI: 10.3109/07420528.2014.956362

[52] Nakahata Y, Grimaldi B, Sahar S, Hirayama J, Sassone-Corsi P. Signaling to the circadian clock: Plasticity by chromatin remodeling. Current Opinion in Cell Biology. 2007;**19**:230-237. DOI: 10.1016/j.ceb.2007.02.016

[53] Westerman K, Sebastiani P, Jacques P, Liu S, DeMeo D, Ordovás JM. DNA methylation modules associate with incident cardiovascular disease and cumulative risk factor exposure. Clinical Epigenetics. 2019;**11**:142. DOI: 10.1186/s13148-019-0705-2

[54] Azzi A, Dallmann R, Casserly A, Rehrauer H, Patrignani A, Maier B, et al. Circadian behavior is light-reprogrammed by plastic DNA methylation. Nature Neuroscience. 2014;**17**:377-382. DOI: 10.1038/nn.3651

[55] Feinberg AP. Phenotypic plasticity and the epigenetics of human disease. Nature. 2007;**447**:433-440. DOI: 10.1038/nature05919

[56] Leproult R, Holmbäck U, Van Cauter E. Circadian misalignment augments markers of insulin resistance and inflammation, independently of sleep loss. Diabetes. 2014;**63**:1860-1869. DOI: 10.2337/db13-1546

[57] Gemma C, Sookoian S, Dieuzeide G, García SI, Gianotti TF, González CD, et al. Methylation of TFAM gene promoter in peripheral white blood cells is associated with insulin resistance in adolescents. Molecular Genetics and Metabolism. 2010;**100**:83-87. DOI: 10.1016/j.ymgme.2010.02.004

[58] Zhu Y, Stevens RG, Hoffman AE, Tjonneland A, Vogel UB, Zheng T, et al. Epigenetic impact of long-term shiftwork: Pilot evidence from circadian genes and whole-genome methylation analysis. Chronobiology International. 2011;**28**:852-861. DOI: 10.3109/07420528.2011.618896

[59] Ripperger JA, Merrow M. Perfect timing: Epigenetic regulation of the circadian clock. FEBS Letters. 2011;**585**:1406-1411. DOI: 10.1016/j.febslet.2011.04.047

[60] Bozek K, Relógio A, Kielbasa SM, Heine M, Dame C, Kramer A, et al. Regulation of clock-controlled genes in mammals. PLoS One. 2009;**4**:e4882. DOI: 10.1371/journal.pone.0004882

[61] Dong C, Yoon W, Goldschmidt-Clermont PJ. DNA methylation and atherosclerosis. The Journal of Nutrition. 2002;**132**:2406S-2409S. DOI: 10.1093/jn/132.8.2406s

[62] Oka D, Yamashita S, Tomioka T, Nakanishi Y, Kato H, Kaminishi M, et al. The presence of aberrant DNA methylation in noncancerous esophageal mucosae in association with smoking history: A target for risk diagnosis and prevention of esophageal cancers.

Cancer. 2009;**115**:3412-3426. DOI: 10.1002/cncr.24394

[63] Samblas M, Milagro FI, Gómez-Abellán P, Martínez JA, Garaulet M. Methylation on the circadian gene BMAL1 is associated with the effects of a weight loss intervention on serum lipid levels. Journal of Biological Rhythms. 2016;**31**:308-317. DOI: 10.1177/0748730416629247

[64] Škrlec I, Milić J, Cilenšek I, Petrovič D, Wagner J, Peterlin B. Circadian clock genes and myocardial infarction in patients with type 2 diabetes mellitus. Gene. 2019;**701**:98-103. DOI: 10.1016/J.GENE.2019.03.038

[65] Škrlec I, Milić J, Heffer M, Peterlin B, Wagner J. Genetic variations in circadian rhythm genes and susceptibility for myocardial infarction. Genetics and Molecular Biology. 2018;**41**:403-409. DOI: 10.1590/1678-4685-gmb-2017-0147

[66] Sharma P, Kumar J, Garg G, Kumar A, Patowary A, Karthikeyan G, et al. Detection of altered global DNA methylation in coronary artery disease patients. DNA and Cell Biology. 2008;**27**:357-365. DOI: 10.1089/dna.2007.0694

[67] Jiang D, Sun M, You L, Lu K, Gao L, Hu C, et al. DNA methylation and hydroxymethylation are associated with the degree of coronary atherosclerosis in elderly patients with coronary heart disease. Life Sciences. 2019;**224**:241-248. DOI: 10.1016/j.lfs.2019.03.021

[68] Jiang YZ, Jiménez JM, Ou K, McCormick ME, Di Zhang L, Davies PF. Hemodynamic disturbed flow induces differential DNA methylation of endothelial Kruppel-like factor 4 promoter in vitro and in vivo. Circulation Research. 2014;**115**:32-43. DOI: 10.1161/CIRCRESAHA.115.303883

[69] Ward-Caviness CK, Agha G, Chen BH, Pfeiffer L, Wilson R, Wolf P, et al. Analysis of repeated leukocyte DNA methylation assessments reveals persistent epigenetic alterations after an incident myocardial infarction. Clinical Epigenetics. 2018;**10**:161. DOI: 10.1186/s13148-018-0588-7

[70] Baccarelli A, Wright R, Bollati V, Litonjua A, Zanobetti A, Tarantini L, et al. Ischemic heart disease and stroke in relation to blood DNA methylation. Epidemiology. 2010;**21**:819-828. DOI: 10.1097/EDE.0b013e3181f20457

[71] Nakatochi M, Ichihara S, Yamamoto K, Naruse K, Yokota S, Asano H, et al. Epigenome-wide association of myocardial infarction with DNA methylation sites at loci related to cardiovascular disease. Clinical Epigenetics. 2017;**9**:54. DOI: 10.1186/s13148-017-0353-3

[72] Castro R, Rivera I, Blom HJ, Jakobs C, Tavares de Almeida I. Homocysteine metabolism, hyperhomocysteinaemia and vascular disease: An overview. Journal of Inherited Metabolic Disease. 2006;**29**:3-20. DOI: 10.1007/s10545-006-0106-5

[73] Gómez-Uriz AM, Goyenechea E, Campión J, De Arce A, Martinez MT, Puchau B, et al. Epigenetic patterns of two gene promoters (TNF-α and PON) in stroke considering obesity condition and dietary intake. Journal of Physiology and Biochemistry. 2014;**70**:603-614. DOI: 10.1007/s13105-014-0316-5

[74] Jones MJ, Goodman SJ, Kobor MS. DNA methylation and healthy human aging. Aging Cell. 2015;**14**:924-932. DOI: 10.1111/acel.12349

[75] Sahar S, Sassone-Corsi P. The epigenetic language of circadian clocks. Handbook of Experimental Pharmacology. 2013:29-44. DOI: 10.1007/978-3-642-25950-0_2

[76] Cantó C, Auwerx J. Caloric restriction, SIRT1 and longevity. Trends in Endocrinology and Metabolism. 2009;**20**:325-331. DOI: 10.1016/j.tem.2009.03.008

[77] Doi M, Hirayama J, Sassone-Corsi P. Circadian regulator CLOCK is a histone acetyltransferase. Cell. 2006;**125**:497-508. DOI: 10.1016/j.cell.2006.03.033

[78] Etchegaray JP, Lee C, Wade PA, Reppert SM. Rhythmic histone acetylation underlies transcription in the mammalian circadian clock. Nature. 2003;**421**:177-182. DOI: 10.1038/nature01314

[79] Masri S, Zocchi L, Katada S, Mora E, Sassone-Corsi P. The circadian clock transcriptional complex: Metabolic feedback intersects with epigenetic control. Annals of the New York Academy of Sciences. 2012;**1264**:103-109. DOI: 10.1111/j.1749-6632.2012.06649.x

[80] Masri S, Sassone-Corsi P. The circadian clock: A framework linking metabolism, epigenetics and neuronal function. Nature Reviews. Neuroscience. 2013;**14**:69-75. DOI: 10.1038/nrn3393

[81] Naruse Y, Oh-hashi K, Iijima N, Naruse M, Yoshioka H, Tanaka M. Circadian and light-induced transcription of clock gene Per1 depends on histone acetylation and deacetylation. Molecular and Cellular Biology. 2004;**24**:6278-6287. DOI: 10.1128/mcb.24.14.6278-6287.2004

[82] Haigis MC, Guarente LP. Mammalian sirtuins—Emerging roles in physiology, aging, and calorie restriction. Genes & Development. 2006;**20**:2913-2921. DOI: 10.1101/gad.1467506

[83] Nakahata Y, Kaluzova M, Grimaldi B, Sahar S, Hirayama J, Chen D, et al. The NAD+-dependent deacetylase SIRT1 modulates CLOCK-mediated chromatin remodeling and circadian control. Cell. 2008;**134**:329-340. DOI: 10.1016/j.cell.2008.07.002

[84] Nakahata Y, Sahar S, Astarita G, Kaluzova M, Sassone-Corsi P. Circadian control of the NAD+ salvage pathway by CLOCK-SIRT1. Science. 2009;**324**:654-657. DOI: 10.1126/science.1170803

[85] Ramsey KM, Yoshino J, Brace CS, Abrassart D, Kobayashi Y, Marcheva B, et al. Circadian clock feedback cycle through NAMPT-mediated NAD+ biosynthesis. Science. 2009;**324**:651-654. DOI: 10.1126/science.1171641

[86] Asher G, Gatfield D, Stratmann M, Reinke H, Dibner C, Kreppel F, et al. SIRT1 regulates circadian clock gene expression through PER2 deacetylation. Cell. 2008;**134**:317-328. DOI: 10.1016/j.cell.2008.06.050

[87] Longo VD, Kennedy BK. Sirtuins in aging and age-related disease. Cell. 2006;**126**:257-268. DOI: 10.1016/j.cell.2006.07.002

[88] Zhang P, Yu Y, Qin Y, Zhou Y, Tang R, Wang Q, et al. Alterations to the microbiota–colon–brain axis in high-fat-diet-induced obese mice compared to diet-resistant mice. The Journal of Nutritional Biochemistry. 2019;**65**:54-65. DOI: 10.1016/j.jnutbio.2018.08.016

[89] Feng D, Liu T, Sun Z, Bugge A, Mullican SE, Alenghat T, et al. A circadian rhythm orchestrated by histone deacetylase 3 controls hepatic lipid metabolism. Science. 2011;**331**:1315-1319. DOI: 10.1126/science.1198125

[90] Fontaine C, Dubois G, Duguay Y, Helledie T, Vu-Dac N, Gervois P, et al. The orphan nuclear receptor rev-Erbα is a peroxisome proliferator-activated receptor (PPAR) γ target gene and promotes PPARγ-induced adipocyte

differentiation. The Journal of Biological Chemistry. 2003;**278**:37672-37680. DOI: 10.1074/jbc.M304664200

[91] Preitner N, Damiola F, Luis-Lopez-Molina L, Zakany J, Duboule D, Albrecht U, et al. The orphan nuclear receptor REV-ERBα controls circadian transcription within the positive limb of the mammalian circadian oscillator. Cell. 2002;**110**:251-260. DOI: 10.1016/S0092-8674(02)00825-5

[92] Akashi M, Takumi T. The orphan nuclear receptor RORα regulates circadian transcription of the mammalian core-clock Bmal1. Nature Structural & Molecular Biology. 2005;**12**:441-448. DOI: 10.1038/nsmb925

[93] Matsushima S, Sadoshima J. The role of sirtuins in cardiac disease. American Journal of Physiology-Heart and Circulatory Physiology. 2015;**309**:H1375-H1389. DOI: 10.1152/ajpheart.00053.2015

[94] Williams SM, Golden-Mason L, Ferguson BS, Schuetze KB, Cavasin MA, Demos-Davies K, et al. Class I HDACs regulate angiotensin II-dependent cardiac fibrosis via fibroblasts and circulating fibrocytes. Journal of Molecular and Cellular Cardiology. 2014;**67**:112-125. DOI: 10.1016/j.yjmcc.2013.12.013

[95] Wada TT, Araki Y, Sato K, Aizaki Y, Yokota K, Kim YT, et al. Aberrant histone acetylation contributes to elevated interleukin-6 production in rheumatoid arthritis synovial fibroblasts. Biochemical and Biophysical Research Communications. 2014;**444**:682-686. DOI: 10.1016/j.bbrc.2014.01.195

[96] Wang Y, Miao X, Liu Y, Li F, Liu Q, Sun J, et al. Dysregulation of histone acetyltransferases and deacetylases in cardiovascular diseases. Oxidative Medicine and Cellular Longevity. 2014;**2014**:1-11. DOI: 10.1155/2014/641979

[97] Xie M, Kong Y, Tan W, May H, Battiprolu PK, Pedrozo Z, et al. Histone deacetylase inhibition blunts ischemia/reperfusion injury by inducing cardiomyocyte autophagy. Circulation. 2014;**129**:1139-1151. DOI: 10.1161/CIRCULATIONAHA.113.002416

[98] Pitchiaya S, Heinicke LA, Park JI, Cameron EL, Walter NG. Resolving subcellular miRNA trafficking and turnover at single-molecule resolution. Cell Reports. 2017;**19**:630-642. DOI: 10.1016/j.celrep.2017.03.075

[99] Cheng HYM, Papp JW, Varlamova O, Dziema H, Russell B, Curfman JP, et al. microRNA modulation of circadian-clock period and entrainment. Neuron. 2007;**54**:813-829. DOI: 10.1016/j.neuron.2007.05.017

[100] Ahlin F, Arfvidsson J, Vargas KG, Stojkovic S, Huber K, Wojta J. MicroRNAs as circulating biomarkers in acute coronary syndromes: A review. Vascular Pharmacology. 2016;**81**:15-21. DOI: 10.1016/j.vph.2016.04.001

[101] Wagschal A, Najafi-Shoushtari SH, Wang L, Goedeke L, Sinha S, Delemos AS, et al. Genome-wide identification of microRNAs regulating cholesterol and triglyceride homeostasis. Nature Medicine. 2015;**21**:1290-1297. DOI: 10.1038/nm.3980

[102] Goedeke L, Rotllan N, Canfrán-Duque A, Aranda JF, Ramírez CM, Araldi E, et al. MicroRNA-148a regulates LDL receptor and ABCA1 expression to control circulating lipoprotein levels. Nature Medicine. 2015;**21**:1280-1288. DOI: 10.1038/nm.3949

[103] Tan X, Zhang P, Zhou L, Yin B, Pan H, Peng X. Clock-controlled mir-142-3p can target its activator, Bmal1. BMC Molecular Biology. 2012;**13**:27. DOI: 10.1186/1471-2199-13-27

[104] Shende VR, Goldrick MM, Ramani S, Earnest DJ. Expression and rhythmic modulation of circulating microRNAs targeting the clock gene Bmal1 in mice. PLoS One. 2011;**6**:e22586.DOI: 10.1371/journal.pone.0022586

[105] Bartman CM, Oyama Y, Brodsky K, Khailova L, Walker L, Koeppen M, et al. Intense light-elicited upregulation of miR-21 facilitates glycolysis and cardioprotection through Per2-dependent mechanisms. PLoS One. 2017;**12**:e0176243. DOI: 10.1371/journal.pone.0176243

[106] Eckle T, Hartmann K, Bonney S, Reithel S, Mittelbronn M, Walker LA, et al. Adora2b-elicited Per2 stabilization promotes a HIF-dependent metabolic switch crucial for myocardial adaptation to ischemia. Nature Medicine. 2012;**18**:774-782. DOI: 10.1038/nm.2728

[107] Ji X, Takahashi R, Hiura Y, Hirokawa G, Fukushima Y, Iwai N. Plasma miR-208 as a biomarker of myocardial injury. Clinical Chemistry. 2009;**55**:1944-1949. DOI: 10.1373/clinchem.2009.125310

[108] Brainard J, Gobel M, Bartels K, Scott B, Koeppen M, Eckle T. Circadian rhythms in anesthesia and critical care medicine: Potential importance of circadian disruptions. Seminars in Cardiothoracic and Vascular Anesthesia. 2015;**19**:49-60. DOI: 10.1177/1089253214553066

[109] Brainard J, Gobel M, Scott B, Koeppen M, Eckle T. Health implications of disrupted circadian rhythms and the potential for daylight as therapy. Anesthesiology. 2015;**122**:1170-1175. DOI: 10.1097/ALN.0000000000000596

[110] Ritchie H, Stothard E, Wright K. Entrainment of the human circadian clock to the light-dark cycle and its impact on patients in the ICU and nursing home settings. Current Pharmaceutical Design. 2015;**21**:3438-3442. DOI: 10.2174/13816128216661507 06111155

[111] Foster RG, Peirson SN, Wulff K, Winnebeck E, Vetter C, Roenneberg T. Sleep and circadian rhythm disruption in social jetlag and mental illness. Progress in Molecular Biology and Translational Science. 2013;**119**:325-346. DOI: 10.1016/B978-0-12-396971-2.00011-7

[112] Depner CM, Stothard ER, Wright KP. Metabolic consequences of sleep and circadian disorders. Current Diabetes Reports. 2014;**14**. DOI: 10.1007/s11892-014-0507-z

Chapter 4

Overview of the Global Prevalence and Diagnostic Criteria of Takotsubo Syndrome

Shogade Taiwo and Akpabio Akpabio

Abstract

Takotsubo syndrome (TTS) is an acute and reversible abnormal condition of the heart also known as stress cardiomyopathy, apical ballooning syndrome, or broken heart syndrome. It is an uncommon disease that mostly occurs among Asians though studies have shown its occurrence in other parts of the world. The typical takotsubo syndrome patient has a unique circumferential left ventricular contraction abnormality that extends beyond a coronary artery supply territory and appears to follow the anatomical cardiac sympathetic innervation.

The syndrome predominantly affects postmenopausal women and is often preceded by severe emotional or physical stress. The high risk of misdiagnosis on account of the similar clinical presentation between acute coronary syndrome (ACS) and TTS patients makes it imperative to do a detailed diagnostic work up of suspected patients.

Diagnosis of TTS is made by elevation of cardiac enzymes, abnormal electrocardiogram (ECG), visualization of abnormal myocardial wall motion, and demonstration of normal coronary arteries. Often, cardiac wall motion abnormalities resolve in weeks, and therapy is only necessary in hemodynamic unstable patients and if severe complications, such as arrhythmias, heart failure, thromboembolism, cardiac arrest, and cardiac wall rupture, occur. A universally acceptable guideline on TTS is necessary for its early diagnosis and optimal management.

Keywords: prevalence, diagnostic criteria, takotsubo syndrome, acute coronary syndrome

1. Introduction

Takotsubo syndrome (TTS) also known as left ventricular apical ballooning syndrome (LVBS), transient apical ballooning, broken heart syndrome or stress cardiomyopathy is an acute and reversible wall motion abnormality classically of the left ventricular myocardium, commonly but not exclusively seen among the Asian population. Takotsubo syndrome was first diagnosed in Hiroshima City Hospital Japan, in 1983 [1]. Sato and Dote in 1990 and 1991 introduced the term takotsubo (tako = octopus, tsubo = a pot) to describe the left ventricular silhouette during systole in five patients presenting with clinical features of myocardial infarction but without obstructive coronary artery disease [2].

(The syndrome is characterized by regional left ventricular wall motion abnormality (LVWMA) with a peculiar circumferential pattern resulting in a conspicuous ballooning of the left ventricle during systole as seen in **Figure 1a** and **b**. The LVWMA extends beyond a single coronary artery supply region and is reversible with almost complete resolution of ventricular dysfunction in hours to weeks depicted in **Figure 1c** and **d**). The LVWMA may be localized to the apical, midapical, midventricular, midbasal, or basal segments of the left ventricle [4].

However TTS gained international attention in the early 2000s, when the first diagnostic criteria: including apical dyskinesia/akinesia with basal hyperkinesia, absence of obstructive coronary artery disease (CAD) on coronary angiography, new electrocardiographic abnormalities, modest elevation in serum cardiac troponin in the absence of pheochromocytoma, and myocarditis, were published [5].

Recently, the Heart Failure Association of the European Society of Cardiology in a position statement from the task force on TTS introduced the terms primary and secondary TTS. They reported that "Acute cardiac symptoms are the primary reason for seeking medical care in primary TTS while in secondary TTS, the syndrome occurs in patients already hospitalized for a medical or surgical condition" [6].

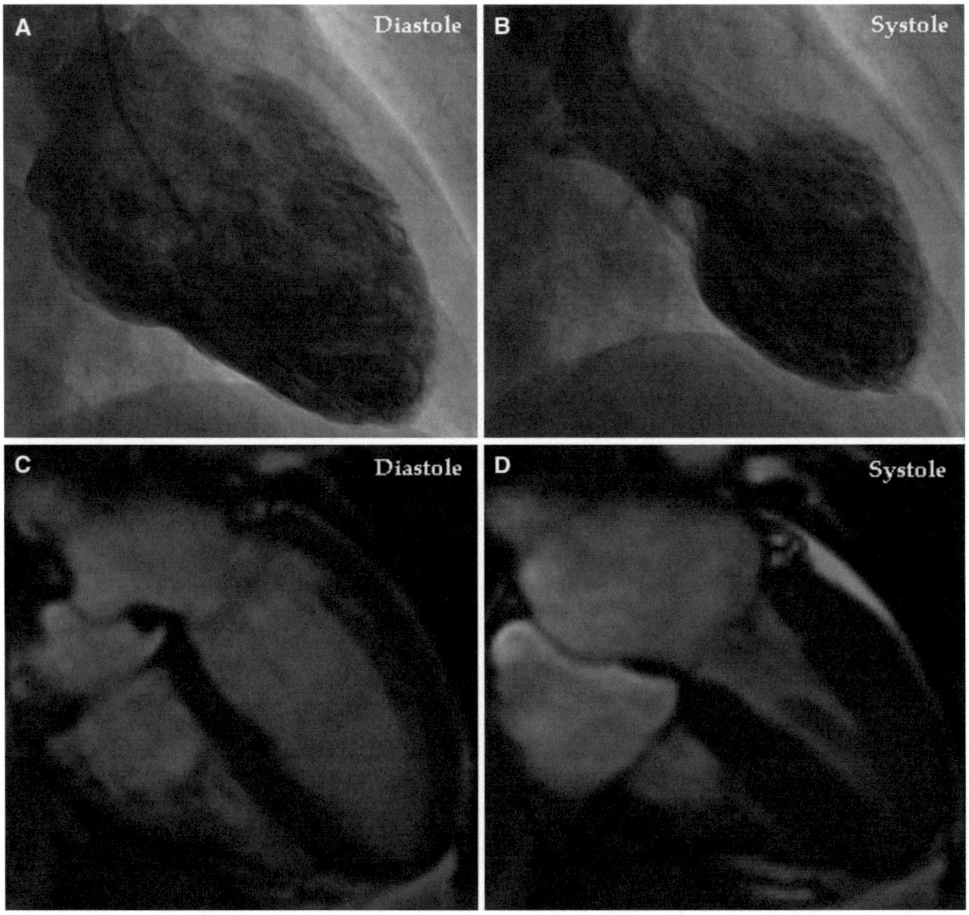

Figure 1.
Left ventriculography during the acute stage of takotsubo syndrome shows typical midapical ballooning during systole (a) diastole, (b) systole. Cardiac magnetic resonance imaging 4 days after left ventriculography shows complete normalization of the left ventricular function (c) diastole, (d) systole. The figure is reproduced with permission from Y-Hassan et al. [3].

2. Global prevalence

The prevalence of TTS has been reported to be approximately 2% of all patients presenting with clinical manifestation of ACS and up to 10% if only women are considered [7]. More than 85% of the patients with TS are said to be postmenopausal women (aged 65–70 years) thus suggesting a possible hormonal response [6]. In Western countries, there is a female-to-male ratio of 9:1 [8], in contrast, men are more affected than women, for unknown reasons in Japan [9]. The syndrome has also been reported in all age groups and even in children [6].

Since the introduction of the term takotsubo in 1990 [4], TTS has increasingly gained more recognition in almost all countries of the world. The syndrome has been reported in a variety of races, the incidence and prevalence are rising in the Western countries due to greater awareness and widespread access to early invasive coronary angiography, but the syndrome is infrequently seen among African and Hispanics descents which maybe be due to poor awareness of the disease [10].

Minhas et al. reported from study done among North American population almost 20 times increase in the incidence of TTS from 2006 to 2012 (**Figure 2**) [11]. Similarly, a study by Murugiah et al. showed that hospitalization rates for TTS are increasing, in that study the incidence of primary TTS increased from 2.3 to 7.1 hospitalizations per 100,000 person-years in 2007 to 2012. The corresponding incidence for secondary TTS increased from 3.4 hospitalizations per 100,000 person-years in 2007 to 10.3 in 2012 [12].

2.1 Pathogenesis/pathophysiology

The proposed mechanism for the pathogenesis and pathophysiology of TS are complex and multifactorial which include acute reversible myocardial ischemia resulting from multivessel coronary artery spasm, microvascular dysfunction, left ventricular outflow tract obstruction (LVOTO), blood-borne catecholamine induced myocardial toxicity, epinephrine-induced switch in the intracellular signal

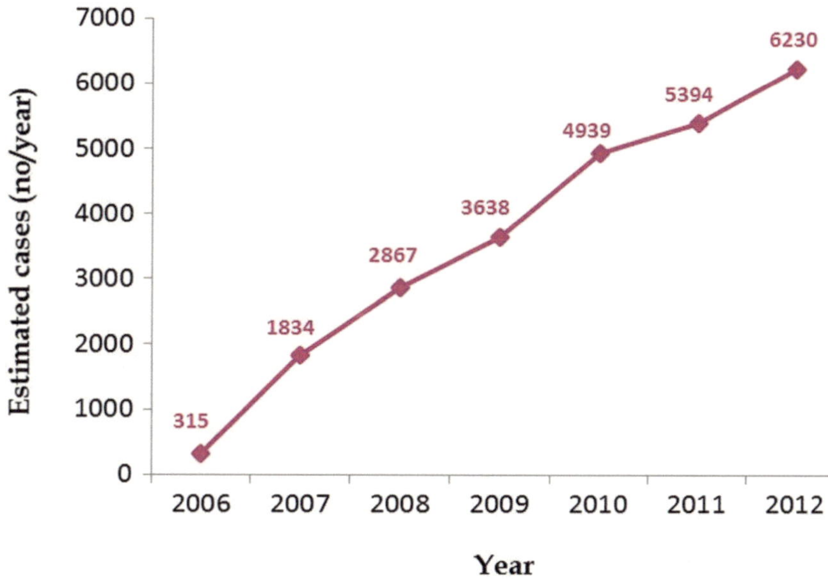

Figure 2.
Trends in reported incidence of takotsubo syndrome from 2006 to 2012. Modified with permission from a table by Minhas et al. [11].

trafficking from Gs (stimulatory) to Gi (inhibitory) protein signaling through the B2 adrenoreceptor (B2AR) and sympathetic nervous system hyperactivation including local cardiac sympathetic disruption and norepinephrine excess and spillover [6].

2.2 Clinical presentation

Patients with TTS can present with acute chest pain, dyspnea, and syncope. They may also be completely asymptomatic and diagnosis made based on incidental abnormal electrocardiographic (ECG) or imaging features [13]. Furthermore, a minority of TTS patients may present with symptoms due to complications such as heart failure, pulmonary edema, cardiogenic shock, cardiac arrest, or stroke [14]. Takotsubo syndrome is often known to be preceded by a stressor; usually emotional in females or physical in males though no stressor may be identified in up to 30% of cases [14].

A strong association of subarachnoid hemorrhage and status epilepticus with TTS as well as a less strong association with seizures, transient global amnesia, meningoencephalitis, migraine headache, intracerebral hemorrhage and ischemic stroke was reported by Morris et al. [15]. In order to detect triggers in some cases, it is mandatory to scrutinize the individual's history for such events, often time relatives or close friends may need to be consulted in instances that patients are reluctant to talk about stressful events.

With the present Covid-19 pandemic it will not be unusual if there is a surge in the global incidence of TTS which could be as a result of, physical stressors: the direct impacts of the covid-19 infection on the heart and other organs of the body or emotional stressors: in form of emotional distress arising from direct or indirect effects of the covid 19 infection. Covid 19 infection have been associated with stress cardiomyopathy especially among postmenopausal females, Minhas et al. reported the case of a 58 year old female Caucasian who presented with symptoms of corona virus infection and subsequently developed mixed shock with echocardiography findings classic for TTS [16].

Morner and colleagues suggested that the presence of a preexisting subclinical cardiomyopathy may be a co-pathophysiological factor; they reported a patient with background hypertrophic cardiomyopathy (HCM) who developed heart failure with echocardiographic confirmed large left ventricular aneurysm after gastrointestinal surgery. Therefore, such background condition ought to be identified and monitored closely because it may impact negatively on the outcome of the syndrome. Thyroid dysregulation and pheochromocytoma are also known stressor in the pathogenesis of TTS [17, 18].

2.3 Imaging modalities

Transthoracic echocardiography (TTE): provides a quick method of demonstrating the left ventricular wall-motion abnormalities which usually extend beyond the distribution of a single coronary artery. Typically seen in TTS is hypokinesis or akinesis of the apical- and mid-segment of the left ventricle (LV) with characteristic hyperkinetic basal segment. Other variants include basal segment akinesia with midventricular and apical sparing, as well as the focal variant, characterized by focal wall motion abnormalities. Transthoracic echocardiography also helps in following up patients and assessing progress by estimating the LV ejection fraction (LVEF). Mean LVEF of affected patients are in the range of 20–49% [19].

Left ventricular ejection fraction though commonly assessed by echocardiography, can also be estimated by means of cardiac magnetic resonance imaging

(CMRI), or left ventriculography. Cardiac MRI offers unique advantage of safety, detailed anatomical visualization, and tissue characterization data, CMRI is essential for the exclusion of other entities particularly myocarditis and myocardial infarction with nonobstructive coronary arteries (MINOCA) [20].

Cardiac MRI is increasingly being preferred as a diagnostic technique uniquely suited for diagnosing TTS by accurately identifying reversible injury to the myocardium by the presence of inflammation/edema and the absence of necrosis/fibrosis, quantifying ventricular function as well as visualizing regional wall-motion abnormalities. Importantly cardiac MRI helps differentiate TTS which is characterized by absence of delayed gadolinium hyper-enhancement from myocardial infarction and myocarditis in which delayed enhancement occurs.

In 2011, CMR diagnostic criteria for TTS were established which includes:

1. The presence of wall motion abnormalities

2. Edema of dysfunctional segments on T2 weighted sequences

3. Absence of late gadolinium enhancement (LGE)

The absence of LGE suggests that there is no fibrosis or increased extracellular space. However, in some cases up to 9%, some spots of fibrosis are found, and these have been associated with worst prognosis [21].

Studies based on positron emission tomography (PET) and myocardial SPECT have shown a discrepancy between normal perfusion and reduced glucose utilization in TTS, commonly known as "inverse flow metabolism mismatch". In the acute phase, TTS may be clinically indistinguishable from acute MI but, by means of PET, it has been successfully distinguished from acute MI [22]. Undoubtedly, coronary angiography is essential for the diagnosis of TTS by demonstrating a completely normal coronary arteries or rarely noncritical stenosis. It's important to note that left ventriculography is perhaps the best imaging modality for demonstrating the pathognomonic wall motion abnormalities and evaluating LV ejection fraction.

Data obtained from several registries including the international Takotsubo (InterTAK) Registry, a multicenter, prospective, retrospective, and observational study, which was conducted in more than 35 cardiovascular centers in 15 European countries, has enabled a diagnostic algorithm to be formulated. The diagnosis of TTS, which must be based on the absence of culprit coronary disease or presence of mild forms of coronary atherosclerosis. Therefore, TTS is gradually being better investigated and understood, and the number of diagnoses is increasing, as evidenced in the disease being included in the recent 4th universal definition of myocardial infarction by the European Society of Cardiology (ESC) [23].

2.4 Electrocardiogram

Electrocardiogram (ECG) is important in making a diagnosis of TTS, ECG is very useful in differentiating TTS from is closest differential, acute myocardial infarction. **Table 1** depicts the differences between the two conditions. ST-segment elevation and T-wave inversion are the commonest abnormalities seen on the initial ECG, which have been found to commonly involve the precordial leads and to be maximal in leads V2-V3. Unlike patients with ST-elevation myocardial infarction (STEMI) from left anterior descending (LAD) coronary artery occlusion, patients with TTS had significantly lower amplitude of ST-segment elevations. Similarly, T- wave inversions tend to occur in the days and weeks following presentation as the ST segments normalize, thus ECG cannot reliably differentiate TTS from other

Takotsubo syndrome	Acute anterior myocardial infarction
1. ST-segment elevation is detectable on precordial leads V1–V4 and limb leads I and aVL.	1. ST-segment elevation is mainly localized in V2–V5 leads and in limb leads II and aVR
2. Absence of reciprocal changes in inferior leads	2. There is presence of reciprocal changes in lateral and inferior leads
3. ST-segment elevation occurs more frequently in aVR	3. ST-segment elevation occurs more frequently in V1
4. There is absence of Q-wave	4. There is presence of Q-wave
5. ST-segment depressions occur in 10% of cases	5. ST-segment depression occurs in 30% of cases
6. Significantly lower amplitude of ST-segment elevation	6. Higher amplitude of ST-segment elevation

Table 1.
Electrocardiographic differences between takotsubo syndrome and acute myocardial infarction [24].

conditions with ST segments elevation. Chest radiograph, which is readily available and affordable, though often normal may demonstrate pulmonary edema in patients with the syndrome.

2.5 Biochemical profiles of takotsubo syndrome

Serum troponin is usually positive in the acute phase, but its values tend to be low when compares with the extent of myocardial dysfunction. The troponin level in TTS is commonly believed to be lower than in acute myocardial infarction (MI), though the InterTAK Registry has shown no difference between the two conditions. On the contrary, the hs-TnT/CKMB ratio has been found to be significantly higher in TTS when compares with STEMI and NSTEMI [25].

Increased levels of serum NT-proBNP can be demonstrated during the course of TTS. Nef and colleagues found that serum levels of NT-proBNP on admission were correlated to the severity of post-TTS complications during hospitalization, the higher the serum levels of NT-proBNP were on admission, the more clinical complications such as pulmonary edema and malignant ventricular arrhythmia present [26].

Recently, a two-part International expert consensus document on Takotsubo syndrome was published, providing a detailed characterization of TTC that allows clinicians to understand this cardiac dysfunction with a multidisciplinary view. There have been several attempts to create effective diagnostic criteria for TTS. The most widely used since 2018 has been the European Society of Cardiology (ESC) International Takotsubo Diagnostic Criteria (InterTAK Diagnostic Criteria) [27], which implements a diagnostic algorithm and assigns a score to TTS. InterTAK Diagnostic Score considers the following variables and gives each one a specific score: female sex; emotional and physical stress; absent ST depression; psychiatric disorders; neurologic disorders; and QTc prolongation. If the score is ≤70 points, the probability of having TTS is intermediate or low, whereas a score ≥70 indicates a high probability (**Table 2**).

Coronary angiography and left ventriculography are indicated in patients with a low probability of TTS and suspicion of ACS, while in patients with a high score, transthoracic echocardiography (TTE) should be performed. Wall motion abnormalities on TTE helps to decide the next step; if the typical presentation with circumferential ballooning pattern is absent, coronary angiography with left ventriculography is the next choice. In normal coronaries and typical ballooning, myocarditis must be excluded. The algorithm includes some red flags of

InterTak diagnostic score
Female sex 25 points
Emotional stress 24 points
Physical stress 13 points
No ST depression 12 points
Psychiatric disorders 11 points
Neurologic disorders 9 points
QTc prolongation 6 points
Score >70 points: high probability of TTS
Score ≤70 points: low/intermediate probability of TTS

Table 2.
Diagnostic criteria used to distinguish takotsubo syndrome (TTS) from acute coronary syndrome (ACS).

myocarditis (signs and symptoms of viral infection, elevated ESR and/or PCR, and pericardial effusion); in the presence of the above, myocarditis should be excluded by Cardiac MRI.

2.6 Treatment

Supportive treatment is mainly indicated in the acute phase while promptly diagnosing and treating complications appropriately. In mild cases, in addition to supportive treatment bisoprolol and aspirin may be considered. However, for patients with complications standard treatment for the complications should be commenced such as antiarrhythmic drugs for arrhythmias, anticoagulation for those with documented thrombus in the left ventricle or embolic phenomena or until resolution of LVWMA.

The suggested treatment in cardiogenic shock due to left ventricular outflow tract obstruction (LVOTO) is intravenous fluid and parenteral beta-blocker which increases cardiac filling and suppresses the basal hypercontractility thereby reducing LVOTO or phenylephrine if patient is intolerant to intravenous fluid and betablocker. In primary failure, venoarterial extracorporeal membrane oxygenation, left ventricular assist device or levosimendan should be considered as bridge to recovery [28].

2.7 Complications

Though initially believed to be a benign condition, outcomes in patients with TTS can be influenced negatively owing to the various in-hospital complications that may arise as a result of electrical and hemodynamic instability, such as cardiac arrhythmias, cardiogenic shock, ventricular thrombus, pulmonary edema, ventricular septal defect, free-wall rupture and arterial thromboembolism. Male patients have been shown to have three times higher mortality rate due to major adverse cardiac and cerebrovascular events [27].

2.8 Prognosis of takotsubo syndrome

Takotsubo syndrome has been known to recur, recurrence rate varies widely between 1.5% and 6.1% during 6 years follow up period. Notably female patients showed higher recurrence rate of TTS compared to male [29, 30]. A significantly higher recurrence rate of 17.7% have been reported in patients with pheochromocytoma-triggered TTS [18]. While some studies reported more male mortality compared to female [31]. Patel et al. found in their analysis no significant sex difference in respect to overall mortality rates of TTS patients aged ≥50 years [32].

Battrawy et al. reported from the multicenter GEIST (German Italian Stress Cardiomyopathy) Registry a recurrence rate of 4% at a median follow-up of 830 days among 749 patients. A variable TTS pattern at recurrence is common in up to 20% of recurrence cases. In this study it was observed that many patients that presented initially with involvement of only the left ventricle (LV), some years later developed right ventricular or biventricular involvement [30].

3. Conclusion

In conclusion, TTC is an acute and reversible cardiac disease, which commonly affects females of post-menopausal age and is often triggered by emotional or physical factors. Initially thought to be limited to the Asian population, it is also found in other parts of the world. This syndrome is associated with acute dysfunction of the central and autonomic nervous systems.

In order to better understand TTC, research on better diagnostic tools and therapeutic options need to be done. The recently published consensus document on TTS enhances clinical characterization of the syndrome and is hereby recommended.

Conflict of interest

Dr. Shogade Tolulope and Dr. Akpabio Akpabio declare no conflicts of interest.

Author details

Shogade Taiwo* and Akpabio Akpabio
University of Uyo Teaching Hospital, Uyo, Nigeria

*Address all correspondence to: docttaiwo@yahoo.com

References

[1] Sato H. Tako-tsubo-like left ventricular dysfunction due to multivessel coronary spasm. In: Kodama K, Haze K, Hori M, editors. Clinical Aspect of Myocardial Injury: From Ischemia to Heart Failure. Tokyo, Japan: Kagakuhyoronsha Publishing Co; 1990. p. 56-64

[2] YH S, Yamasaki K. History of takotsubo syndrome: Is the syndrome really described as a disease entity first in 1990? Some inaccuracies. International Journal of Cardiology. 2013;**166**:736-737

[3] Y-Hassan S, Tornvall P. Epidemiology, pathogenesis, and management of takotsubo syndrome. Clinical Autonomic Research. 2018;**28**:53-65. DOI: 10.1007/s10286-017-0465-z

[4] YH S, De Palma R. Contemporary review on the pathogenesis of takotsubo syndrome: The heart shedding tears: Norepinephrine churn and foam at the cardiac sympathetic nerve terminals. International Journal of Cardiology. 2016;**228**:528-536

[5] Prasad A, Lerman A, Rihal C. Apical ballooning syndrome (tako-tsubo or stress cardiomyopathy): A mimic of acute myocardial infarction. American Heart Journal. 2008;**155**(3):408-417

[6] Lyon AR, Bossone E, Schneider B, Sechtem U, Citro R, Underwood S, et al. Current state of knowledge on takotsubo syndrome: A position statement from the taskforce on takotsubo syndrome of the heart failure Association of the European Society of cardiology. European Journal of Heart Failure. 2016;**18**:8-27. DOI: 10.1093/eurheartj/ehy885

[7] Akashi YJ, Nef HM, Lyon A. Epidemiology and pathophysiology of takotsubo syndrome. Nature Reviews. Cardiology. 2015;**12**:387-397

[8] Schneider B, Athanasiadis A, Stöllberger C, et al. Gender differences in the manifestation of tako-tsubo cardiomyopathy. International Journal of Cardiology. 2013;**166**(3):584-588

[9] Aizawa K, Suzuki T. Takotsubo cardiomyopathy. Heart Failure Clinics. 2013;**9**(2):243-247. DOI: 10.1093/eurheartj/ehy686

[10] Nascimento FO, Larrauri-Reyes MC, Santana OP-C, M; Lamas G. Comparison of stress cardiomyopathy in Hispanic and non-Hispanic patients. Revista Espanola de Cardiologia (Engl Ed). 2013;**66**:67-68

[11] Minhas AS, Hughey AB, Kolias T. Nationwide trends in reported incidence of takotsubo cardiomyopathy from 2006 to 2012. The American Journal of Cardiology. 2015;**116**:1128-1131

[12] Murugiah K, Wang Y, Desai NR, Spatz ES, Nuti SV, Dreyer R, et al. Trends in short- and long-term outcomes for takotsubo cardiomyopathy among medicare fee-for-service beneficiaries, 2007 to 2012. JACC: Heart Failure. 2016;**4**:197-205

[13] Ghadri JR, Wittstein IS, Prasad A, et al. International expert consensus document on Takotsubo syndrome (part II): Diagnostic workup, outcome, and management. European Heart Journal. 2018;**39**(22):2047-2062

[14] Templin C, Ghadri JRDJ, et al. Clinical features and outcomes of takotsubo (stress) cardiomyopathy. The New England Journal of Medicine. 2015;**373**(10):929-938

[15] Morris NA, Chatterjee A, Adejumo OL, Chen M, Merkler AE, Murthy S, et al. The risk of takotsubo cardiomyopathy in acute neurological disease. Neurocritical Care.

2018;**30**:171-176. DOI: 10.1007/s12028-018-0591-z

[16] Minhas A, Scheel P, Garibaldi B, Liu G, Horton M, Jennings M, et al. Takotsubo syndrome in the setting of COVID-19. Journal of the American College of Cardiology: Case Rep. 2020;**2**:1321-1325. DOI: 10.1016/j-jaccas.2020.04.023

[17] Rueda D, Aguirre R, Contardo D, Finocchietto P, Hernandez S, di Fonzo H. Takotsubo myocardiopathy and hyperthyroidism: A case report and literature review. American Journal of Case Reports. 2017;**18**:865-870

[18] YH S. Clinical features and outcome of pheochromocytoma- induced takotsubo syndrome: Analysis of 80 published cases. The American Journal of Cardiology. 2016;**117**:1836-1844

[19] Citro R, Rigo CC, D'Andrea A, et al. Echocardiographic correlates of acute heart failure, cardiogenic shock, and inhospital mortality in tako-tsubo cardiomyopathy. JACC: Cardiovascular Imaging. 2014;**7**(2):119-129

[20] Placido ER, Cunha Lopes B, Almeida AG, Rochitte C. The role of cardiovascular magnetic resonance in takotsubo syndrome. Journal of Cardiovascular Magnetic Resonance. 2016;**18**(1):68

[21] Wu KC, Weiss RTD, et al. Late gadolinium enhancement by cardiovascular magnetic resonance heralds an adverse prognosis in nonischemic cardiomyopathy. Journal of the American College of Cardiology. 2008;**51**(25):2414-2421

[22] Testa M, Feola M. Usefulness of myocardial positron emission tomography/nuclear imaging in takotsubo cardiomyopathy. World Journal of Radiology. 2014;**6**(7):502-506

[23] Thygesen K, Alpert JJA, et al. Fourth universal definition of myocardial infarction (2018). European Heart Journal. 2019;**40**:237-269

[24] Frangieh AH, Obeid SGJ, et al. ECG criteria to differentiate between Takotsubo (stress) cardiomyopathy and myocardial infarction. Journal of the American Heart Association. 2016;**5**(6):e003418

[25] Pirlet C, Pierard L, Legrand V, Gach O. Ratio of highsensitivity takotsubo, troponin to creatine kinase-MB in syndrome. International Journal of Cardiology. 2017;**243**:300-305

[26] Nef, HM; Mollmann, M; Troidl, C; Weber, M; Hamm C and EA. "Tako-tsubo cardiomyopathy: NT-proBNP as a reliable parameter of a favourable prognosis?" International Journal of Cardiology 2008;124(2):237-238

[27] Ghadri JR, Wittstein IA, Prasad A, et al. International expert consensus document on Takotsubo syndrome (part I): Clinical characteristics, diagnostic criteria, and pathophysiology. European Heart Journal. 2018;**39**(22):2032-2046

[28] Santoro F, Ieva R, Ferraretti A, Ienco V, Carpagnano G, Lodispoto M, et al. Safety and feasibility of levosimendan administration in takotsubo cardiomyopathy: A case series. Cardiovascular Therapeutics. 2013;**31**:e133-e137

[29] El-Battrawy I, Ansari U, Behnes M, Hillenbrand D, Schramm KHD, et al. Clinical and echocardiographic analysis of patients suffering from recurrent Takotsubo cardiomyopathy. Journal of Geriatric Cardiology. 2016;**13**:888-893. DOI: 10.11909/j.issn.1671-5411.2016.11.002

[30] El-Battrawy I, Santoro F, Stiermaier T, Möller C, Guastafierro F,

Novo Guasta G, et al. Incidence and clinical impact of recurrent Takotsubo syndrome. Journal of American Heart Association. 2019;**ke010753**:1-7. DOI: 10.1161/JAHA.118.010753

[31] Konstantinos G, El-Battrawy I, Schramm K, Uzair A, Hoffmann U, Martin B, et al. Comparison and outcome analysis of patients with Takotsubo cardiomyopathy triggered by emotional stress or physical stress. Frontiers in Psychology. 2017;**8**:527-531. DOI: 10.3389/fpsyg.2017.00527

[32] Patel SM, Chokka RG, Prasad KPA. Distinctive clinical characteristics according to age and gender in apical ballooning syndrome (Takotsubo/stress cardiomyopathy): An analysis focusing on men and young women. Journal of Cardiac Failure. 2013;**19**:306-310. DOI: 10.1016/j.cardfail.2013.03.007

Chapter 5

Gender Differences in Clinical Outcomes of Patients with Coronary Artery Disease after Percutaneous Coronary Intervention

Yaya Guo, YanPing Bai, Yan Gao, Chenxia Wang and Zhilu Wang

Abstract

With the increasing incidence of coronary artery disease, the percutaneous coronary intervention (PCI) has become one of the most effective treatments for coronary artery disease. After more than 40 years of clinical application, development and research, and continuous improvement, it has been widely used around the world. In recent years, due to the continuous innovation of drug-eluting stents, equipment, drugs, and interventional technology, the indications for treatment have been continuously broadened, many heart centers can deal with complete revascularization for high-risk indicated patient session, and the efficacy has been further improved. However, studies have shown that there are gender differences in the clinical prognosis of patients with coronary artery disease after percutaneous coronary intervention, which are affected by many related risk factors of gender differences, but there is lack of systematic and comprehensive review of relevant factors. The purpose of this review is to evaluate the possible causes of gender differences in the clinical outcomes of patients after percutaneous coronary intervention and to put forward recommendations for primary prevention and secondary prevention.

Keywords: coronary artery disease, percutaneous coronary intervention, gender, differences

1. Introduction

Coronary artery disease is the most common cardiovascular disease caused by myocardial ischemia, hypoxia, and necrosis due to coronary stenosis, spasm, or occlusion. Since the first application of percutaneous coronary intervention (PCI) to myocardial infarction by Gruentzig in 1977, it has become the most common method to recover myocardial reperfusion under various states, significantly improving the survival and quality of life of patients with coronary artery disease [1]. Notably, PCI has been considered as the cornerstone of management for

IntechOpen

patients with or without ST elevation acute coronary syndromes [2–4]. In the past two decades, with the emergence of drug-eluting stent, the indication of PCI in high-risk patients with coronary artery disease has been tremendously broadened. In recent years, the progress of interventional techniques has also fundamentally changed the treatment of coronary artery disease. Moreover, since balloon angioplasty has been used in patients with coronary artery disease, the influence of gender on clinical outcomes after PCI has been continuously investigated. In particular, previous studies have reported that the incidence of adverse outcomes in female patients with coronary artery disease after PCI is higher than that in male patients with those after PCI, including short- and long-term mortality, major adverse cardiovascular events (MACE), and revascularization. On the one hand, some studies have shown that gender differences in clinical outcomes persist after adjusting for multivariate factors, such as age, prior peripheral vascular disease, prior myocardial infarction, prior PCI, and chronic renal failure [5–8]. On the other hand, other studies have demonstrated that gender is not an independent factor in the clinical outcome [9–11]. Due to the protection of estrogen, a large number of studies have revealed that the onset age of female patients with coronary artery disease is approximately 5–10 years later than that of male patients with those. Additionally, the prevalence of hypertension, diabetes mellitus, and hyperlipidemia was higher in female individual than that in male individual, while the prevalence of former or current smokers was more in male individual. Therefore, the purpose of the present review is to summarize the gender differences in clinical studies of patients with coronary artery disease after PCI and to put forward suggestions for improving primary and secondary prevention strategies.

2. Representative researches

In a Japanese observational study including 43,231 patients with non-ST-segment elevation acute coronary syndrome who underwent PCI from January 2014 to December 2014, the authors concluded that female patients had a higher risk of hospital complications than male patients, especially bleeding [5]. Another large-scale cohort study involving 95,030 male and 35,955 female patients from a clinical registry of PCI procedures revealed that female gender remained as an independent predictor for mortality of patients with coronary artery disease underwent PCI after multivariable adjustment from January 2006 to February 2011 [6]. A multi-center study from the United Kingdom and Sweden, which included 338,462 male and 119,799 female patients, indicated that female patients with coronary artery disease after PCI had a higher all-cause mortality than male patients with those and the age was also a strong predictor of mortality [7]. Moreover, a retrospective cohort study from Germany showed that female patients with ST-segment elevation myocardial infarction undergoing PCI harbored a 20% higher age-adjusted risk of death and ischemic cardiac and cerebrovascular events [8].

A systematic review involving 21 studies with 21,666 patients from the Netherlands showed that crude short- and long-term mortality was higher in female patients with ST-segment elevation myocardial infarction than that in male patients with those. However, the abovementioned gender differences generally disappeared after adjusting for baseline characteristics [12]. A comprehensive meta-analysis from the United States reported that there were gender differences in patients with coronary artery disease who underwent PCI, including short- and long-term mortality. Nevertheless, these differences were also gradually weakened after adjusting for the clinical differences and/or hospitalization course [13]. Although there were no significant gender differences in long-term mortality after adjustment, the short-term mortality of female patients with coronary artery disease undergoing primary angioplasty was still higher than that of male patients with those. Meanwhile, a meta-analysis involving 48 studies from Italy to explore the gender differences in clinical outcomes for patients with ST-segment elevation myocardial infarction who underwent PCI [14] indicated that female patients with ST-segment elevation myocardial infarction undergoing PCI had higher rates of bleeding and stroke and the early mortality was lower than that of male patients with those, but not in the mid-term.

Both previous qualitative and quantitative studies have suggested that there are gender differences in clinical outcomes of patients with coronary artery disease after PCI, which are mainly reflected in the fact that the mortality rate of female patients with those is higher than that of male patients with those; however, the above systematic review and meta-analysis results were only limited to patients with ST-segment elevation myocardial infarction who underwent PCI. In order to determine the prognosis other than mortality, a systematic review was performed, which suggested that the prognosis of male patients with coronary artery disease after PCI was better than that of female patients with those, including mortality, MACE, and short-term revascularization, except for long-term revascularization [15]. Based on the results of previous studies, it is necessary to analyze the possible causes of these gender differences.

3. Related factors of gender differences

3.1 Risk factors

It is clear that the elderly patients not only have a higher risk of cardiovascular disease but also have a higher risk of mortality. The major reason for the delayed onset of female patients with coronary artery disease is the protective effect of estrogen, which can be delayed to female patients with postmenopause. Estrogen can directly protect myocardial cells, reduce myocardial apoptosis, and prevent plaque rupture through sarcKATP channels and β-estrogen receptor [16, 17]. Nevertheless, female patients with coronary artery disease were facing the same risk factors as male patients with those. Female patients with coronary artery disease frequently had hypertension in clinical practice, which can damage endothelial cells, lead to endothelial dysfunction, and accelerate atherosclerosis. Meanwhile, hypertension is associated with chronic alterations of renin-angiotensin-aldosterone system and overexpression of angiotensin II receptor 1/renin-angiotensin-aldosterone system, which can increase myocardial fibrosis, cardiomegaly, extracellular matrix, and diastolic dysfunction. Besides, elevated blood pressure can also increase infarct size of patients with myocardial infarction [18]. In addition, previous studies have shown that more female patients with cardiovascular disease had diabetes mellitus and dyslipidemia, which can impair the endothelial cells of coronary artery and strengthen the functions of coagulation factor VIII and platelets, which can thereby further accelerate the occlusion of the coronary artery and arteriosclerosis. It has been shown that hyperuricemia and hyperhomocysteinemia are independent predictors of female patients with coronary artery disease. Uric acid crystals can deposit on the vessel wall, which can promote inflammation and atherosclerosis [19]. Hyperhomocysteinemia can affect the functions of vascular endothelial cells and lipid metabolism and increase platelet aggregation and adhesion [20, 21]. All of these risk factors may contribute to the occurrence of adverse prognosis events in female patients with coronary artery disease after PCI.

3.2 Anatomy and pathophysiology

Some studies have elucidated that gender differences in the prognosis of patients with coronary artery disease after PCI are due to the fundamental differences in physiology, pathophysiology, pathological anatomy, and other aspects between male and female. Anatomically, the coronary arteries of female patients with coronary artery disease are smaller than that of male patients with those, and the smaller blood vessels can cause higher risks of bleeding complications and vascular damage [22]. In general, male patients with coronary artery disease are prone to complex lesions, such as left main artery lesions, chronic total occlusion lesions, and long lesions, while female patients with coronary artery disease tend to have small vessel lesions, which are more likely to show no significant stenosis of the coronary artery during coronary angiography [23]. Meanwhile, coronary microvascular reactivity and myocardial response to ischemia are also different between male and female individuals. It is suggested that the hemodynamic state of female patients with coronary artery disease is worse than that of male patients with those, which leads to differences of cell cycle process and apoptosis-related protein levels of cardiac fibroblasts between different genders [24]. In addition, female patients with myocardial infarction often show atypical symptoms [25]. As a result, such patients will not be paid much attention to, and physicians may be misled or underestimate the possibility of acute coronary syndrome, thereby prolonging the time from myocardial infarction to revascularization [26]. These pathophysiology and anatomy differences are irreversible factors. If the physiological and pathological characteristics of female patients with coronary artery disease can be identified in time, appropriate coronary intervention strategies will be selected to reduce complications and improve their clinical prognosis.

3.3 Ischemia-reperfusion time

According to the statistics of the time from the onset of coronary artery disease to reperfusion ischemia time, the interval of female patients was longer than that of male patients, including the prehospital delay and the time from door to balloon [27–30]. A study by Lichtman et al. has revealed that the cardiovascular risk of female patients with coronary artery disease, especially young female patients with those, is not easy to be accurately assessed, which may lead to be delayed diagnosis of acute myocardial infarction, thereby affecting treatment and prognosis [31]. Another registration study from one of 11 centers in Switzerland providing primary PCI around the clock, which has demonstrated that female patients with acute myocardial infarction between 2005 and 2010 may be discriminated when they receive PCI [32]. It is speculated that this situation may also exist in other countries. The prognosis of female patients with coronary artery disease who are discriminated in clinic is partly poor. Moreover, a study from the United States has found that female patients with coronary artery disease were less likely to undergo PCI than male patients with those and more female patients with those had delayed time of ischemia-reperfusion [33]. These controllable factors can lead to the failure of female patients with coronary artery disease to improve myocardial ischemia effectively in a short period of time, which is one of the important factors of poor prognosis. The duration of ischemia-reperfusion may be longer in female patients with these atypical symptoms than in male patients, which is another factor of higher mortality and MACE in female patients with coronary artery disease after PCI.

3.4 MACE

MACE is one of the factors that significantly affect the prognosis for patients with coronary artery disease after PCI. Previous study has indicated that the incidence of MACE is lower in male patients with coronary artery disease after PCI than that in female patients with those [9, 10, 23, 34]. A prospective, multicenter, cohort study by Glaser et al. has exhibited that female patients with non-ST-segment elevation acute coronary syndrome undergoing PCI at the age of 65 was more likely to have MACE than male patients with those at the same time [28]. Further analysis has shown that the incidence of congestive heart failure was higher in female patients with ST-segment elevation myocardial infarction than that in male patients with those, and the former was more likely to have cardiogenic shock when myocardial infarction occurred [5–7]. High incidence of ventricular septal rupture and severe mitral regurgitation during cardiogenic shock can be considered as important factors affecting the poor prognosis of female patients with myocardial infarction in the hospital. In a word, the above pathological factors can lead to the high incidence of MACE in female patients with coronary artery disease after PCI.

3.5 Revascularization

A study has demonstrated that the low incidence of revascularization in female patients with coronary artery disease may also be attributed to the lower follow-up rate, atypical symptoms, difficulty identifying myocardial ischemia, unwillingness to undergo invasive investigations, and prejudice against female patients [9]. In addition, the mortality of female patients with coronary artery disease was higher during the short- and long-term follow-up compared with male patients with those, which may also reduce the chance of revascularization [23, 34]. Furthermore, male patients with coronary artery disease who underwent PCI often have more complex lesions, which may be also an independent predictor of revascularization [23]. In terms of pathophysiology, the male subjects are more likely to have atherosclerotic plaque rupture, platelet-rich thrombus, and micro-embolism [35], while the platelets are more sensitive to aggregation stimulation in female patients, and this pathophysiological difference may also increase the risk of male patients with coronary artery disease who underwent PCI or CABG [36]. Moreover, some studies have shown that male patients with coronary artery disease have a higher PCI or CABG history than the female with those, which may be another reason for the higher incidence of overall revascularization in male patients with those [7, 8].

3.6 Other risk factors

Earlier evidence has supported that the female individuals would experience depression after the initial diagnosis of coronary artery disease and acute cardiac events, leading to all-cause mortality and the risk of MACE in the following months [37, 38]. Breast cancer is one of the most important causes of female individual death worldwide. However, the administration of estrogen receptor modulators in anti-breast cancer treatments may increase the incidence of coronary artery disease [39]. The incidence of autoimmune diseases for female individuals is also high, especially systemic lupus erythematosus, which is more common in female individuals. The pathogenic antibodies of the disease can cause antiphospholipid antibody syndrome (thrombosis, thrombocytopenia), thereby involving coronary artery and even resulting in acute myocardial infarction [40]. Therefore, it is important to prevent and reduce the incidence of female high-risk diseases and to reduce the mortality and MACE of female patients with coronary artery disease after PCI.

4. Primary and secondary prevention

For population with high risk of cardiovascular events in the future and population who have already suffered from coronary artery disease, it is very important to implement the primary and secondary prevention of coronary artery disease. At present, various academic institutions around the world have formulated relevant suggestions, scientific statements, expert consensus documents, and clinical practice guidelines and put forward many measures for the primary and secondary prevention for patients with coronary artery disease and its PCI. However, the latest study shows that there are still significant gender differences for the primary and secondary prevention of cardiovascular disease. Compared with male patients, female patients with high risk of cardiovascular disease in the next 10 years are difficult to control their blood pressure, blood lipid, and body weight, while female patients who suffered from cardiovascular disease were worse in taking guideline-directed medications [41]. Therefore, the secondary prevention is particularly important for patients with coronary artery disease after PCI. On the basis of adherence to long-term drug treatment, the risk factors should be managed and controlled, and appropriate exercise should be performed, especially female coronary artery disease patients with higher risk factors and poor prognosis after PCI.

5. Conclusions

PCI has long been the main treatment method for patients with coronary artery disease, which significantly reduces the mortality of myocardial infarction and improves the quality of life of patients. However, compared with male patients with coronary artery disease, female patients with those have a higher MACE and mortality after PCI, while male patients with those have advantages in revascularization. Hypertension, diabetes mellitus, and dyslipidemia are the traditional risk factors of arteriosclerosis disease, which seriously affect the occurrence and development of coronary artery disease. Female patients with coronary artery disease are faced with more cardiovascular risk factors and adverse factors affecting the prognosis of PCI, which is a major challenge for female patients with PCI. In addition, it is necessary to pay attention to the management of non-cardiovascular risk factors for postmenopausal female. Meanwhile, psychological diseases should be identified and intervened in patients with coronary artery disease in time. Finally, it should be emphasized that the prevention and treatment of coronary artery disease should not be ignored for individuals with more than 65 years and population with vulnerable region of medical resources.

Author details

Yaya Guo[1†], YanPing Bai[1†], Yan Gao[1†], Chenxia Wang[1†] and Zhilu Wang[2*]

1 Department of Cardiology, Affiliated Hospital of Yan'an University, Yan'an, Shaanxi, China

2 Department of Cardiology, The First Hospital of Lanzhou University, Lanzhou, Gansu, China

*Address all correspondence to: wangzhl@lzu.edu.cn

† These authors are contributed equally to this work.

References

[1] Stason WB, Sanders CA, Smith HC. Cardiovascular care of the elderly: Economic consideration. Journal of the American College of Cardiology. 1987;**10**:18A-21A

[2] Amsterdam EA, Wenger NK, Brindis RG, et al. AHA/ACC Guideline for the Management of Patients With non-ST-elevation Acute Coronary Syndromes: Executive Summary: A Report of the American College of Cardiology/American Heart Association Task Force on Practice Guidelines. Circulation. 2014;**130**(25):2354-2394

[3] Levine GN, Bates ER, Blankenship JC, et al. 2015 ACC/AHA/SCAI focused update on primary percutaneous coronary intervention for patients with ST-elevation myocardial infarction: An update of the 2011 ACCF/AHA/SCAI guideline for percutaneous coronary intervention and the 2013 ACCF/AHA guideline for the management of ST-elevation myocardial infarction. Journal of the American College of Cardiology. 2016;**67**(10):1235-1250

[4] Benjamin EJ, Virani SS, Callaway CW, et al. Heart disease and stroke statistics-2018 update: A report from the American heart association. Circulation. 2018;**137**(12):e67-e492

[5] Numasawa Y, Inohara T, Ishii H, et al. Comparison of outcomes of female versus male with non-ST-elevation acute coronary syndromes undergoing percutaneous coronary intervention (from the Japanese Nationwide Registry). American Journal of Cardiology. 2017;**119**(6):826-831

[6] Lempereur M, Magne J, Cornelis K, et al. Impact of gender difference in hospital outcomes following percutaneous coronary intervention. Results of the Belgian Working Group on Interventional Cardiology (BWGIC) registry. EuroIntervention. 2014;**12**(2):e216-e223

[7] Kunadian V, Qiu W, Lagerqvist B, et al. Gender differences in outcomes and predictors of all-cause mortality after percutaneous coronary intervention (data from United Kingdom and Sweden). American Journal of Cardiology. 2017;**119**(2):210-216

[8] Heer T, Hochadel M, Schmidt K, et al. Sex differences in percutaneous coronary intervention—Insights from the coronary angiography and PCI registry of the German Society of Cardiology. Journal of the American Heart Association. 2017;**6**(3):e004972

[9] Mrdovic I, Savic L, Asanin M, et al. Sex-related analysis of short- and long-term clinical outcomes and bleeding among patients treated with primary percutaneous coronary intervention: An evaluation of the RISK-PCI data. The Canadian Journal of Cardiology. 2013;**29**:1097-1103

[10] Fath-Ordoubadi F, Barac Y, Abergel E, et al. Gender impact on prognosis of acute coronary syndrome patients treated with drug-eluting stents. American Journal of Cardiology. 2012;**110**:636-642

[11] Takagi K, Chieffo A, Shannon J, et al. Impact of gender on long-term mortality in patients with unprotected left main disease: The Milan and New-Tokyo (MITO) Registry. International Journal of Cardiology. 2014;**177**:1131-1133

[12] van der Meer MG, Nathoe HM, van der Graaf Y, et al. Worse outcome in female with STEMI: A systematic review of prognostic studies. European Journal of Clinical Investigation. 2015;**45**(2):226-235

[13] Bavishi C, Bangalore S, Patel D, et al. Short and long-term mortality in female and male undergoing primary angioplasty: A comprehensive meta-analysis. International Journal of Cardiology. 2015;**198**:123-130

[14] Conrotto F, D'Ascenzo F, Humphries KH, et al. A meta-analysis of sex-related differences in outcomes after primary percutaneous intervention for ST-segment elevation myocardial infarction. Journal of Interventional Cardiology. 2015;**28**(2):132-140

[15] Yaya G, Fahui Y, Chunlei F, et al. Gender difference in clinical outcomes of the patients with coronary artery disease after percutaneous coronary intervention: A systematic review and meta-analysis. Medicine. 2018;**97**(30):e11644

[16] Boese AC, Kim SC, Yin KJ, et al. Sex differences in vascular physiology and pathophysiology: Estrogen and androgen signaling in health and disease. American Journal of Physiology. Heart and Circulatory Physiology. 2017;**313**(3):H524-H545

[17] Gabel SA, Walker VR, London RE, et al. Estrogen receptor beta mediates gender differences in ischemia/reperfusion injury. Journal of Molecular and Cellular Cardiology. 2005;**38**(2):289-297

[18] Saluveer O, Redfors B, et al. Hypertension is associated with increased mortality in patients with ischaemic heart disease after revascularization with percutaneous coronary intervention—A report from SCAAR. Blood Pressure. 2017;**26**(3):166-173

[19] Yoshitata K, Tamiko Y, Akiko O, et al. Soluble uric acid promotes atherosclerosis via AMPK (AMP-activated protein kinase)-Mediated Inflammation. Arteriosclerosis, Thrombosis, and Vascular Biology. 2020;**40**(3):570-582

[20] Schaffer A, Verdoia M, Cassetti E, et al. Relationship between homocysteine and coronary artery disease: Results from a large prospective cohort study. Thrombosis Research. 2014;**134**:288-293

[21] Liu Y, Tian T, Zhang H, et al. The effect of homocysteine-lowering therapy with folic acid on flow-mediated vasodilation in patients with coronary artery disease: A meta-analysis of randomized controlled trials. Atherosclerosis. 2014;**235**:31-35

[22] Numasawa Y, Kawamura A, Kohsaka S, et al. Anatomical variations affect radial artery spasm and procedural achievement of transradial cardiac catheterization. Heart and Vessels. 2014;**29**(1):49-57

[23] Yang J, Zhang F, Qian J, et al. Sex-based influence on clinical outcomes after drug-eluting stent implantation in real-world patients: Insight from the FOCUS registry. Annals of Medicine. 2017;**49**(3):185-195

[24] Zhao X, Eghbali-Webb M. Gender-related differences in basal and hypoxia-induced activation of signal transduction pathways controlling cell cycle progression and apoptosis, in cardiac fibroblasts. Endocrine. 2002;**18**(2):137-145

[25] Dreyer RP, Beltrame JF, Tavella R, et al. Evaluation of gender differences in door-to-balloon time in ST-elevation myocardial infarction. Heart, Lung & Circulation. 2013;**22**:861-869

[26] Wei TF, Zhao B, Liu PL, et al. Impact of symptom onset to first medical contact time on the prognosis of patients with acute ST-segment elevation myocardial infarction. Zhonghua Xin Xue Guan Bing Za Zhi. 2017;**45**(5):393-398

[27] Ferrante G, Presbitero P, Corrada E, et al. Sex-specific benefits

of sirolimus-eluting stent on long-term outcomes in patients with ST-elevation myocardial infarction undergoing primary percutaneous coronary intervention: Insights from the Multicenter evaluation of single high-dose bolus tirofiban versus abciximab with sirolimus-eluting stent or bare-metal stent in acute myocardial infarction study trial. Journal of the American Heart Association. 2012;**163**:104-111

[28] Wijnbergen I, Tijssen J, van't Veer M, et al. Gender differences in long-term outcome after primary percutaneous intervention for ST-segment elevation myocardial infarction. Catheterization and Cardiovascular Interventions. 2013;**82**:379-384

[29] Velders MA, Boden H, van Boven AJ, et al. Influence of gender on ischemic times and outcomes after ST-elevation myocardial infarction. American Journal of Cardiology. 2013;**111**:312-318

[30] Laufer-Perl M, Shacham Y, Letourneau-Shesaf S, et al. Gender-related mortality and in-hospital complications following ST-segment elevation myocardial infarction: Data from a primary percutaneous coronary intervention cohort. Clinical Cardiology. 2015;**38**(3):145-149

[31] Lichtman JH, Leifheit-Limson EC, Watanabe E, et al. Symptom recognition and healthcare experiences of young women with acute myocardial infarction. Circulation. Cardiovascular Quality and Outcomes. 2015;**8**(1):31-38

[32] Pilgrim T, Heg D, Tal K, et al. Age- and gender-related disparities in primary percutaneous coronary interventions for acute ST-segment elevation myocardial infarction. PLoS One. 2015;**10**(9):e0137047

[33] D'Onofrio G, Safdar B, Lichtman JH, et al. Sex differences in reperfusion in young patients with ST-segment-elevation myocardial infarction: Results from the VIRGO study. Circulation. 2015;**131**(15):1324-1332

[34] Idris H, French JK, Shugman IM, et al. Influence of age and gender on clinical outcomes following percutaneous coronary intervention for acute coronary syndromes. Heart, Lung & Circulation. 2017;**26**(6):554-565

[35] Wiviott SD, Cannon CP, Morrow DA, et al. Differential expression of cardiac biomarkers by gender in patients with unstable angina/non-ST-elevation myocardial infarction: A TACTICS-TIMI 18 (treat angina with aggrastat and determine cost of therapy with an invasive or conservative strategy-thrombolysis in myocardial infarction 18) substudy. Circulation. 2004;**109**:580-586

[36] Jacobs AK. Coronary intervention in 2009: Are women no different than men? Circulation. Cardiovascular Interventions. 2009;**2**(1):69-78

[37] Hess CN, Mccoy LA, Duggirala HJ, et al. Sex-based differences in outcomes after percutaneous coronary intervention for acute myocardial infarction: A report from TRANSLATE-ACS. Journal of the American Heart Association. 2014;**3**(1):e000523

[38] Mallik S, Spertus JA, Reid KJ, et al. Depressive symptoms after acute myocardial infarction: Evidence for highest rates in younger women. Archives of Internal Medicine. 2006;**166**(8):876-883

[39] Jameera Begam A, Jubie S, Nanjan MJ. Estrogen receptor agonists/antagonists in breast cancer therapy: A critical review. Bioorganic Chemistry. 2017;**71**:257-274

[40] Kokosi M, Lams B, Agarwal S. Systemic lupus erythematosus and antiphospholipid antibody

syndrome. Clinics in Chest Medicine. 2019;**40**(3):519-529

[41] Shijun X, Xin D, Lizhu G, et al. Sex differences in primary and secondary prevention of cardiovascular disease in China. Circulation. 2020;**14**(1):530-539

Chapter 6

Obesity Acceptance: Body Positivity and Clinical Risk Factors

Ketrell L. McWhorter

Abstract

Most people are aware of how they look and, whether poor or positive, have an opinion about their image. Social media influencers, pressure from societal norms, media images, and even friends and family can impact body image. Body positivity has undoubtedly gone mainstream. Included in this movement are obesity acceptance and its demarginalization. However, the acceptance of overweight and obesity may undermine the decades-long progress made toward reducing risk factors for cardiovascular disease (CVD). Obesity is a global epidemic disease with risk factors that include hypertension, inflammation, heart attack, stroke, and diabetes. Obesity is also associated with obstructive sleep apnea. Positive body image is an important component of overall health. However, also maintaining a proper clinical definition and self-perception of what constitutes "normal" weight, coupled with weight management, regular exercise, and monitoring blood pressure and blood sugar, will continue progress toward reducing the risk of cardiovascular disease.

Keywords: obesity, overweight, weight gain, weight reduction, diet, body image, self-image, cardiovascular disease, hypertension, heart disease, stroke, diabetes

1. Introduction

Obesity is a chronic disease with risk factors that include positive energy balance, resulting primarily from "obesogenic" changes that include economic growth, abundance, inexpensive and nutrient-poor food, industrialization, and sedentary lifestyles [1]. Comorbidities and sequelae associated with obesity include hypertension (HTN), inflammation, dyslipidemia, infertility, certain cancers, heart attack, stroke, type 2 diabetes, and obstructive sleep apnea [1, 2]. Weight stigmatization and its associated mental and behavioral consequences, economic burden, and premature death are also associated with obesity.

Historically, obesity went hand in hand with a poor sense of self-perception. Most people are aware of how they look, and whether poor or positive, have an opinion about their body image. Social media influencers, pressure from societal norms, and media images, as well as friends and family, all have an impact on body image. Over the past decade, the body positivity movement has undoubtedly gone mainstream. Often synonymous with this movement is fat acceptance, a movement focused on the demarginalization of the overweight or obese (OW/obese) population. Also mentioned in discussions of fat acceptance and fat rights activism is Health at Every Size® (HAES) as a public health approach to obesity. Yet, the acceptance of overweight and obesity in the absence of prevention or weight reduction threatens to undermine the decades-long progress made toward mitigating risk for cardiovascular disease (CVD).

Positive body image is indeed a necessary component of overall health and an important factor in determining one's ability to reach weight loss goals. An imperative complement to these movements, however, is adequate health literacy, or an ability to read, comprehend, and use information in a manner that promotes and maintains good health [3]. It is only with proper knowledge of what constitutes a clinical definition of "normal" weight versus higher weights associated with increased CVD risk, coupled with mindful weight management, regular exercise, monitoring blood pressure (BP), and maintenance of blood sugar, that will continue progress toward reducing CVD risk.

2. Obesity

2.1 The obesity pandemic

Over the past 40 years, there has been a sharp rise in worldwide obesity with prevalence nearly tripling since 1975 [4]. According to the World Health Organization (WHO), overweight and obesity are defined as having abnormal or excessive fat accumulation that may impair health [4]. Studies show the global obesity epidemic is worsening. In 2016, nearly 2 billion adults over 18 years worldwide were overweight and of these, over 650 million were obese [4].

Prevalence of obesity and severe obesity in the U.S. continue to rise [5]. Currently, the rates of obesity exceed 30% in most sex and adult age groups, whereas its prevalence has reached 17% among children and adolescents, defined as a BMI exceeding the 95th percentile [6]. In 2017–2018, it was estimated that 42.4% of U.S. adults aged 20 and over were obese (**Figure 1**) and 9.2% were severely obese [7] (**Figure 2**), and these may be underestimated. In a study comparing rates of obesity diagnosis to national rates of obesity based on BMI data from the Behavioral Risk Factor Surveillance System, the authors found that obesity is largely underdiagnosed and undertreated in clinical settings [8].

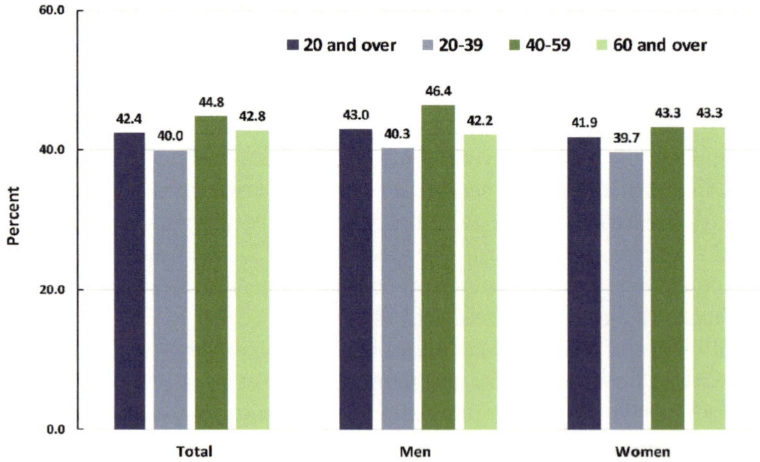

Figure 1.
Prevalence of obesity among adults aged 20 and over, by sex and age: United States, 2017–2018. Notes: Estimates for adults aged 20 and over were age-adjusted by the direct method to the 2000 U.S. Census population using the age groups 20–39, 40–59, and 60 and over. Crude estimates are 42.5% for total, 43.0% for men, and 42.1% for women. ***Figure 1*** *is adapted from data table at: https://www.cdc.gov/nchs/data/databriefs/db360_tables-508.pdf#1 [Accessed: 13 August 2020]. Source: National Center for Health Statistics (NCHS), National Health and Nutrition Examination Survey, 2017–2018.*

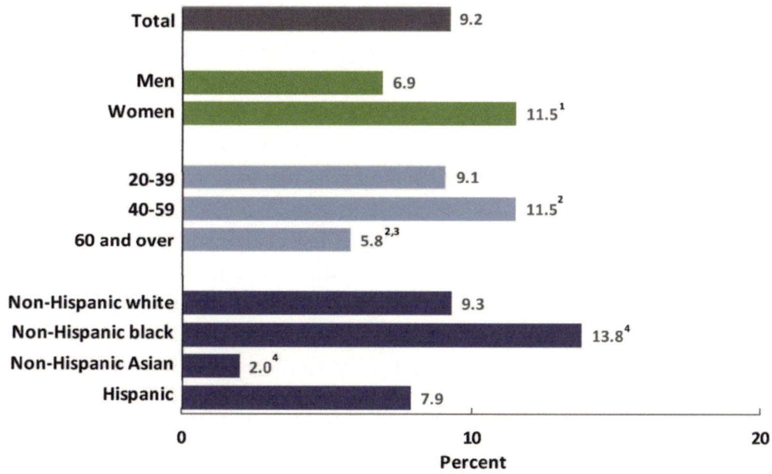

Figure 2.
Age-adjusted prevalence of severe obesity among adults aged 20 and over, by sex, age, and race and Hispanic origin: United States, 2017–2018. [1]Significantly different from men. [2]Significantly different from adults aged 20-39. [3]Significantly different from adults ages 40-59. [4]Significantly different from all other race and Hispanic-origin groups. Notes: Estimates for adults aged 20 and over were age-adjusted by the direct method to the 2000 U.S. Census population using the age groups 20–39, 40–59, and 60 and over. Crude estimates are 9.0% for total, 6.8% for men, and 11.1% for women. ***Figure 2*** *is adapted from data table at: https://www.cdc.gov/nchs/data/databriefs/db360_tables-508.pdf#3 [Accessed: 03 August 2020]. Source: Figure adapted from National Center for Health Statistics (NCHS), National Health and Nutrition Examination Survey, 2017–2018.*

Over the past 20 years, mean weight, waist circumference (WC), and BMI among U.S. adults over aged 20 increased across all age groups for non-Hispanic white and Mexican-American men and women, and for non-Hispanic black women [9]. Men had more obesity among those aged 20–39 and 40–59 than women in the same respective age groups, and less obesity among those 60 and over compared to women of the same age group [7]. However, none of the reported differences were significant. On the contrary, during this same time period, women reportedly had a higher overall prevalence of severe obesity than men, with significant differences in age groups race/ethnicity, and sex [7] (**Figure 2**).

2.2 Body mass index and other body composition methods

BMI is a useful inexpensive tool that has long been used to assess overweight, obesity, and risk for diseases that occur resulting from excess body fat. The internationally accepted standard cut-off points for defining a healthy or unhealthy weight is when body mass index (BMI) is 25 kg/m^2. The prevailing BMI classifications are underweight (BMI < 18.5 kg/m^2), normal weight (BMI of 18.5–24.9 kg/m^2), overweight (BMI of 25.0–29.9 kg/m^2), obesity$_{\text{Class I}}$ (BMI of 30.0–34.9 kg/m^2), obesity$_{\text{Class II}}$ (BMI of 35.0–39.9 kg/m^2), and extreme obesity$_{\text{Class III}}$ (BMI ≥ 40.0 kg/m^2) [5].

BMI is not without its limitations, often overestimating body fat in individuals with more muscle tissue, while underestimating body fat in individuals who have lost muscle [10]. Another challenge with using BMI as an adiposity metric is that it is unable to estimate percent body fat nor can it differentiate fat distribution for a given BMI, which can vary across age groups, sex, and race/ethnicity [11–13]. Results from some epidemiological investigations have even justified implementing adjustments to the cut-off values for classifying obesity and elevated WC among racial/ethnic populations [5, 14]. Lastly, using BMI percentile cutoffs to determine obesity and morbid obesity becomes especially problematic among children as it fails to consider large head size and high torso-to-leg ratio in the pediatric population [15]. The variation of high BMIz values, due to sex and age, make it very difficult to interpret the high BMIz levels (and changes in these levels) among children with severe obesity, possibly leading to incorrect conclusions [16]. Despite its limitations, BMI is used in most clinical settings and is correlated to more direct measures of body fat, such as underwater weighing and dual energy X-ray absorptiometry [17].

When predicting cardiometabolic disease, many studies demonstrate the use of WC, a measure of visceral adipose tissue and commonly used to calculate waist-to-hip ratio, as a preferred approach over BMI for estimating body fat [5, 18]. A WC ≥ 102 cm in men and ≥ 88 cm in women can be an indicator of increased risk for type 2 diabetes, HTN, and CVD, even among individuals with normal weight [19]. Other studies have suggested a combination of adiposity metrics more efficiently identifies all CVD risk factors [20], while some have found the use of either BMI or WC as the index of adiposity identifying the same persons, with equal utility [21].

Many sophisticated direct volumetric techniques are available for body composition assessment that vary in sensitivity and specificity. For example, some more expensive methods include tracer dilution, bioelectrical impedance plethysmography, densitometry, dual-energy X-ray absorptiometry (DEXA), and air displacement plethysmography [22]. Still, other tools that can better visualize and quantify tissues, organs, muscle, and adipose tissue include imaging techniques such as nuclear magnetic resonance and computed tomography [14, 22]. However, in most clinical settings, BMI along with other simple, non-invasive anthropometric measures are used.

2.3 Factors driving obesity

On a physiological level, obesity is the result of an energy imbalance between calories consumed and the calories expended, creating an energy surplus and a state of positive energy balance resulting in excess body weight [1]. Obesity also arises from poor health behaviors (e.g., poor sleep habits, diet, physical activity), genetic and epigenetic factors, gut microbiota, and a failure of health care professionals to advise people with obesity on appropriate courses of action for weight reduction [13, 23, 24]. Other "obesogenic" environmental drivers of obesity include marketing of inexpensive nutrient-poor foods, sedentary places of employment, industrialization, mechanized transportation, and urbanization [1].

An indirect driver of increasing BMI is the increasing trend in mean body weight without corresponding increases in height over time. According to the National Health Statistics Report, there is a rising trend in BMI with no significant change in height, with even slight decreases in height among some racial/ethnic groups [9]. For example, among all men, mean height significantly increased from 1999 to 2000 (175.6 cm) to 2003 to 2004 (176.6 cm) and subsequently decreased until 2015–2016 (175.4 cm) [9]. Among all male racial/ethnic groups, only non-Hispanic black men experienced a significant decrease in mean height from 1999 to 2000 (176.0 cm) to 2015 to 2016 (175.5 cm). In contrast, among all women, no significant linear trends were observed over the same time period or for any racial/ethnic subgroup [9].

2.4 Obesity-related health risks and comorbidities

It is widely recognized that cardiovascular risk and metabolic complications are due to a constellation of obesity, physical inactivity, and primary HTN [25]. Compared to those with a healthy or normal weight, people with obesity are at especially increased risk for many adverse health outcomes, including high BP, higher levels of low-density lipoprotein cholesterol, lower levels of high-density lipoprotein (HDL) cholesterol, type 2 diabetes, stroke, sleep apnea, and poor quality of life [7, 24, 26] (**Figure 3**). Obesity has also been linked to cancers of the esophagus, colon and rectum, liver, gallbladder and biliary tract, pancreas, breast, uterus, ovary, kidney, and thyroid. [26]. Individuals with severe obesity are further susceptible to obesity-related complications, such as coronary heart disease and end-stage renal disease [7].

A systematic evaluation of the health effects of high BMI revealed that in 2015, excess body weight accounted for about 4 million deaths worldwide, with an additional 120 million disability-adjusted life-years [26]. Higher BMI classified as overweight and not obese is also associated with mortality. Over one-third of global deaths and disability-adjusted life-years were related to BMI classified as overweight (less than 30 kg/m^2) [26].

In a U.S. study using National Health and Nutrition Examination Survey data examining the prevalence of 11 common chronic conditions, obesity experienced the largest significantly increased trend of any condition over the past 25 years (1998–2014) [27]. Due to its pervasiveness and its detrimental impact on morbidity and mortality, obesity is included as a chronic condition in multimorbidity models rather than as a control factor [27].

2.5 Characterization of metabolic profiles

Although obesity, particularly visceral adiposity, is typically associated with metabolic dysfunction and cardiometabolic diseases, there are some obesity

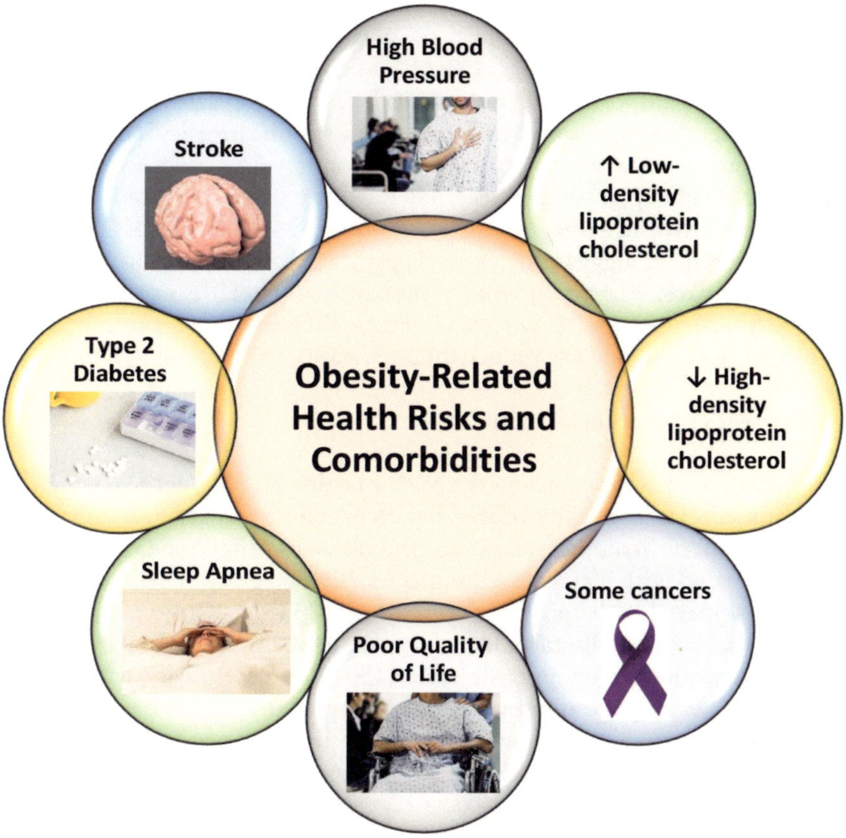

Figure 3.
Obesity-related health risks and comorbidities [7, 24, 26].

phenotypes that appear protected from some of the adverse metabolic effects of excess body fat [28]. Disease risk may not be uniform across all obese phenotypes.

The classification of an individual as "metabolically healthy" is not clearly defined, with 5 to more than 30 definitions documented across studies [28, 29]. In 2009, a harmonized definition for metabolic syndrome (MetS) was derived by The International Diabetes Federation Task Force on Epidemiology and Prevention, the National Heart, Lung, and Blood Institute, American Heart Association, World Heart Federation, International Atherosclerosis Society, and the International Association for the Study of Obesity [30]. According to this definition, participants who met ≥3 of the 5 abnormal criteria, excluding WC, were classified as having MetS and thus metabolically unhealthy and obese (MUO). These five components include high fasting blood glucose, high systolic and diastolic BP, elevated plasma triglyceride levels, low high-density lipoprotein cholesterol levels, and obesity (particularly central adiposity) [28, 30]. Obese participants who met 0, 1, or 2 of these criteria were classified as metabolically healthy but obese (MHO) [28, 31].

A classification of MHO should not be mistaken for metabolically unhealthy normal weight (MUN). These individuals are not phenotypically obese but share a metabolic profile similar to an overt obese person, including hyperinsulinemia, insulin resistance, and a predisposition to type 2 diabetes and premature CVD [32]. Studies suggest that MHO is a transient state and only a precursor to MUO [25, 33]. Data from longitudinal studies suggest that approximately 30% to nearly half of people with MHO transition back to MUO after 4 to 20 years of follow-up [28]. Indeed, in the absence of regular, systematic, and supervised diet and exercise programs, obese individuals with MHO profiles experience subsequent declines in cardiometabolic health [34].

Differences in metabolic profiles of those with MHO versus MUO could be due to phenotypic characteristics that lower risk of MetS, such as lower visceral adiposity, higher birth weight, adipose cell size characteristics, and genetic markers of adipose cells [35]. Alternatively, differentiation of these metabolic profiles has been attributed to variations in physical activity and cardiorespiratory fitness levels [28, 31], diet (e.g., lower intake of sugar, sugar-sweetened beverages, and saturated fat in MHO than MUO), and lower adiponectin concentrations in MUO than MHO [28].

Recent studies have suggested that MHO profiles may not indicate a lower risk for mortality, particularly when compared to metabolically healthy normal weight [33], and lifestyle interventions (e.g., weight management and physical activity) should continue to be recommended to reduce total mortality in all obese individuals [35].

2.6 Other considerations of obesity

Obesity has a profound impact on the cost of health care. Direct costs refer to money consumed to treat obesity-related health problems such as hospitalization, medical consultations in outpatient clinics, and obesity-related medications [36]. Obesity is associated with increases in annual health-care costs of 36% and medication costs of 77% compared with being of normal weight [37]. In 2014, a pooled estimate of annual medical costs attributable to obesity was $1901 in USD (ranging from $1239–$2582), accounting for approximately $150 billion nationally, with variations in costs primarily driven by age and severity of obesity-related comorbid condition [6].

There are long-term negative economic consequences and indirect costs of obesity. Indirect costs refer to lost productivity or costs to the economy outside of the health sector. Childhood obesity is associated with truancy from school, even after controlling for key covariates [37]. According to the National Longitudinal Survey on Youth 1979 data, higher BMI in late-teen years was associated with 3.5% lower hourly wages for men and women [38]. Obese adolescents were also more likely to be the victim of bullying (e.g., name-calling, teasing, physical abuse) and isolation during adolescence [37], which can result in an economic cost associated with (untreated) mental and behavioral health. If obesity could be addressed in early life by reducing the number overweight and obese 16 and 17-year-olds by 1%, then the number of adults with obesity would reduce by 52,812, and lifetime medical costs would decrease by $586 million [37].

Obesity is also a matter of national security. The impact of obesity on the U.S. military has largely been unreported [39]. Since 2002, there has been a 61% rise among active duty forces, with obesity-related healthcare spending and costs to replace personnel unfit to serve exceeding $1.5 billion USD [39]. The military is facing significant recruiting challenges, with nearly 25% of young adults and over 70% of citizens in most states ineligible to serve due to higher BMI [39]. Other obesity-related issues faced by the military include lost work among those in active duty totaling 656,000 days, violent intentions and behavior, food demand and insecurity, impaired responses to infectious diseases, and vulnerability to injury and death [40].

Currently, there are no accepted standards for what constitutes a health-related threat to national security. Focusing only on the harms of obesity to the wellbeing of the population at large, not just to individuals with obesity, carries with it a risk of perpetuating weight stigmatization [40]. However, framing obesity as a national security threat has significant public health importance, provided importance is placed on gathering quantitative and qualitative data that characterizes the threat, and correlation and causation relationships are properly differentiated [40].

3. Cardiometabolic research

3.1 Strides

Over the last 40 years, the decline in mortality from CVD in the U.S. has been a public health success story. In the U.S., coronary heart disease as a leading cause of death has fallen 60% from its peak in the mid-1960s, with similar declines observed in nearly all regions of the world, especially in high-income countries [41]. However, if we place a narrower focus on racial/ethnic subgroups, or select populations from developing countries, we find that progress has not been equally shared [41, 42].

The sharp decline in mortality rates has been fueled by swift progress in prevention and treatment efforts. These efforts include rapid declines in cigarette smoking, improved methods for treating and controlling HTN, the use of statins to lower circulating cholesterol levels, and limiting or preventing infarction through the use of sophisticated methods [43]. Other factors have resulted in decreases in the rate of CVD despite increases in BMI, such as improved treatment or changes in other risks [26]. Clinical interventions have also proven effective in treating and controlling major risk factors of CVD, such as high systolic BP, cholesterol, and fasting plasma glucose [26].

3.2 Setbacks

3.2.1 Medicalizing obesity

The medical profession and social constructionists profess different concepts of illness. The medical model approaches disease as a biological condition, universal and unchanging, independent of time or place; in contrast, social constructionists define illness as the social and cultural meaning of that condition [44].

The idea of obesity as a social and cultural construct has contributed to its shift from being viewed as a comorbidity that ultimately leads to more complex diseases to its own treatment as a chronic disease with a complex etiology. In 2013, the American Medical Association officially recognized obesity as a complex chronic or non-communicable disease requiring medical attention [5, 13, 45]. The medicalization of obesity has presented a setback in the progress toward combating obesity and its resulting morbidities. Treating obesity as a health outcome rather than a comorbid condition leading to a chronic disease influences policies to focus on medical solutions (e.g., gastric bypass surgeries or pharmacological treatment of obesity-related comorbidities) rather than social and environmental factors as primary drivers of obesity, such as health illiteracy, the role of nutrition-deficient product promotion by the food industry, or healthy food access in areas with high rates of OW/obesity [44]. Other observers have raised similar concerns, not only emphasizing medicalization's overexpansion of medicine's domain, but also proclaiming it to be a mechanism by which the pharmaceutical industry can increase markets [46]. These medical policy changes will thus further contribute to rising health care costs. The Food and Drug Administration similarly expresses concern that proposed obesity drugs themselves increase cardiovascular or other risks and may require changes to clinical research protocols [46]. By treating the medical and social narratives of obesity as mutually exclusive, we may indeed see a resurgence of CVD in the near future.

3.2.2 Constructionist view of the obesity pandemic

The concept of health, illness, and disease are defined differently based on various factors in society. A medical practitioner may define health in very different terms than social or cultural definitions. However, all modern concepts of health recognize health as more than the absence of disease, pointing toward a greater capacity of the individual for self-realization and self-fulfillment [47].

According to the WHO, health is a state of complete physical, mental and social well-being and not merely the absence of disease or infirmity [48]. Other definitions of health can be found in three main models that include social, biomedical, and functional aspects. The social model places its focus on the social determinants of health and illness and argues that the way society is structurally organized affects the etiology of health and illness [49]. It highlights changes that need to be made by society, including health disparities by social class, occupation, race/ethnicity, gender, and income, in order to make the population healthier [49]. The biomedical model of health, currently dominant in medical practice, focuses on biological determinants playing a key role in explaining disease as a condition, primarily caused by external (e.g., physical, chemical, and microbiologic factors) or internal (e.g., vascular, immunologic, and metabolic) factors [50]. In this model, the physical or biological aspects of disease and illness serves as the focal endpoint and is associated with the diagnosis, cure, and treatment of disease. Lastly, functional medicine model focuses more on the dynamic functional processes that result in a person's disease and less with disease as the endpoint [51].

There are skeptics, primarily influenced by the social model of health, who assert the obesity epidemic, and even the idea of health itself, is socially constructed. Holland et al. view obesity as a construct propagated by scientific discourse, which functions within a context of social surveillance and bio-power, even though they acknowledge obesity rates as "social facts" and being obese as a reality [52]. The Association for Size Diversity and Health, an international professional organization and strong proponent of the HAES® movement, asserts that, "health exists on a continuum that varies with time and circumstance for each individual. Health should be conceived as a resource or capacity available to all regardless of health condition or ability level, and not as an outcome or objective of living [53]."

Natalie Boero characterizes the obesity epidemic as a "postmodern epidemic," or "epidemics in which unevenly medicalized phenomena lacking a clear pathological basis get cast in the language and moral panic of "traditional" epidemics [54]." The "postmodern" and constructed labels given to the obesity epidemic are said to be justified due to there being no known discrete cause of obesity, having been attributed to a wide range of factors, from genetic predisposition, to socioeconomic factors (e.g., food quality/scarcity), to the built environment. Adding to this argument is the idea that obesity research tends to conflate overweight and obesity, largely attributable to a critical reliance on a fluid metric (due to its changing categories) to diagnose health [54] and issues with participant selection in study populations [55].

The constructionist view of obesity, largely endorsed by sociologists and members of fat activism, and those that treat obesity as a biomedical fact and health risk, undoubtedly occupy two poles of obesity scholarship. Both hold influence on how the public views and treats OW/obesity. Yet, how can we continue our public health campaign of reducing obesity while avoiding what members of the fat acceptance movement label as "fat shaming"? Is there still a platform wherein OW/obesity and its health ramifications can be publicly discussed from a biomedical perspective while also avoiding weight stigmatization? Until these questions are addressed, the contention between these two groups will remain and the growing popularity of body positivity and fat activism, without regard for the health risks that accompany obesity, will render the public health message of the health advantages of preventing or treating obesity largely ignored.

4. Body image

Body image involves a person's perceptions, thoughts, behaviors, and feelings regarding his or her appearance. There are several aspects of body image that can be explored: perceptual, attitudinal, and psychological [56]. Perceptual body image investigates the accuracy of body size estimations relative to its actual size. Attitudinal body image assesses an overall subjective satisfaction of the body, personal feelings and beliefs about the body, and avoidance of exposure of the body to others [56]. Finally, psychological measures combine one or more of these components. In all aspects, body image is a subjective concept and experience.

Any aspect of body image an individual has of his or her body is pivotally determined by interactions within obesogenic environments [57], (social) media [58], fitness imagery [59], and sociocultural experiences [59–61]. For example, in a study examining the impact of different forms of inspirational fitness ("fitspiration") images on women's image of their bodies, the authors found that exposure to "fitspiration" images led to decreased body satisfaction and increased negative mood over time [59].

Body image satisfaction also exhibits elasticity and can change throughout developmental periods. For example, adolescents display body image elasticity as they undergo the significant physical and psychological changes of puberty [56]. Other examples of groups who may pay special attention to body-related imagery and display sensitivity to media cues are pregnant women, bodybuilders, athletes, and people with eating disorders. Research suggests there are also qualitative differences in body image that vary between men and women, by age group, sexual orientation, and race/ethnicity [56, 62].

5. Weight stigmatization

5.1 The role of culture and society

Western societies, particularly those with affluence in the twenty-first century, have generally associated thinness with happiness, success, youthfulness, and social acceptance [56]. Most citizens of the Western world view fatness as a negative that is to be avoided. There has been a cultural prejudice and stigma toward those with overweight or obesity [60]. However, weight stigmatization has itself become a public health concern due to the associated psychological and physical health consequences to OW/obese individuals. The psychological and social stigmata associated with being OW/obese often makes this population vulnerable to discrimination in their personal and work lives [5]. Often blamed for their weight, the OW/obese are labeled as lazy, weak-willed, out of control, and lacking motivation [2, 56, 60]. The prevailing message in the media is that the cause and cure for obesity lies within the individual [60]. In a study examining obesity perception among policymakers from over 10 developed countries, over 90% saw lack of personal motivation as having a "strong" or "very strong" impact on obesity [23].

Nevertheless, weight stigmatization has been a long-standing approach to reducing obesity. However, it has not proven to be a motivator for weight loss [60]. There are studies that show stigmatizing weight is counterproductive. Individuals who experience weight stigma or perceived weight discrimination are at increased risk for anxiety, depression, bulimia, body dissatisfaction, low self-esteem and other psychological disorders [24]. Other findings have shown that even after controlling for key covariates such as BMI, age, and sex, these psychological outcomes remain, indicating that overweight perception rather than obesity is associated with psychological distress [63].

Weight stigma perpetuates unhealthy behaviors, including increased eating, reduced self-regulation, and avoidance of exercise [64]. Further, chronic stress resulting from weight stigma contributes to the development and/or pathophysiology of obesity, independent of adiposity [64]. Stress has been found to induce high levels of cortisol (an obesogenic hormone), leading to increased activity of the sympathetic nervous system (SNS) and release of corticotrophin-releasing hormone. Chronically elevated SNS activity could deregulate hypothalamic-pituitary-adrenal axis activity, thus further contributing to the etiology of obesity [65].

5.2 Weight bias in clinical settings

Reducing obesity rates has become a target for public health action, due to the link between obesity and a range of chronic diseases and premature mortality. However, critics of this view suggest that obesity has been primarily framed within a medical narrative, thus generating greater social anxiety and fears of "fatness" [66]. Some argue that dominant medical narratives are responsible for the discourse circulating around the idea of fatness as a pathology and a moral failing [66], further asserting that all the statistics on fat people being unhealthy are baseless due to the failure of society to delineate between fat and fat stigma [67]. The supposed bias of physicians has increasingly come under scrutiny. Physicians are said to notoriously view fat patients as noncompliant, or unwilling to follow their directions [67]. Some medical and allied health professionals have been overtly labeled "fat phobic" and showing weight bias. Weight bias is defined as having a widespread stereotypical and prejudicial attitude, assumption, belief, or judgment toward fat people [68, 69]. Studies show widespread weight bias among medical professionals [70], medical students and physician assistants [71], and exercise and nutrition professionals [72], with no clearly defined approach to reduce these biases among students and professionals across various health disciplines [69]. There have even been reports of obese women avoiding routine gynecological exams, despite having higher rates of gynecological cancers than nonobese women, due to weight stigmatization and the corresponding negative attitudes of health care professionals toward overweight people [44]. The obesity problem we are facing is only exacerbated when participants express reluctance to address weight concerns with their health care providers for fear they will not be taken seriously [70], or avoid seeing their primary care physician or specialist entirely.

6. Body positivity

There has been a growing awareness of the psychosocial harms of weight stigmatization and fat shaming. Our culture is moving more toward body positivity, self-empowerment, inclusivity, and encouraging individuals to take pride in and accept their bodies, despite having BMI's that classify them as clinically OW/obese. Popularized through Instagram, with over 11 million posts tagged with #bodypositive, 4 million for #bodypositivity, and more than 1 million for #bopo [73]. Indeed, an internet search of body positivity will yield more than 112 million results [73]. Body positivity aims to challenge dominant body image ideals, promote acceptance and respect of all bodies, irrespective of shape, size, and features, focusing more on appreciating the functionality and health of the body rather than only its appearance [73] (**Figure 4**).

Positive body image is indeed a key factor in determining one's ability to reach weight loss goals. However, setting positive weight loss goals is an assumption in traditional approaches to weight loss [74]. Other assumptions include 1) the notion that adiposity increases risk of morbidity and mortality, 2) maintaining weight loss can be achieved through proper diet and exercise, which will prolong life, 3) obese individuals can improve health only through weight loss, 4) and finally, the high

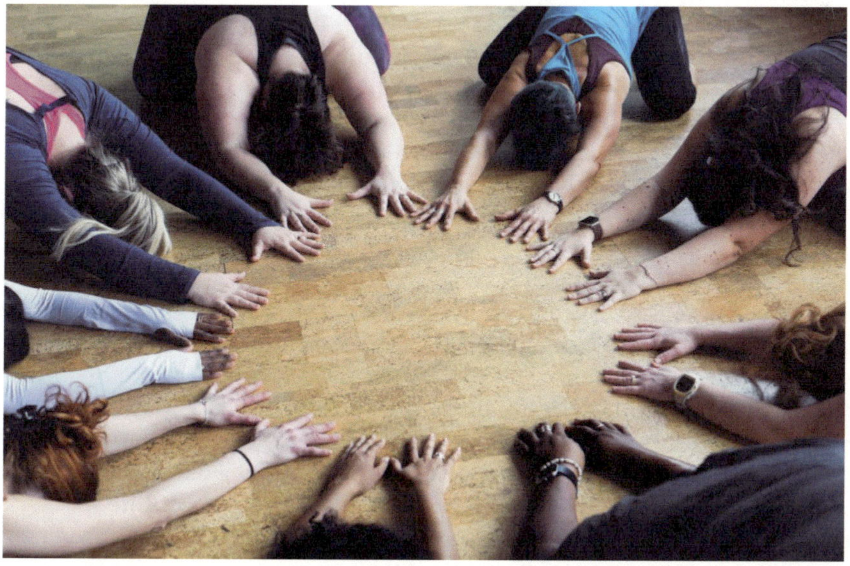

Figure 4.
A group of women at a fitness facility stretch to hold a child's pose with their hands all reaching in to form a circle. Body positivity promotes strength and fitness coming in many forms, no matter the body shape or size (photo by: Sarah Pflug. Available from: https://burst.shopify.com/photos/ladies-stretch-circle?c=yoga [Accessed: 13 August 2020]).

economic burden on the health care system incurred by obesity-related costs can be mitigated by obesity treatment and prevention [74].

Many people who pursue weight-loss programs are seemingly motivated to lose weight to be normal, wear smaller clothes, and avoid weight stigmatization and discrimination rather than by the dangers of obesity or its associated health risks [54]. OW/obese individuals are now being more positively represented in the media, movies, and even in arenas where they have historically been absent or ignored, such as in the fitness and fashion industries, or as role models in music and entertainment. However, visual normalization of larger bodies, that is, more habitual visual exposure to people with excess weight, may further contribute to the higher prevalence of overweight and obesity, particularly among those with lower levels of education and income [75].

7. Fat acceptance and health at every size movements

7.1 Fat acceptance

Established in 1969, the National Association to Advance Fat Acceptance (NAAFA) is a fat-rights organization congealed out of early protests of fat activists (**Figure 5**). Established as a support movement, the organization protests discrimination in the workplace and lack of fat acceptance in society [76]. The organization is dedicated to protecting the rights and improving the quality of life for fat people [77].

Fat acceptance and body positivity have become synonymous terms of late. Arguing that the former term is rooted in the latter term, some claim that fat acceptance is threatening to destroy the body positive movement. They contend that those originally intended to benefit from body positivity were individuals like cancer survivors who have suffered physical disfigurement, people with physical disabilities, and members of underrepresented racial/ethnic groups frequently ignored by the media. These individuals have no control over primarily physical factors that have set them apart.

Parallels have been drawn between fatness and smoking (i.e. an unhealthy and deadly condition brought on by behaviors, but difficult to change once the behavior is set in motion) [78]. It follows that those with no apparent medical reason for OW/obesity (e.g., medications, Cushing's syndrome, polycystic ovary syndrome), on some level, choose to be OW/obese. Conversely, there are those that believe the idea that fat is permanently changeable to be a myth, citing studies that report participants gaining more weight than originally lost within three years of ending a diet [67].

Culture, society, (social) media, and reality TV have all influenced obesity perception, outpacing influential and well-established clinical definitions and medical advice warning of the cardiometabolic risks of obesity. For example, the terms "fat," "curvy," "plus-sized," and "full-figured" are more frequently used among plus-size fashion bloggers, reclaiming the use of the word "fat," and lessening the weight stigma around obesity [79]. OW/obese people can now be found on the glossy covers of magazines and amassing followers on social media outlets such as blog sites, Instagram, YouTube, TikTok, Tumblr, Twitter, and other online spaces. Under the guise of glamor and glitz, OW/obese social media and reality TV influencers advertise "fit, fabulous, and fat" lifestyles, which only serve to contradict public health messaging discouraging unhealthy lifestyles. While fat activists and the fat acceptance movement are working to reduce weight stigmatization, their influence on the public, particularly those with central adiposity, can potentially undermine the recognition of being overweight and its health consequences [75].

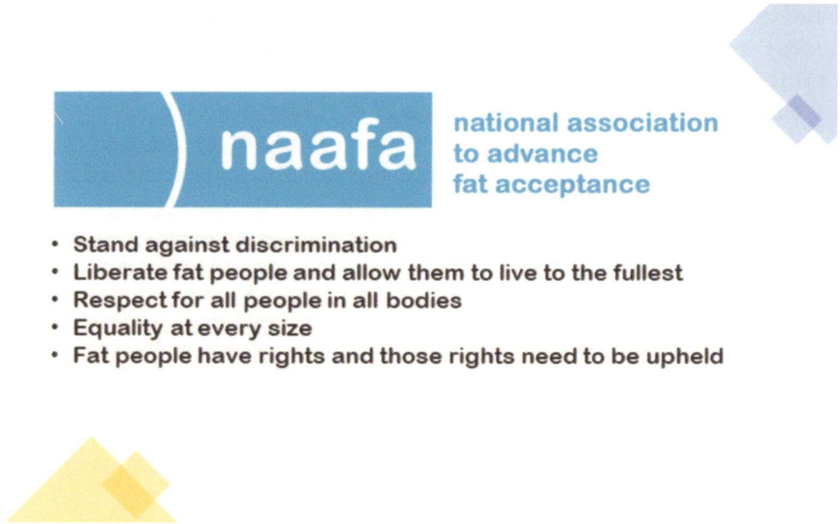

Figure 5.
The National Association to Advance Fat Acceptance (NAAFA) is an all-volunteer, multigenerational fat-rights organization seeking to change the narrative around fatness, fight for fat-rights, and increase respect for all people, regardless of body type or size. Available from: https://naafa.org/ [Accessed: 13 August 2020].

Civil lawmakers are also shifting the narrative to more acceptance and inclusivity as it relates to OW/obese perception. Antidiscrimination law theorizes unfairness based on government classifications of a group of people who are singled out and burdened without sufficiently good reason or in employment decisions based on protected traits outlined in Title VII of the 1964 Civil Rights Act. Fat advocates have become familiar with the difficulty of seeking legal arguments for fat rights protection under Title VII while also arguing that obesity is a medicalized impairment and disability [78].

7.2 Health at every size

Like the fat acceptance movement, HAES® is a weight-neutral approach that advocates the idea that health can be achieved and sustained, independent of weight status. The HAES® approach advocates intuitive eating, which involves listening to and acting on internal hunger and satiety cues and preferences. A HAES® approach attempts to addresses weight bias and stigma in individuals living with obesity, and is touted as a promising public health approach instead of focusing on weight status as an ultimate health outcome [74]. Proponents of HAES® assert that the long-term sustainability of traditional medical or behaviorally based interventions (e.g., pharmacological, surgical, and behavioral) for obesity has been disappointing. HAES® is emerging as standard practice in the eating disorders field [80] whose principles are professed by an array of civil rights groups and international professional organizations dedicated to promoting fat acceptance and fighting weight discrimination [80].

There is evidence supporting the notion of fit at every size. Higher fitness levels among the MHO are associated with fewer metabolic complications and lower prevalence of MetS at any age and across different weight status groups [31]. However, as previously mentioned, MHO has been shown to be a transient state to MUO [25, 33].

It is important to emphasize that health is a continuum on which every person lies, with one end of the spectrum representing morbidity/mortality and the other health and vitality. There is a size threshold, albeit non-discrete, over which a person crosses over into a state of increased risk of, or overt illness. Established comorbidities and sequelae frequently accompany sustained obesity, despite practicing intuitive eating, that reduce quality of life, not the least of which include increased risk of musculoskeletal pathology [81], arthritis/joint pain, respiratory conditions/diseases (e.g., sleep apnea, asthma), depression/anxiety, inability to participate in certain activities, and physical disability [1]. Additionally, the association between intuitive eating and diet quality remains unclear in epidemiologic literature. Nevertheless, HAES® holds value in its deemphasis on restrictive dieting, which has been associated with increased psychological stress, increased cortisol levels, and subsequent weight gain [65].

Despite years of empirical medical and comprehensive epidemiological research, many fat activists take pride in maintaining higher BMI and embracing their size, all while holding in contempt any efforts to increase health and wellness. Permeating through activism, academia, fashion, and even sports, the HAES® approach appears to promote not only acceptance, but pride in the esthetic of the fat body. Members of this movement seek to bring people of larger size back from the margins of society, fiercely labeling those who oppose their ideas as "body-shamers" and "fat phobic" perpetuators of societal norms.

While the OW/obese may find intuitive eating and HAES® approaches successful, there still remains a tremendous (mental) health care cost of obesity-related illnesses. These costs are a real economic impact to society. Years of medical and scientific research has provided irrefutable evidence of the deadly cost of condoning preventable OW/obesity and unhealthy lifestyles of over 650 million OW/obese worldwide. Simultaneously, the medical and public health community must not use the campaign to reduce fat as justification for prejudice and oppression. OW/obese individuals have a right to make their own choices; but health literacy and knowledge of the correct information and use of that information to make informed health decisions is of utmost public health concern.

8. Preventing the reversal of progress made in CVD research

8.1 Health behaviors

At the primary level of prevention, modifying health behaviors, such as incorporating healthy eating and fitness habits into everyday lifestyles, can reduce metabolic risk factors (e.g., cholesterol levels, blood sugar levels, and BP) [25, 82]. The benefits of both reducing sedentary behavior together with increasing physical activity, especially in the elderly, is associated with a reduced risk for type 2 diabetes, compared with those physically inactive [82]. Lowering body fat, even if from obesity to overweight, can result in a reduction in metabolic abnormalities and lower levels of systemic inflammation, and lower BP [25]. The Look AHEAD study examined the effects of an intensive lifestyle intervention and found that lifestyle interventions can produce long term weight loss and improvement in fitness and sustained beneficial effects on CVD risk factors [83].

8.2 Health literacy

While self-acceptance and positive self-perception are certainly noble attributes, scientific knowledge of well-established risks of clinical obesity, particularly excess central body fat, cannot go unheeded. Health literacy, in combination with body positivity, may prevent reversal of the strides made in the reduction of CVD.

Health literacy is the degree to which individuals are able to access, understand, and use or process basic health information and services, thereby promoting good health for themselves, their families, and their communities [3]. Insufficient health literacy has been associated with poorer outcomes prior to and following coronary events, excess body weight, higher morbidity and mortality rates, healthcare use, and costs [84, 85] (**Figure 6**). Increasing health literacy will contribute to greater ability to read food labels, determine energy content, and make better food choices complementary to a healthy, physically active lifestyle. Health literacy should be evaluated as part of secondary prevention programs aiming to reduce CVD risk, such as dropout rates in cardiac rehabilitation [84].

With the power to fundamentally change the way the population regards obesity and its health risks, health literacy has the potential to profoundly reduce barriers to health delivery, reduce health care costs, and improve overall health status.

8.3 Social media

Social media is a crowded space that is filled with competing health messages. These platforms play a principal role in attempting to change health behavior and prevent or improve CVD health outcomes. Social media messages have influenced the health care decision making among patients, not all of whom always check the authenticity of information received. For example, in a study exploring the impact of health-related information sharing and the influence of social media on people's online health information-seeking behavior, the authors found that social media users received health information (80–90%), and admitted to starting (47%), and stopping medication (42%) after reading messages received on a social media platform [86]. Taking this into account, public health practitioners must focus their resources on platforms to counter sociological agendas. For example, most tenets of fat acceptance, body positivity (independent of weight status), and HAES® openly contradict health guidelines that are based on years of medical research. They must increase the amount of available information on CVD health, reinforce its salience

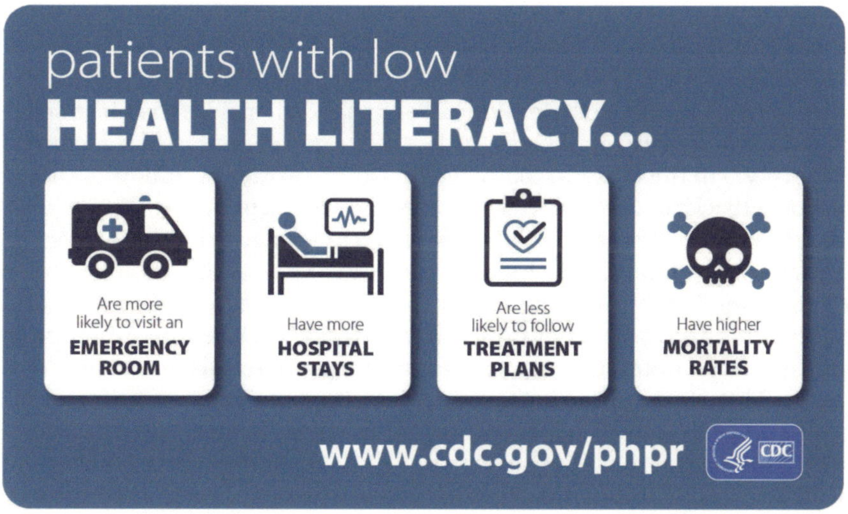

Figure 6.
Adverse health risks for patients with low health literacy (source: Centers for Disease Control and Prevention (CDC), Center for Preparedness and Response. Available from: https://www.cdc.gov/cpr/infographics/healthliteracy.htm [Accessed: 03 August 2020]).

as a CVD risk factor and public health problem, attract the attention of the OW/obese population, and offer practical solutions [87].

Medical advice must be translated into lay terms, adjusting for multiple levels of health literacy. Messages must include health incentives that are relatable to their audience. A successful public health campaign will include communication that is sensitive to the body positivity movement, one that encourages self-acceptance, and supports the mental health of this population. Incorporating elements from the social, biomedical, and functional models of health may elucidate why reducing body fat is beneficial for cardiometabolic health.

8.4 Clinical settings

In clinical settings, it is imperative that medical professionals, including physician assistants [71] and exercise and nutrition professionals [72], increase their awareness of their own weight bias, as well as that of their colleagues. Creating a welcoming setting where the OW/obese do not feel stigmatized will open more opportunities for doctor-patient educational discourse on the health benefits of reducing body weight, restructure how they are clinically monitored, and reduce bias while profiling their CVD risk.

The biomedical model has been the dominant approach in medicine. However, in its organ-oriented approach and its failing to take psychosocial aspects of disease into account, its efficacy in the advent of chronic disease prevalence has become questionable [50]. There is an increasing recognition of the influential role of culture and society in our perception of health and healthy behaviors. Rather than medical practitioners taking the historic biomedical model approach to obesity in clinical settings, a more effective approach will be to incorporate ideas from the social model (e.g., screening for social and environmental contributors to obesity), together with concepts from the functional model (e.g., examining functional health of the OW/obese). Building bridges across models will advance our prevention efforts and holistic treatment in this population.

9. Chapter conclusion

Obesity is still a pervasive problem, confirming its intractability. Obesity is a well-known risk factor for CVD, which is still a leading cause of morbidity and mortality in the U.S. and most developed countries. Yet, strides have been made in reducing CVD mortality rates. Over the last 40 years, we have seen a decline in mortality from CVD in the U.S. and many regions of the world. In response, there have been major setbacks to this progress, namely the fat acceptance and body positivity movements. Principally rooted within sociological frameworks, these movements appear inattentive to the established adverse health risks of maintaining an OW/obese status; nor do they promote efforts to modify health behaviors that reduce obesity and thus decrease risk of type 2 diabetes and CVD. Yet these emerging views are gaining momentum, revealing key changes in trends in fat identity and fat acceptance. These trends have key public health implications with a direct impact on a generation who daily engages with social media influencers who promote such messages. The parallel trend of the body positivity movement, in the absence of weight status consideration, threatens to reverse decades of progress made toward reducing coronary heart disease and its comorbidities.

The urgency of reducing obesity as a public health message continues. The body positivity and fat activism communities must reconcile with medical and public health professionals to equally address both the mental health benefits of self-acceptance and positive body image, while also bearing in mind the short- and long-term health advantages of preventing or treating obesity. Both groups must weigh in and not compete to win on framing the narrative of obesity. The future of cardiovascular health relies upon this collaboration.

Author details

Ketrell L. McWhorter
School of Science, Health and Mathematics, Asbury University, Wilmore, Kentucky, United States

*Address all correspondence to: ketrell.mcwhorter@asbury.edu

References

[1] Hruby A, Hu FB. The epidemiology of obesity: A big picture. Pharmaco Economics. 2015;**33**(7):673-689

[2] Upadhyay J et al. Obesity as a disease. Medical Clinics. 2018;**102**(1):13-33

[3] World Health Organization. The mandate for health literacy. In: 9th Global Conference on Health Promotion, Shanghai 2016. Geneva, Switzerland: World Health Organization; 2017. Available from: www.who.int/healthpromotion/conferences/9gchp/health-literacy/en/

[4] World Health Organization. Obesity and Overweight. Geneva, Switzerland: World Health Organization; 2020. Available from: www.who.int/en/news-room/fact-sheets/detail/obesity-and-overweight

[5] Purnell JQ. Definitions, classification, and epidemiology of obesity. In: Feingold KR, Anawalt B, Boyce A, et al., editors. Endotext [Internet]. South Dartmouth (MA): MDText.com, Inc.; 2000. Available from: https://www.ncbi.nlm.nih.gov/books/NBK279167/.[Updated: 12 April 2018]

[6] Kim DD, Basu A. Estimating the medical care costs of obesity in the United States: Systematic review, meta-analysis, and empirical analysis. Value in Health. 2016;**19**(5):602-613

[7] Hales CM, Carroll MD, Fryar CD, Ogden CL. Prevalence of Obesity and Severe Obesity among Adults: United States, 2017-2018. NCHS Data Brief, No 360. Hyattsville, MD: National Center for Health Statistics; 2020

[8] Ciciurkaite G, Moloney ME, Brown RL. The incomplete medicalization of obesity: Physician office visits, diagnoses, and treatments, 1996-2014. Public Health Reports. 2019;**134**(2):141-149

[9] Fryar CD, Kruszon-Moran D, Gu Q, Ogden CL. Mean body weight, height, waist circumference, and body mass index among adults: United States, 1999-2000 through 2015-2016. National Health Statistics Reports; No 122. Hyattsville, MD: National Center for Health Statistics; 2018

[10] National Heart Lung and Blood Institute. Assessing Your Weight and Health Risk. USA: U.S. Department of Health and Human Services, National Heart Lung and Blood Institute; 2020. Available from: www.nhlbi.nih.gov/health/educational/lose_wt/risk.htm

[11] Watson RM et al. Influence of age, ethnicity and sex on body composition thresholds for the accumulation of visceral adipose tissue in adults. American Journal of Sports Science. 2019;**7**(3):111-120

[12] Heymsfield SB et al. Why are there race/ethnic differences in adult body mass index-adiposity relationships? A quantitative critical review. Obesity Reviews : An Official Journal of the International Association for the Study of Obesity. 2016;**17**(3):262-275

[13] Romieu I et al. Energy balance and obesity: What are the main drivers? Cancer Causes & Control: CCC. 2017;**28**(3):247-258

[14] Timothy Garvey W. The diagnosis and evaluation of patients with obesity. Current Opinion in Endocrine and Metabolic Research. 2019;**4**:50-57

[15] Moffat T. The "childhood obesity epidemic": Health crisis or social construction? Medical Anthropology Quarterly. 2010;**24**(1):s-21

[16] Freedman DS et al. The Limitations of transforming very high body Mass indexes into z-scores among 8.7 million 2- to 4-year-old Children. The Journal of Pediatrics. 2017;**188**:50-56.e1

[17] Centers for Disease Control and Prevention. Body Mass Index: Considerations for Practitioners. Atlanta, GA: Department of Health and Human Services; 2020. Available from: https://stacks.cdc.gov/view/cdc/25368

[18] Bener A et al. Obesity index that better predict metabolic syndrome: body mass index, waist circumference, waist hip ratio, or waist height ratio. Journal of Obesity. 2013;**2013**:269038

[19] National Heart Lung and Blood Institute. Losing Weight, Body Mass Index. USA: U.S. Department of Health and Human Services: National Heart Lung and Blood Institute; 2020. Available from: www.nhlbi.nih.gov/health/educational/lose_wt/BMI/bmi_dis

[20] Lam BCC et al. Comparison of body mass index (BMI), body adiposity index (BAI), waist circumference (WC), waist-to-hip ratio (WHR) and waist-to-height ratio (WHtR) as predictors of cardiovascular disease risk factors in an adult population in Singapore. PLoS One. 2015;**10**(4):e0122985

[21] Abbasi F, Blasey C, Reaven GM. Cardiometabolic risk factors and obesity: Does it matter whether BMI or waist circumference is the index of obesity? The American Journal of Clinical Nutrition. 2013;**98**(3):637-640

[22] Kuriyan R. Body composition techniques. The Indian Journal of Medical Research. 2018;**148**(5):648-658

[23] Cooper K, C3 Collaborating for Health. Obesity: Perception and Policy—Multi-Country Review and Survey of Policymakers. London, UK: European Association for the Study of Obesity; 2014

[24] Williams EP et al. Overweight and obesity: Prevalence, consequences, and causes of a growing public health problem. Current Obesity Reports. 2015;**4**(3):363-370

[25] Corres P et al. A Metabolically healthy profile is a transient stage when exercise and diet are not supervised: Long-term effects in the EXERDIET-HTA study. International Journal of Environmental Research and Public Health. 2020;**17**(8):2830

[26] Afshin A et al. Health effects of overweight and obesity in 195 countries over 25 years. The New England Journal of Medicine. 2017;**377**(1):13-27

[27] King DE, Xiang J, Pilkerton CS. Multimorbidity trends in United States adults, 1988-2014. Journal of American Board of Family Medicine. 2018;**31**(4):503-513

[28] Smith GI, Mittendorfer B, Klein S. Metabolically healthy obesity: Facts and fantasies. The Journal of Clinical Investigation. 2019;**129**(10):3978-3989

[29] Liu C et al. The prevalence of metabolically healthy and unhealthy obesity according to different criteria. Obesity Facts. 2019;**12**(1):78-90

[30] Alberti KG et al. Harmonizing the metabolic syndrome: A joint interim statement of the International Diabetes Federation Task Force on Epidemiology and Prevention; National Heart, Lung, and Blood Institute; American Heart Association; World Heart Federation; International Atherosclerosis Society; and International Association for the Study of Obesity. Circulation. 2009;**120**(16):1640-1645

[31] Ortega FB et al. The intriguing metabolically healthy but obese phenotype: Cardiovascular prognosis and role of fitness. European Heart Journal. 2013;**34**(5):389-397

[32] Mathew H, Farr OM, Mantzoros CS. Metabolic health and weight: Understanding

metabolically unhealthy normal weight or metabolically healthy obese patients. Metabolism - Clinical and Experimental. 2016;**65**(1):73-80

[33] Mongraw-Chaffin M et al. Metabolically healthy obesity, transition to metabolic syndrome, and cardiovascular risk. Journal of the American College of Cardiology. 2018;**71**(17):1857

[34] Hwang YC et al. Visceral abdominal fat accumulation predicts the conversion of metabolically healthy obese subjects to an unhealthy phenotype. International Journal of Obesity (2005). 2015;**39**(9):1365-1370

[35] Primeau V et al. Characterizing the profile of obese patients who are metabolically healthy. International Journal of Obesity. 2011;**35**(7):971-981

[36] Abdelaal M, le Roux CW, Docherty NG. Morbidity and mortality associated with obesity. Annals of Translational Medicine. 2017;**5**(7):161-161

[37] Apovian CM. Obesity: Definition, comorbidities, causes, and burden. The American Journal of Managed Care. 2016;**22**(7 Suppl):s176-s185

[38] Han E, Norton EC, Powell LM. Direct and indirect effects of body weight on adult wages. Economics and Human Biology. 2011;**9**(4):381-392

[39] Christeson W, Clifford K, Taggart A. Retreat is not an option: healthier schools meals protect our children and our country. Washington, D.C.: Mission Readiness; 2017. Available from: http://missionreadiness.s3.amazonaws.com/wp-content/uploads/MR-NAT-Retreat-Not-an-Option.pdf [Accessed: 16 July 2020]

[40] Voss JD, Pavela G, Stanford FC. Obesity as a threat to national security: the need for precision engagement. International Journal of Obesity. 2019;**43**(3):437-439

[41] Jones DS, Greene JA. The decline and rise of coronary heart disease: Understanding public health catastrophism. American Journal of Public Health. 2013;**103**(7):1207-1218

[42] Carnethon Mercedes R et al. Cardiovascular health in African Americans: A scientific statement from the American Heart Association. Circulation. 2017;**136**(21):e393-e423

[43] Mensah GA et al. Decline in cardiovascular mortality: Possible causes and implications. Circulation Research. 2017;**120**(2):366-380

[44] Conrad P, Barker KK. The social construction of illness: Key insights and policy implications. Journal of Health and Social Behavior. 2010;**51**(1_suppl):S67-S79

[45] Stanford FC, Tauqeer Z, Kyle TK. Media and its influence on obesity. Current Obesity Reports. 2018;**7**(2):186-192

[46] Blackburn GL. Medicalizing obesity: Individual, economic, and medical consequences. Virtual Mentor. 2011;**13**(12):890-895. Published 2011 Dec 1. DOI: 10.1001/virtualmentor.2011.13.12.pfor1-1112

[47] Svalastog AL et al. Concepts and definitions of health and health-related values in the knowledge landscapes of the digital society. Croatian Medical Journal. 2017;**58**(6):431-435

[48] World Health Organization. Constitution. Geneva, Switzerland: World Health Organization; 2020. Available from: www.who.int/about/who-we-are/constitution

[49] Adibi H. Health: Its implications within the biomedical and social models of health—A critical review.

Cyber Journals: Multidisciplinary Journals of Science and Technology. 2014;**4**(2):16-23

[50] Havelka M, Despot Lučanin J, Lučanin D. Biopsychosocial model—The integrated approach to health and disease. Collegium Antropologicum. 2009;**33**(1):303-310

[51] Bland J. Defining function in the functional medicine model. Integrative Medicine (Encinitas, Calif.). 2017;**16**(1):22-25

[52] Holland KE et al. Our girth is plain to see': An analysis of newspaper coverage of Australia's Future 'Fat Bomb. Health, Risk & Society. 2011;**13**(1):31-46

[53] Association for Size Diversity and Health. HAES® Principles. ASDAH, Association for Size Diversity and Health; 2020. Available from: www.sizediversityandhealth.org/content.asp?id=152

[54] Boero N. Killer Fat: Media, Medicine, and Morals in the American "Obesity Epidemic". New Brunswick/New Jersey/London: Rutgers University Press; 2012. Available from: http://www.jstor.org/stable/j.ctt5hjf6p [Retrieved: 4 September 2020]

[55] Boero N. Obesity in the media: Social science weighs in. Critical Public Health. 2013;**23**(3):371-380

[56] Grogan S. Body Image: Understanding Body Dissatisfaction in Men, Women and Children. 3rd ed. London/New York: Routledge/Taylor & Francis Group; 2016

[57] Yayan EH, Çelebioğlu A. Effect of an obesogenic environment and health behaviour-related social support on body mass index and body image of adolescents. Global Health Promotion. 2018;**25**(3):33-42

[58] Chen I et al. A qualitative study of obesity perceptions in social media through Twitter's tweets. International Journal of Management, Economics and Social Sciences (IJMESS). 2018;**7**(Special Issue):40-57

[59] Prichard I et al. The impact of different forms of# fitspiration imagery on body image, mood, and self-objectification among young women. Sex Roles. 2018;**78**(11-12):789-798

[60] Puhl RM, Heuer CA. Obesity stigma: Important considerations for public health. American Journal of Public Health. 2010;**100**(6):1019-1028

[61] Fardouly J et al. Social comparisons on social media: The impact of Facebook on young women's body image concerns and mood. Body Image. 2015;**13**:38-45

[62] Male vs. Female Body Image. Bradley University. Available from: www.bradley.edu/sites/bodyproject/male-body-image-m-vs-f/

[63] Atlantis E, Ball K. Association between weight perception and psychological distress. International Journal of Obesity. 2008;**32**(4):715-721

[64] Tomiyama AJ et al. Associations of weight stigma with cortisol and oxidative stress independent of adiposity. Health Psychology : Official Journal of the Division of Health Psychology, American Psychological Association. 2014;**33**(8):862-867

[65] Lucassen EA, Cizza G. The hypothalamic-pituitary-adrenal axis, obesity, and chronic stress exposure: Sleep and the HPA axis in obesity. Current Obesity Reports. 2012;**1**(4):208-215

[66] Murray S. Pathologizing "fatness": Medical authority and popular culture. Sociology of Sport Journal. 2008;**25**(1):7-21

[67] McMichael L. Acceptable Prejudice?: Fat, Rhetoric and Social Justice. Pearlsong Press; 2013

[68] Bacon JG, Scheltema KE, Robinson BE. Fat phobia scale revisited: The short form. International Journal of Obesity. 2001;**25**(2):252-257

[69] Alberga AS et al. Weight bias reduction in health professionals: A systematic review. 2016

[70] Puhl RM, Heuer CA. The stigma of obesity: A review and update. Obesity. 2009;**17**(5):941

[71] Wolf C. Physician assistants' attitudes about obesity and obese individuals. Journal of Allied Health. 2012;**41**(2):45E-48E

[72] Panza GA et al. Weight bias among exercise and nutrition professionals: A systematic review. Obesity Reviews. 2018;**19**(11):1492-1503

[73] Cohen R, Newton-John T, Slater A. The case for body positivity on social media: Perspectives on current advances and future directions. Journal of Health Psychology. 2020:1359105320912450

[74] Penney TL, Kirk SF. The Health at Every Size paradigm and obesity: Missing empirical evidence may help push the reframing obesity debate forward. American Journal of Public Health. 2015;**105**(5):e38-e42

[75] Muttarak R. Normalization of plus size and the danger of unseen overweight and obesity in England. Obesity. 2018;**26**(7):1125-1129

[76] Rasmussen DW. The Rights/Development Nexus: Sen, Olson, and the Obesity Rights Movement*. Social Science Quarterly. 2019;**100**(3):923-935

[77] NAAFA. About Us. 2020: Las Vegas, NV: Naafa; 2020. Available from: naafa.org/about-us

[78] Kirkland A. Think of the hippopotamus: Rights consciousness in the fat acceptance movement. Law and Society Review. 2008;**42**(2):397-432

[79] Limatius H. Fat, curvy or plus-size? A corpus-linguistic approach to identity construction in plus-size fashion blogs. In: Search of Meaning: Literary, Linguistic, and Translational Approaches to Communication. Tampere, Finland: Tampere University; 2018. pp. 12-38

[80] Bacon L, Aphramor L, Weight S. Evaluating the evidence for a paradigm shift. Nutrition Journal. 2011;**10**(1):9

[81] Browning RC, Kram R. Effects of obesity on the biomechanics of walking at different speeds. Medicine & Science in Sports & Exercise. 2007;**39**(9):1632-1641

[82] González K, Fuentes J, Márquez JL. Physical inactivity, sedentary behavior and chronic diseases. Korean Journal of Family Medicine. 2017;**38**(3):111-115

[83] Look ARG, Wing RR. Long-term effects of a lifestyle intervention on weight and cardiovascular risk factors in individuals with type 2 diabetes mellitus: Four-year results of the Look AHEAD trial. Archives of Internal Medicine. 2010;**170**(17):1566-1575

[84] Magnani JW et al. Health literacy and cardiovascular disease: Fundamental relevance to primary and secondary prevention: A scientific statement from the American Heart Association. Circulation. 2018;**138**(2):e48

[85] Michou M, Panagiotakos BD, Costarelli V. Low health literacy and excess body weight: A systematic review. Central European Journal of Public Health. 2018;**26**(3):234-241

[86] Iftikhar R, Abaalkhail B. Health-seeking influence reflected by online

health-related messages received on social media: Cross-sectional survey. Journal of Medical Internet Research. 2017;**19**(11):e382

[87] Randolph W, Viswanath K. Lessons learned from public health mass media campaigns: Marketing health in a crowded media world. Annual Review of Public Health. 2004;**25**:419-437

Chapter 7

Genetic Determinant of Familial Dilated Cardiomyopathy and Genotype-Targeted Therapeutic Strategy

Jing Zhong, Li-Ping Li, Jian-Feng Zhou and Yong-He Ding

Abstract

Dilated cardiomyopathy (DCM) is a myocardium disease characterized by left ventricular dilation and systolic dysfunction. Genetic susceptibility contributes significantly to the disease progression in familial DCM. Mutations in more than fifty different genes have been identified to cause DCM, accounting for up to 50% of familial DCM cases. Elucidation of genetic basis for the remaining familial DCM probands promises to substantially increase the efficiency of genetic testing for early disease diagnosis and intervention. Dissecting genetic pathways linked to DCM and related pathogenic mechanisms can provide valuable insights into the understanding of disease pathophysiology that can be leveraged for development of genotype-targeted therapeutic strategy. Here, we review genetic variants, with a focus on affected genes most commonly implicated in DCM, and highlight their underlying pathophysiological mechanisms of action. We discuss recent progress on gene-based therapeutic strategy which holds the opportunities to implement individualized medicine and ultimately to improve patient outcome in the future.

Keywords: dilated cardiomyopathy, genetic determinant, genetic testing, gene therapy, pathophysiology

1. Introduction

Heart failure afflicts about 26 million patients worldwide. The estimated economic burden related to heart failure is 120 billion US dollars [1]. Dilated cardiomyopathy (DCM), referred to a group of heart muscle disorders characterized by heart chamber dilation and systolic dysfunction, is a common cause of heart failure. DCM is the most common form of non-ischemic cardiomyopathy and the most common indication in patients who need heart transplantation [2, 3]. In the pediatric, nearly 50% of patients dying suddenly or undergoing cardiac transplantation are affected by cardiomyopathy, predominantly by DCM [4]. In the young, DCM is the most frequent cause of heart failure [5]. In the adult, it is the second most common cause of heart failure (after the coronary heart disease), underlying about one third of all heart failure cases [1]. While the true prevalence for DCM in general population is not fully defined yet due to lack of well-designed large-scale population based studies, its estimated prevalence ranges from 1 in 2500 to 1 in 250 people [6]. The annual incidence of DCM is approximately 7 cases per 10,000 individuals, and males are about 3 times more frequently affected than females [2, 7, 8].

Classically, DCM is defined based on two major criteria: 1) left LV fractional shortening <25% (> 2 standard deviations [SD]) and/or LV ejection fraction <45% (>2 SD); and 2) LV end-diastolic diameter greater than 117% of the predicated value corrected for age and body surface area. DCM is diagnosed when any other known cause of myocardial diseases are excluded [9]. The updated definitions of DCM are left ventricular or biventricular systolic dysfunction and dilatation that are not explained by abnormal loading conditions or coronary artery disease [10].

DCM is caused by a variety of etiologies, including acquired, genetic and/or mixed origins. Acquired risk factors such as infection, myocarditis, drug toxin, autoimmune response, excess alcohol consumption and metabolic disorders are recognized to cause DCM. Primary DCM results when all these acquired factors are exclude, which can be either idiopathic or familial. Familial DCM (FDC) is classified when two or more family members are diagnosed in first-degree relatives. The prevalence of familial DCM differs in different patient cohorts, estimated to range from 20–50% of all DCM cases. The remaining DCM cases are thus classified as idiopathic [6, 11]. However, the frequency of familial DCM is believed to be underestimated, due to the limitation of large pedigree and family's availability for diagnostic screening. Genetic factors which predispose to DCM have been increasingly recognized. Since the discovery of the first disease causative gene to cardiomyopathy [12], to date, more than 50 genes have been identified to associate with DCM and the number is still increasing. Genetic mutations in all these genes combined can explain about 40–50% of familial DCM cases, underpinning the genetic determinant of this disease [6]. The familial DCM appears to be inherited as a monogenic trait and is mainly transmitted in an autosomal dominant inheritance pattern, manifesting incomplete, age-related penetrance and variable expression. Other patterns such as autosomal recessive, X-linked and mitochondrial inheritance also occurs in a small portion of the familial DCM cases [6, 13].

Current management of DCM is mainly focused on treating patients with symptoms following the standard guidelines, similar to treating other forms of heart failure with reduced ejection fraction (EF). The guideline driven therapies mostly adapt a "one-size-fits-all" approach that uses β-adrenergic blockers, angiotensin-converting enzyme inhibitors, or angiotensin receptor blockers to improve cardiac function and symptom by reducing congestion and management of arrhythmia [14, 15]. Recently, several new additions of armamentarium are also implemented in the treatment options [16–18]. Despite of advances in these treatment protocols, DCM remains one of the major reasons for patients needed for heart transplantation, and the morbidity and mortality rate of DCM still remains unacceptably high. Thus, the current management of DCM with the "one-size-fits-all" strategy is challenged. More novel and effective and individualized treatment options are desirable.

Considering the genetic determinant of DCM, and up to 50% of familial DCM patients have a genetic origin, genotype-targeted therapies, by directly targeting at the specific gene mutations, have emerged as promising strategies toward development of more effective and individualized treatment. In this chapter, we firstly review definitive genes linked to DCM and classify them based on their intracellular localization (**Figure 1**), with a major focus on genes most commonly implicated in DCM, and highlight their underlying pathophysiological mechanism of action if known (**Table 1**). Next, we discuss progress and challenges on the emerging genotype-based therapeutic strategies for effective and individualized medicine explored in the treatment of DCM (**Table 2**), which hold the opportunities to ultimately improve patient outcome in the future.

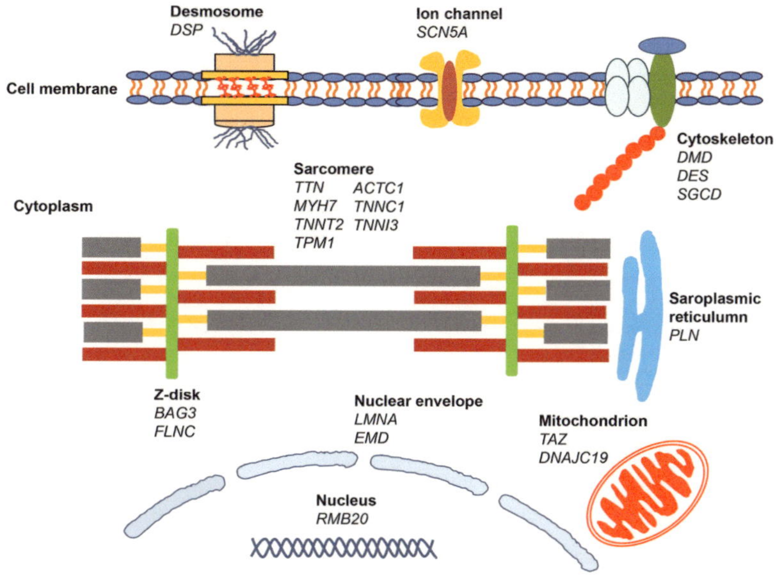

Figure 1.
Subcellular localization of the protein encoded by dilated cardiomyopathy disease genes. The graphic shows schematic representations and approximate intracellular localization of the encoded proteins by genes strongly implicated in dilated cardiomyopathy disease.

Gene	Protein	Function	Frequency and overlapping phenotype	Inheritance pattern
Sarcomere				
ACTC1	Alpha cardiac actin	Structural component of thin filament	<1% of DCM; HCM, LVNC	Autosomal dominant
MYH7	Beta-myosin heavy chain	Cardiac muscle contraction	5% of DCM; HCM, ACM, LVNV	Autosomal dominant
TNNC1	Cardiac troponin C	Cardiac muscle contraction	<1% of DCM; HCM, LVNC	Autosomal dominant
TNNI3	Cardiac troponin I	Cardiac muscle contraction	<1% of DCM; HCM	Autosomal recessive
TNNT2	Cardiac troponin T	Cardiac muscle contraction	3% of DCM; HCM, ACM, LVNC	Autosomal dominant
TPM1	Tropomyosin alpha-1 chain	Cardiac muscle contraction	1–2% of DCM; HCM, LVNC	Autosomal dominant
TTN	Titin	Sarcomere scaffold	15–25% of DCM; HCM	Autosomal dominant
Cytoskeleton				
DES	Desmin	Contractile force transduction	<1% of DCM; Desminopathies	Autosomal dominant
DMD	Dystrophin	Contractile force transduction	<1% of DCM; Duchenne/Becker muscular dystrophy	X-linked
SGCD	δ-sarcoglycan	Structural component of dystrophin-glycoprotein complex	<1% of DCM; HCM, LGMD2E	Autosomal recessive
Nuclear envelope				
EMD	Emerin	Nuclear membrane anchorage	<1% of DCM; EMDM	X-linked

Gene	Protein	Function	Frequency and overlapping phenotype	Inheritance pattern
LMNA	Lamin A/C	Nuclear envelope structure	6% of DCM; EMDM, LGMD1B	Autosomal dominant
Nucleus				
RBM20	RNA-binding protein 20	Regulator of cardiac gene splicing	2% of DCM	Autosomal dominant
Ion channel				
SCN5A	Sodium voltage-gated channel alpha subunit 5	Sodium channel protein	2–3% of DCM; LQTs Brugada syndrome	Autosomal dominant
Z-disk				
BAG3	BCL2-associated athanogene 3	Co-chaperone, inhibition of apoptosis	3% of DCM; Myofibrillar myopathy	Autosomal dominant
FLNC	Flamin-C	Actin filament crosslinking	<1% of DCM; HCM, RCM	Autosomal dominant
Desomosome				
DSP	Desmoplakin	Structural component of desomosome, cell–cell mechanotransmission	2% of DCM; ACM	Autosomal recessive
Mitochondrion				
DNAJC19	DnaJ heat shock protein family homolog, C19	Protein transporter	<1% of DCM; 3-Methylglutaconic aciduria, type V	Autosomal recessive
TAZ	Tafazzin	Phospholipid transacylase	<1% of DCM; HCM, Barth syndrome	X-linked
Sarcoplasmic reticulum				
PLN	Cardiac phospholamba	Regulator of calcium pump	<1% of DCM; HCM, ACM	Autosomal dominant

ACM, Arrhythmogenic cardiomyopathy; DCM, dilated cardiomyopathy; EDMD, Emery–Dreifuss muscular dystrophy; LVNC, left ventricular noncompaction; HCM, hypertrophic cardiomyopathy; LGMD, limb-girdle muscular dystrophy; LQTs, long QT syndrome; RCM, restrictive cardiomyopathy.

Table 1.
Genes linked to dilated cardiomyopathy with strong evidence.

Gene	Variant type	Clinical phenotype	Molecular pathophysiology	Genotype-based therapy	Reference
DMD	Nonsense Deletion	DCM, DMD, Becker muscular dystrophy, premature death	Absence of functional dystrophin protein, replacement of muscle by fibrotic and adipose tissue, contraction weakness	1) Exon skipping; 2) Mini dystrophin gene replacement; 3) CRISPRA/Cas9 genome editing; 4) Stop codon readthrough	[60–62, 67, 71–73, 80]
LMNA	Nonsense Deletion	DCM with high penetrance, high risk of arrhythmia, early lethality	Lamins A and C proteins haploinsufficiency, nuclear malformations, biomechanical defects, activation of p38 kinase pathway	1) Preventive therapy, lower the threshold for cardiac defibrillator implantation; 2) p38 inhibition; 3) Trans-splicing; 4) Stop codon readthrough	[29, 30, 58, 75, 79]

Gene	Variant type	Clinical phenotype	Molecular pathophysiology	Genotype-based therapy	Reference
TTN	Truncating	DCM, HCM, ventricular arrhythmias	Titin protein haploinsufficiency, sarcomere insufficiency, metabolic and energetic adaption, increased sensitivity to mechanical stress	Exon-skipping	[82]
PLN	Missense Deletion	Ventricular dilation, contractile dysfunction and ventricular arrhythmias, heart failure by middle age	Abnormal PLN protein subcellular localization, calcium handling defects, electrical instability	TALEN genome editing	[22, 84]
SGCD	Deletion	DCM, HCM	δ-sarcoglycan protein deficiency, sarcolomma instability, increased myocyte apoptosis, reduced expression of miRNA-669a	1) Gene replacement; 2) microRNA overexpression	[83, 88, 89]

Table 2.
Examples of gene-targeted therapeutic strategies.

2. Genetic causes of familial DCM

Extensive studies on genetic basis of DCM underscored profound heterogeneous nature of DCM disease. DCM variants mutate genes encoding a broad spectrum of proteins with distinct functions and intracellular localization have been identified (**Figure 1** and **Table 1**). For example, mutations in genes encoding sarcomere protein involving in mechanosensing and force transmission, encoding nuclear envelope proteins required for the protection of biochemical forces, encoding desmosomal proteins required for maintaining the structural integrity of desomosome, encoding ion channels and molecules involving in calcium handling, encoding chaperone proteins, transcription factors and RNA-binding proteins have all been identified to cause DCM. Specific variants in these genes may alter various signaling pathways and cellular structures in cardiomyocyte that can disrupt the mechanism of cardiac muscle contraction and function, leading to common phenotypes of DCM.

2.1 Sarcomere genes

Sarcomere is the basic contractile unit mainly composed of thin and thick filaments. Mutations in sarcomere genes are one of the most important causes of DCM, which have been identified in about one third of DCM [19–21]. In addition to cause DCM, mutations in sarcomere genes often lead to overlapping phenotypes of hypertrophic cardiomyopathy (HCM), another major genetic type of cardiomyopathy characterized by ventricular wall thickness and diastolic dysfunction. Genes with definitive evidence, supported by studies from multiple centers/groups, with both clinical linkage data and confirmative data from animal models, include *ACTC1, MYH7, TNNT2, TNNC1, TRM1,TTN*. Among which, *TTN, MYH7* and *TTNT2* are most commonly implicated in DCM, accounting for about 25%, 5% and 3% of familial DCM, respectively.

TTN gene encodes the titin, the largest known protein in human, consisting of 364 exons and about 35,000 amino acids that spans about a half of the sarcomere. It has long been recognized as a sarcomere scaffolding protein that serves as a blue print for sarcomerogenesis and myofibrillar assembly. In addition, titin also serves as a molecular spring that provides passive tension to regulate sarcomere contraction. With the advent of next-generation sequencing, human genetic analysis had revealed that *TTN*-truncating variants (*TTNtvs*) represent the most prevalent gene mutations in DCM patients, accounting for up to 25% of familial DCM cases [19]. Notebly, *TTNtvs* are also found in about 1% of general population [22, 23]. While not all of these healthy individuals with the *TTNtvs* are expected to develop DCM, they showed significantly increased left ventricular volumes and mild reduction of contractility [23]. Initially, it was hypothesized that *TTNtvs* caused DCM through a dominant negative mechanism [24]. This hypothesis is compromised by that truncated titin peptides were not detected from DCM hearts that harbored *TTNtvs*. Instead, there is evidence to support that premature truncations in the *TTN* transcripts trigger nonsense-mediated decay in rat models with *TTNtvs* [23]. Together with recently cumulative data derived from studies in human induced pluripotent stem cell-derived cardiomyocytes (iPSC-CMs) and human cardiac tissues, the hypothesis of haploinsufficiency mechanisms is now more widely recognized [25].

MYH7 encodes the beta isoform of myosin heavy chain (MHC-β) that is predominantly expressed in the heart. MHC-β is a major component of the thick filament responsible for hydrolyzing ATP to produce force for cardiac muscle contraction. The Arg403Gln missense mutation of *MYH7* was first identified to cause HCM back to 1990 [12]. Since then, many *MYH7* variants were identified to associate with both HCM and DCM, accounting for approximately 40% of HCM and 5% of DCM cases, respectively. The definitive mechanisms underlying how *MYH7* mutations cause different types of cardiomyopathies remain to be elusive. Clinically, HCM is often characterized by hypercontractility. In contrast, DCM is characterized by hypocontractility. Mutations in myosin head domain consume more energy, leading to hypercontractility. One observation is that the *MYH7* variants associated with HCM are located more in the region encoding the myosin head domain, while *MYH7* mutations causal to DCM appear to disperse across the entire gene. The Arg403Gln variant causal to HCM, for example, increased energy usage due to impaired catalytic cycle of ATP hydrolysis, resulting in increased contractility [26]. In contrast, mutations associated with DCM showed an increased tension cost, with more energy consumption, have reduced force-generating capacity, thus causes a hypocontractility, leading to DCM [27, 28]. For example, the ASN1918LYS variant, causal to DCM, is located to the coiled-coil rod region, which is hypothesized to impair the incorporation of myosin into the myofilaments.

TNNT2 encodes the cardiac muscle isoform of troponin T (cTnT). cTnT is one of the major tropomyosin-binding subunits of troponin on the thin filament that regulates cardiac muscle contraction. *TNNT2* variants are thought to account for approximately 5% of HCM, up to 3% of DCM, and a small fraction of arrhythmogenic cardiomyopathy (ACM). Many mutations in *TNNT2* causing DCM are located in both the middle and C-terminal regions of cTnT. These mutations mostly impair the cTnT's interaction with the thin filament regulatory system, myofilament calcium sensitivity, and/or the myosin ATPase activity, thus cause DCM.

TPM1 encodes the alpha tropomyosin chain protein that belongs to the tropomyosin family of highly conserved thin filament proteins. In association with the troponin complex, tropomyosin mostly participates in the calcium regulation of cardiac muscle contraction and interaction of actin and myosin. Mutations in *TPM1* cause both HCM and DCM phenotypes [29, 30], accounting for about 5% of HCM and 1% of DCM cases, respectively. Functional characterization of *TPM1* mutations associated with both cardiomyopathies has led to a better understanding of the primary effects and consequence triggered by mutations in the long-range communication of the thin filament and specific phenotypes [31].

2.2 Nucleus and nuclear envelope genes

Mutations in gene encoding nucleus or nuclear envelope localized proteins that definitively link to DCM such as *LMNA, EMD* and *RBM20* were reported. *LMNA* is the second most common gene implicated in DCM, and *LMNA* variants account for about 6–10% of genetic DCM [32, 33]. *LMNA* encodes the nuclear envelope localized lamins A and C resulted from differential splicing at the 3′ end. Both lamins A and C are intermediate filament structural proteins, playing major roles in supporting cells with stability and strength. *LMNA* mutations linked to DCM can be both missense and frameshift across the coding region. Both dominant negative and haploinsufficiency mechanisms were proposed for *LMNA* mutations caused DCM. Beyond their roles as structural proteins, both lamins A and C involve in many different cellular process including regulation of gene expression, mechanosensing and nuclear to cytoplasmic transport. Functional study in animal models revealed that ERK1/2, JNK and p38 kinase pathways were drastically activated in *LMNA*-associated DCM. By targeting to the p38 kinase pathway through using a specific p38 kinase inhibitor ARRY-371797, Muchir and colleagues showed that LV dilation and deterioration of EF were effectively blocked, and *LMNA*-related severe biomechanical defects were significantly rescued in neonatal rat ventricular myocytes [34, 35]. Based on their encouraging and other related data, a clinical trial to study the protective effect of ARRY-371797 on patients with symptomatic DCM due to *LMNA* gene mutations was initiated (NCT03439514). This represents one of the first clinical trials involving genotype-specific therapy particularly for DCM.

The RNA binding motif protein 20 (*RBM20)* gene encodes a nucleus localized RNA-binding protein. RBM20 protein mostly functions as a regulator of post-transcriptional splicing of a subset of genes involved in cardiomyopathy, ion-homeostasis, and sarcomere biology [36]. *RBM20* is predominantly expressed in skeletal and cardiac muscles. Loss of function mutations in the *RBM20* were firstly linked to familial DCM and account for 2–5% of DCM cases [37, 38]. Of the many targets regulated by *RBM20*, aberrant splicing of *TTN* is believed to be the main determinant of *RBM20* mutations caused DCM. Calcium/calmodulin-dependent kinase II delta (*CAMK2D*) is another pivotal cardiac gene transcriptionally regulated by *RBM20*. A recent study showed that *RBM20* mutations carriers also had increased risk of malignant ventricular arrhythmias and sudden cardiac death (SCD), likely resultant from disturbed Ca^{2+} handling and arrhythmic Ca^{2+} cycling [39].

2.3 Cytoskeletal protein coding genes

Other genes such as *DES, DMD* and *FLNC* that encode components of cytoskeleton localized proteins are also identified to link to DCM pathogenesis. Pathogenic mutations in these genes causing DCM often accompany with additional phenotypes, most notably skeletal myopathy. *DES* encodes desmin, a muscle-specific component of the intermediate filament presented at the Z-disk and intercalated discs that integrates sarcolemma, Z-disk and nuclear membrane to maintain the structural and functional integrity of sarcomeric contractile apparatus [40].

Mutations in *DES* have been associated with a spectrum of cardiomyopathies, mostly notably DCM, in about 1–2% of cases [41]. Overlapping phenotypes of *DES* mutations including arrhythmia, cardiac conduction diseases, and skeletal myopathy and smooth muscle defects are frequently observed.

Mutations in the gene encoding dystrophin (*DMD*) cause severe muscle weakness and DCM in Duchenne muscular dystrophy (DMD). Because the *DMD* gene is located in the short arm of X chromosome, pathogenic mutations causing DMD mostly affect boys. The frequency of *DMD* caused muscular dystrophy and DCM is rare, with an estimated incidence 1 in 3500 male births worldwide [42]. Dystrophin protein is a key component of dystrophin-glycoprotein complex and plays a critical role in maintaining the structural integrity of sarcolemma during repeated cycles of muscle contraction and relaxation [43]. Mutations in *DMD* result in loss of the dystrophin protein expression that causes primary muscular dystrophy in males presenting with progressive muscle wasting at early childhood. Subsequently, cardiac dysfunction is involved and more than 90% of affected individuals manifest DCM and patient often died of cardiac and respiratory muscle failure [44].

2.4 Z-disk gene

The Z-disk is an anchoring plane for the actin (thin) filaments to attach and stabilize in the sarcomere. Mutations in many Z-disk-associated proteins coding genes result in cardiac disorders. *BAG3* encodes a highly conserved, Z-disk localized co-chaperone protein that is predominantly expressed in heart and skeletal muscle. BAG3 binds to the ATPase domain of the heat shock protein (Hsp) 70 and exerts multiple functions in regulating apoptosis, preserving the integrity of sarcomere, mediating unfolded protein response and autophagy. *BAG3* variants linked to DCM were firstly reported by two independent genome-wide association studies (GWASs). Later on, *BAG3* mutations were identified in 2–7% of DCM cases [45–47]. Genotype–phenotype correlation study revealed that DCM attributed by *BAG3* mutations is characterized by high penetrance in carriers more than 40 years of age. Patients with *BAG3* mutations are at a higher risk of developing a more severe and progressive heart failure compared with patients without *BAG3* mutations [46]. The level of BAG3 protein was reduced by about a half in both animal models of heart failure and DCM patients as well. Based on the evidence that truncation or deletion mutations in *BAG3* are associated with BAG3 haploinsufficiency which co-segregates with affected DCM family members, it was proposed that the decreased levels of BAG3 protein is the cause of DCM. BAG3 is also an independent heart failure risk factors associated with subclinical LV dysfunction. Thus, cumulative data support that *BAG3* as a bona-fide disease susceptibility gene for DCM [48].

2.5 Ion channel gene

Mutations in the ion channel coding gene *SCN5A* are identified to cause DCM with strong supporting evidence. *SCN5A* encodes the sodium channel Nav1.5 that is mainly expressed in the cardiac muscle [49]. Mutations in *SCN5A* are associated primarily with conduction disorder, arrhythmia and DCM. Incidence of pathogenic *SCN5A* variants is estimated to be 2–4% in all DCM cases [50]. Missense mutations such as R222Q variant located in a voltage-sensing domain exert activating effects on sodium channel function and were thought to cause DCM. While guideline-based heart failure therapies have moderate effect, drugs that have sodium channel-blocking properties such as amiodarone or flecainide could substantially reduce DCM phenotype in patients with R222Q carriers [51]. Moreover, a recent report showed that quinidine treatment of a DCM patient with R222Q mutation achieved a rapid and significant reduction of ventricular tachyarrhythmia and an improvement in the myocardial function [52]. These interesting genotype–phenotype association studies thus provide another successful example of elucidation of the genetic basis of familial DCM which can lead to effective genotype-tailored therapeutic strategy.

2.6 Other DCM genes

PLN encodes phosphlamban, a transmembrane protein localized to the sarcoplasmic reticulum. Mutations in *PLN* cause variable DCM phenotype, with underlying mechanisms proposed through inhibiting the sarcoplasmic reticulum Ca2 + -ATPase (SERCA2a) [53]. While founder mutation R14del mutation in *PLN* is associated with severe phenotype with high risk for lethal ventricular arrhythmias and end-stage heart failure in the European [54], a milder phenotype had been reported from others [55], suggesting that genetic background might have a big impact on modifying the disease progression associated with *PLN* mutations caused DCM.

Mutations in genes other encoding the sarcoglycans (α, β, γ, δ) were also identified to cause DCM. The sarcoglycans are transmembrane proteins mainly expressed in heart and skeletal muscle that interact with dystrophin. α-, β-, γ-, and δ-sarcoglycans form the sarcoglycan complex that is key components of the dystrophin-associated glycoprotein complex, conferring structural integrity and stability to the sarcolemma through connecting the muscle fiber cytoskeleton to the extracellular matrix, and protecting muscle fibers from mechanical stress during muscle contraction. Mutations in sarcoglycans coding genes cause primary limb-girdle muscular dystrophy presented with early onset muscle weakness and associate with significant DCM [56]. Notably, mutations in the δ- sarcoglycan coding gene lead to DCM without involvement of obvious muscular dystrophy phenotypes [57].

Mutations in nuclear encoded mitochondrial genes such as *TAZ* and *DNAJC19* were also identified to cause DCM. *TAZ* encodes a mitochondrial localized Tafazzin protein that is predominantly expressed in cardiac and skeletal muscle. Tafazzin functions as a phospholipid transacylase that catalyzes the remodeling of cardiolipin that is required for oxidative phosphorylation. Mutations in the TAZ gene cause X-linked Barth syndrome and DCM, leading to premature death [58]. Mechanistically, mutations in *TAZ* result in Taffazin deficiency and cause mitochondrial dysfunction and impaired mitophagy and increased oxidative stress, leading to DCM [59].

3. Genetic testing

The advent of next-generation sequencing enables cost-effective genetic testing in familial DCM which can define the precise genetic cause of disease. Genetic testing can also help optimize risk stratification and assess prognostics of patients and their relatives. With the identification of a pathogenic mutation and early diagnostic certainty, clinical management of affect individuals could be tailored and patients' survival can be improved. One best example is related to clinical practice of early intervention of DCM patients with *LMNA* mutations. *LMNA*-related DCM usually accompanied by significant conduction system disease, atrial fibrillation, ventricular tachycardia, and sudden cardiac death (SCD). Thus, *LMNA* mutations are often associated with a higher disease penetrance and more severe morbidity and high mortality [60]. Studies in several different cohorts of DCM patients with *LMNA* mutations identified non-missense mutations, LVEF<45% and higher

AV blocker as significant risk factors for disease malignancy [61, 62]. Because of this well-determined genotype–phenotype knowledge, an actionable prognostic genotype–phenotype association, implementation of a lower threshold and earlier implantable cardioverter defibrillator (ICD) therapy than current guidelines recommend in patients with LMNA mutations, was demonstrated to significantly improve patient outcome and survival [63].

Based on the Genetic Testing Registry (https://www.ncbi.nlm.nih.gov/gtr/), there are from 40 to 80 genes included in the testing panels for most commercially available genetic testing for DCM. In familial DCM, the yield of genetic testing, resulting in identification of pathogenic mutations, can thus far reach up to 40%, in a comparable level to that of other inherited cardiac disorders such as HCM and long QT syndrome. The sensitivity of genetic testing is compromised partially due to that not all genes implicated in DCM are included in the gene panels for testing. This is especially the case for those identified from sporadic DCM cases or single family. Furthermore, limited by human genetics approaches that heavily rely on pedigree availability and candidate gene approaches, variants for more than half of familial DCM cases have not been identified yet. As technique advances in genetics of cardiomyopathy, identification of the remaining genetic causes in inherited DCM cases and elucidation of the underlying pathogenic mechanisms leading to the phenotype are evolving rapidly. Targeted gene panels for genetic testing are increasing in an unprecedented scale. With further characterization and functional validation, the ever expanding gene panels of genetic testing promise to increase the rate of positive identification and provide individuals and families with a more comprehensive and conclusive genetic testing.

4. Genotype-targeted therapies

By directly targeting at specific pathogenic mutations causing DCM, genotype-targeted genetic approaches have emerged as promising strategies for effective and individualized therapies to ameliorate disease phenotypes. To carry out genotype-based therapy, many customized genetic strategies were explored. For examples: for loss-of-function mutations that cause reduced or insufficient protein levels, the straightforward gene replacement strategy can be employed. In this scenario, full-length or partial functional cDNA for corresponding mutated gene can be transferred to cardiac tissue to supplement the reduced gene dosage using appropriate gene delivery approach. For mutations that cause dominant-negative effects on a particular gene, exon-skipping or trans-splicing approaches can be considered to remove or modify the mutant transcripts. For pathogenic mutations that cause other protein dysfunction, the highly efficient CRISPRA/Cas9 (Clustered regularly interspaced short palindromic repeats/CRISPR-associated endonuclease) system can be explored to directly correct the mutant variants. In addition, other genotype-based therapeutic strategies such as manipulation of the downstream pathways evoked by specific DCM mutations were also explored. Below, we summarize several examples of gene-targeted therapeutic strategies that produced encouraging results in the treatment of DCM (**Table 2**), which hold the opportunities to ultimately improve patient outcome in the future.

4.1 Dystrophin mutations-targeted gene therapies

Mutations in the dystrophin (*DMD*) gene cause muscular dystrophy patients and X-linked familial DCM in early childhood and patients often die of cardiac and respiratory failure [44]. Currently, there are no effective cures for DMD yet and management of DMD mostly focuses on preserving the limited muscle strength and ameliorating disease symptoms [64]. Mechanistically, dystrophin protein deficiency due to *DMD* gene mutations is the primary cause of DMD and subsequent DCM and heart failure. And the disease severity is mostly correlated with the dystrophin protein level. Thus, a plausible treatment strategy would be to restore the expression level of dystrophin protein [44]. To cure this devastating disease, dystrophin gene-targeted therapeutic strategies such as gene replacement, exon skipping and CRISPRA/Cas9 genome editing techniques are mostly employed, which have shown encouraging results in restoration of dystrophin protein expression and recovery of dystrophin protein function in both animal models and clinical trials.

Gene replacement strategy involves delivering a functioning gene to replace or supplement the mutant gene to the target organ and cells to ease the disease phenotype caused by genetic mutation. This approach often utilizes the adeno-associated virus (AAV) as a vector to mediate gene transfection into the skeletal and cardiac muscle cells. However, as the dystrophin gene has 79 exons and its transcript is about 14 Kb, its size is too large to fit in currently available gene construction vector for gene transfection. Alternatively, a mini- or micro- dystrophin gene coding for a functionally similar to dystrophin but smaller in size was thus used. The authors Wang and colleagues firstly defined the minimal functional region of the dystrophin protein, later referred as mini-dystrophin. The authors then packed this min-dystrophin gene into an AAV vector to mediate muscle transfection and demonstrated the effectiveness of gene delivery and restoration of dystrophin gene function [65]. After this study, several other independent groups latter confirmed the effectiveness of a shortened albeit functional dystrophin gene replacement strategy mediated by the AAV gene delivery system in preservation of cardiac and skeletal muscle function and extending the lifespan in the dystrophic mice [66, 67]. Notably, further studies in animal models of muscular dystrophy and human patients detected certain immunologic responses to the shortened dystrophin peptide, which need to be carefully considered in future clinical application [68–70].

Exon skipping is an RNA-based splice-switching approach that causes cells to "skip" the exon containing the pathogenic variant, resultant in-frame transcripts that produce a shorter peptide, albeit still at least partially functional protein to ameliorate disease phenotypes. This approach was initially developed to mask the pathogenic mutations containing exon 51 using an antisense oligonucleotide (AON), resulting in genetic correction of the open reading frame of the *DMD* gene and partial restoration of dystrophin protein expression and improvement of muscle pathology and function [71–73]. These encouraging studies lead to at least two ongoing clinical trials to evaluate the efficacy and safety of this exon skipping approach targeting to the pathogenic exon 51 or 53 (NCT02255552, NCT02310906).

With the revolutionary development of the CRISPRA/Cas9 genome editing technologies that enable precise and efficient genetic modifications from single-nucleotide alternation, insertion of gene of interest to deletion of chromosomal regions, numerous studies have demonstrated the feasibility and high efficiency of this technique in restoration dystrophin expression and function in skeletal and cardiac muscle, both in vitro and in vivo [74, 75]. For example, a recent study carried out by El Refaey and colleagues packaged SaCas9 (Cas9 from *Staphylococcus aureus*)/gRNA constructs into an AAV serotype rh74 and delivered it to the mdx/$Utr^{+/-}$ dystrophic mice through a retro-orbital approach [76]. The authors showed this CRIPRA-mediated genome editing strategy could efficiently excise the mutant exon 23 of dystrophin in the mice model, resulting in the restoration of the dystrophin protein expression and cardiac myofiber architecture, and significantly improved the cardiac contractility in vivo. A follow up study using this AAV-mediated CRISPR genome editing approach found that restored dystrophin expression and improved cardiac function were consistently detected at up to 19 months [77]. Similarly, Hakim and colleagues modified the dose of AAV.SaCas9 and AAV-9.gRNA vector that directs Cas9 to introns of 22 and 23 and performed the AAV-9 CRISPRA gene therapy in the mdx mice that carry a nonsense mutation in exon 23 of the dystrophin gene [78, 79]. The authors found significantly increased dystrophin restoration and reduced fibrosis in both skeletal and cardiac muscle and improved muscle function and cardiac hemodynamics at up to 18 months.

4.2 *LMNA* mutations-tailored therapeutic strategy

A genetic approach referred as trans-splicing approach was initially carried out to correct *LMNA* mutations in the *Lmna* DelK32 knock-in mouse harboring a *LMNA*-related congenital muscular dystrophy mutation in the exon 1 [80, 81]. The *Lmna* DelK32/DelK32 mice exhibited severe muscular and cardiac defects and early premature death. The trans-splicing approach allows converting the targeted endogenous mutated pre-mRNA to a therapeutic pre–trans-spliced molecule containing the wildtype coding sequence, resulting in a processed mRNA transcript devoid of the exon harboring the pathogenic variant [82, 83]. To perform the trans-splicing rescue in the *Lmna* DelK32 knock-in mouse model, 5'-RNA pre-trans-splicing molecules containing the first five exons of *Lmna* and targeting intron 5 of *Lmna* pre-mRNA were firstly developed. After confirmed the induced trans-splicing events on endogenous *Lmna* mRNA in vitro, AAV mediated delivery system was then evaluated in vivo in the newborn mice. Similarly, trans-splicing events were successfully detected in both skeletal and heart muscle of mice up to 50 days after AAV delivery. However, the tans-splicing occurring efficiency needs to be further improved to exert significant rescue effects on cardiac function and premature death.

To target at the *LMNA* pathogenic variants resulting in deficiency of the protein level, another strategy referred as stop codon readthrough was explored through inactivating the molecules participating in nonsense-mediated decay at the RNA level [84]. This approach applies to the scenario when pathogenic variants result in frameshifts and premature stops, subsequently leading to protein deficiency because of increased nonsense-mediated decay of mutant RNAs. PTC124, also known as ataluren, is a chemical compound that can selectively induce ribosomal readthrough of premature but not normal termination codons [85]. PTC124 was tested in iPSC-CMs derived from patients carrying different nonsense and frameshift mutations in the *LMNA* gene [85]. In one of the three frameshift mutants tested, administration of PTC124 significantly increased the translation of full-length LMNA protein and partially restored the protein function, as shown by reduced cardiomyocyte apoptosis and improved excitation-contraction coupling [84].

4.3 *TTN* truncating variants-targeted gene therapy

While the pathogenicity of *TTN* missense mutations to DCM remains largely undetermined, *TTN* truncating variants (*TTNtvs*) are the most common cause to DCM. To date, experimental evidence generated largely from rodent animal models, human induced pluripotent stem cell-derived cardiomyocyte, and patient tissues mostly support the mechanism of titin protein haploinsufficiency. Correction of the titin protein deficiency by using traditional viral-mediated gene replacement strategy to increase the expression of titin protein, just as that has been successfully employed to restore the dystrophin deficiency, however, is challenging. Because the *TTN* gene spans 294 Kb of genomic region and its spliced transcript is more than 100 Kb, a size that is way bigger than any currently available cargo capacity for AAV mediated gene transfection. Alternatively, exon skipping, a genetic approach that had been initially employed to treat the DMD, through using an AON to mask the pathogenic mutations containing exon 51 or 53 and restoration of DMD phenotype [72], as aforementioned, was explored to treat *TTNtvs* related DCM. Notably, this strategy had been also successfully utilized for treating Mybpc3 mutations caused HCM in a knock-in mouse model [86].

To employ exon skipping strategy for treating *TTNtvs* caused DCM, Gramlich and colleagues targeted to the Ser14450fsX4 variant located in the exon 326 identified in a DCM patient that caused autosomal-dominant truncating frameshift mutation [87]. They used an AON-mediated exon skipping approach to remove the exon 326 in both patient cardiomyocytes in vitro and mouse heart in vivo. In vitro, skipping of the exon 326 containing the Ser14450fsX4 pathogenic variant restored the impaired myofibril assembly and stabilized its structural integrity and normalized expression of sarcomeric protein in the patient-specific cardiomyocytes derived from induced pluripotent stem cells (iPSC-CMs) model. Furthermore, in the corresponding Ttn knock-in mice model, skipping of the exon 326 significantly improved sarcomere formation and contractile function and prevented subsequent development of DCM phenotype. These results provide strong evidence to support that the RNA-based exon skipping strategy could be a potential treatment option for DCM caused by gene variants that are otherwise technically difficult to be delivered due to size limitation for gene replacement therapy.

4.4 Genotype-targeted therapies for other DCM genes

Mutations in the δ- sarcoglycan coding gene (*SGCD*) can lead to DCM without obvious involvement of skeletal muscle disorders [57]. The gene replacement strategy was firstly applied in the treatment of DCM caused by a deletion mutation in the *Sgcd* gene that disrupted the dystrophin-associated glycoprotein complex in a hamster model [88]. The authors Kawada and colleague constructed a recombinant AAV vector containing the full-length cDNA of *Sgcd* gene driven under the cardiac specific expression promoter of CMV and intramurally injected it to the *Sgcd* mutation induced DCM model in the hamster. *They detected* robust expression of the *Sgcd* gene and other types of sarcoglycans as well in the transfected myocardium. The restored expression of *Sgcd* and other sarcoglycans normalized the diameter of transduced cardiomyocytes, improved the contractile function and ultimately prolonged the life span of the animals harboring the *Sgcd* gene mutation. This study provides one of the earliest evidence to employ gene replacement strategy to treat DCM caused by a specific gene mutation with efficient and sustained transfection capability.

An earlier version of genome editing technique referred as transcription activator-affected nuclease (TALEN) was explored to directly correct the *PLN* R14del mutation that is associated with high risk for malignant ventricular arrhythmias and end-stage heart failure in DCM patient carriers [89]. The authors Karakikes and colleague firstly derived iPSC-CMs from a DCM patient harboring the *PLN* R14del mutation, followed by detailed phenotypic characterization of this iPSC-CMs model. Next, the authors made the effort to correct the *PLN* R14del mutation in the iPSC-CMs model using TALEN gene editing strategy. This approach successfully corrected the R14del mutation and attenuated the R14del-associated disease phenotypes in the iPSC-CMs model. Furthermore, the authors engineered an AAV6 vector that enabled knock-down the endogenous *PLN*, while simultaneously overexpress a codon-optimized *PLN*, to effectively reverse the disease phenotype in the iPSC-CMs model as well. Thus, this study provides another successful example to using genome editing approach to directly target at the pathogenic mutations associated with DCM to achieve therapeutic benefit. Notably, while it provides evidence to support the effectiveness of genome editing technique to correct pathogenic variants causing DCM in vitro, germline correction of embryos harboring DCM variants had not been reported yet.

5. Conclusions

The ultimate goal of elucidating genetic basis for DCM is for early disease diagnosis, early disease intervention and treatment. To date, pathogenic mutations in more than 50 genes are associated with DCM. However, these mutations can only explain about 40–50% of familial DCM cases, and the genetic architecture of DCM still remains incompletely understood. Future research directions rely on technique advances for identification of the remaining up to 60% of genetic causes in familial DCM cases. After identifying the genetic causes, functional characterization and validation studies are needed to confirm the pathogenic variants. Extensive studies on delineation of genotype–phenotype relationships are necessary to address currently unmet issues for translational research. Further dissecting genetic pathways linked to DCM and elucidating the pathogenic mechanisms leading to the phenotype can provide valuable insights into the understanding of disease pathophysiology, laying solid foundation for future development of groundbreaking therapeutics.

Gene-based therapies, such as gene replacement, exon skipping and recent evolutionarily developed CRISPRA/Cas9 based genome-editing techniques that directly target at the underlying genetic mutations responsible for the DCM disease progression, have led to several clinical trials which have produced promising results. Thus, the last decade has witnessed encouraging advances in the development of genotype-targeted, personalized therapies. While the progress is promising, several technical issues need to be thoroughly assessed before implementation in clinical practice. For example, current gene delivery system mostly adapt the AAV system because of its many advantages such as long term transgene expression and choice of appropriate serotype for heart enriched expression. One primary limitation for this system, however, is that there exists certain level of anti-AAV antibodies in general human population causing the immunogenicity issue which can potentially lead to development of myocarditis [70, 90–92]. While the efficiency for exogenous delivery of preprocessed RNAs or oligonucleotides for trans-splicing or exon skipping needs to be further improved, a major concern of off-target issue needs to be seriously addressed for the highly efficient AAV9 mediated CRISPR/Cas9 genome editing system. Novel approaches are desirable to comprehensively evaluate any potential off-target mutagenesis in the heart and other tissues for future clinical application.

Conflict of interest

The authors declare no conflict of interest.

Author details

Jing Zhong[1†], Li-Ping Li[1†], Jian-Feng Zhou[2,3] and Yong-He Ding[4*]

1 School of Basic Medicine, The Biomedical Sciences Institute of Qingdao University, Qingdao University, Qingdao, China

2 Key Laboratory of Marine Drugs (Ocean University of China), Chinese Ministry of Education, School of Medicine and Pharmacy, Ocean University of China, Qingdao, China

3 Laboratory for Marine Drugs and Bioproducts, Pilot National Laboratory for Marine Science and Technology (Qingdao), Qingdao, China

4 The Affiliated Hospital of Qingdao University, The Biomedical Sciences Institute of Qingdao University, Qingdao University, Qingdao, China

*Address all correspondence to: dingyonghe@qdu.edu.cn

† Equal contribution.

References

[1] Rosenbaum AN, Agre KE, Pereira NL. Genetics of dilated cardiomyopathy: practical implications for heart failure management. Nat Rev Cardiol. 2020;17(5):286-97. Epub 2019/10/13. doi: 10.1038/s41569-019-0284-0.

[2] Maron BJ, Towbin JA, Thiene G, Antzelevitch C, Corrado D, Arnett D, et al. Contemporary definitions and classification of the cardiomyopathies: an American Heart Association Scientific Statement from the Council on Clinical Cardiology, Heart Failure and Transplantation Committee; Quality of Care and Outcomes Research and Functional Genomics and Translational Biology Interdisciplinary Working Groups; and Council on Epidemiology and Prevention. Circulation. 2006;113(14):1807-16. doi: 10.1161/CIRCULATIONAHA.106.174287.

[3] Redfield MM, Jacobsen SJ, Burnett JC, Jr., Mahoney DW, Bailey KR, Rodeheffer RJ. Burden of systolic and diastolic ventricular dysfunction in the community: appreciating the scope of the heart failure epidemic. JAMA. 2003;289(2):194-202. doi: 10.1001/jama.289.2.194.

[4] McKenna WJ, Maron BJ, Thiene G. Classification, Epidemiology, and Global Burden of Cardiomyopathies. Circ Res. 2017;121(7):722-30. Epub 2017/09/16. doi: 10.1161/CIRCRESAHA.117.309711.

[5] Perez-Serra A, Toro R, Sarquella-Brugada G, de Gonzalo-Calvo D, Cesar S, Carro E, et al. Genetic basis of dilated cardiomyopathy. Int J Cardiol. 2016;224:461-72. Epub 2016/10/25. doi: 10.1016/j.ijcard.2016.09.068.

[6] Hershberger RE, Hedges DJ, Morales A. Dilated cardiomyopathy: the complexity of a diverse genetic architecture. Nat Rev Cardiol. 2013;10(9):531-47. doi: 10.1038/nrcardio.2013.105.

[7] Sweet M, Taylor MR, Mestroni L. Diagnosis, prevalence, and screening of familial dilated cardiomyopathy. Expert Opin Orphan Drugs. 2015;3(8):869-76. doi: 10.1517/21678707.2015.1057498.

[8] Weintraub RG, Semsarian C, Macdonald P. Dilated cardiomyopathy. Lancet. 2017;390(10092):400-14. doi: 10.1016/S0140-6736(16)31713-5.

[9] Mestroni L, Maisch B, McKenna WJ, Schwartz K, Charron P, Rocco C, et al. Guidelines for the study of familial dilated cardiomyopathies. Collaborative Research Group of the European Human and Capital Mobility Project on Familial Dilated Cardiomyopathy. Eur Heart J. 1999;20(2):93-102. Epub 1999/04/01. doi: 10.1053/euhj.1998.1145.

[10] Pinto YM, Elliott PM, Arbustini E, Adler Y, Anastasakis A, Bohm M, et al. Proposal for a revised definition of dilated cardiomyopathy, hypokinetic non-dilated cardiomyopathy, and its implications for clinical practice: a position statement of the ESC working group on myocardial and pericardial diseases. Eur Heart J. 2016;37(23):1850-8. Epub 2016/01/23. doi: 10.1093/eurheartj/ehv727.

[11] Burkett EL, Hershberger RE. Clinical and genetic issues in familial dilated cardiomyopathy. J Am Coll Cardiol. 2005;45(7):969-81. doi: 10.1016/j.jacc.2004.11.066.

[12] Geisterfer-Lowrance AA, Kass S, Tanigawa G, Vosberg HP, McKenna W, Seidman CE, et al. A molecular basis for familial hypertrophic cardiomyopathy: a beta cardiac myosin heavy chain gene missense mutation.

Cell. 1990;62(5):999-1006. doi: 10.1016/0092-8674(90)90274-i.

[13] McNally EM, Mestroni L. Dilated Cardiomyopathy: Genetic Determinants and Mechanisms. Circ Res. 2017;121(7):731-48. doi: 10.1161/CIRCRESAHA.116.309396.

[14] Ponikowski P, Voors AA, Anker SD, Bueno H, Cleland JG, Coats AJ, et al. 2016 ESC Guidelines for the diagnosis and treatment of acute and chronic heart failure: The Task Force for the diagnosis and treatment of acute and chronic heart failure of the European Society of Cardiology (ESC). Developed with the special contribution of the Heart Failure Association (HFA) of the ESC. Eur J Heart Fail. 2016;18(8):891-975. doi: 10.1002/ejhf.592.

[15] Yancy CW, Jessup M, Bozkurt B, Butler J, Casey DE, Jr., Colvin MM, et al. 2017 ACC/AHA/HFSA Focused Update of the 2013 ACCF/AHA Guideline for the Management of Heart Failure: A Report of the American College of Cardiology/American Heart Association Task Force on Clinical Practice Guidelines and the Heart Failure Society of America. J Card Fail. 2017;23(8):628-51. doi: 10.1016/j.cardfail.2017.04.014.

[16] Bozkurt B, Colvin M, Cook J, Cooper LT, Deswal A, Fonarow GC, et al. Current Diagnostic and Treatment Strategies for Specific Dilated Cardiomyopathies: A Scientific Statement From the American Heart Association. Circulation. 2016;134(23):e579-e646. doi: 10.1161/CIR.0000000000000455.

[17] McMurray JJ, Packer M, Desai AS, Gong J, Lefkowitz MP, Rizkala AR, et al. Angiotensin-neprilysin inhibition versus enalapril in heart failure. N Engl J Med. 2014;371(11):993-1004. doi: 10.1056/NEJMoa1409077.

[18] Yancy CW, Januzzi JL, Jr., Allen LA, Butler J, Davis LL, Fonarow GC, et al. 2017 ACC Expert Consensus Decision Pathway for Optimization of Heart Failure Treatment: Answers to 10 Pivotal Issues About Heart Failure With Reduced Ejection Fraction: A Report of the American College of Cardiology Task Force on Expert Consensus Decision Pathways. J Am Coll Cardiol. 2018;71(2):201-30. doi: 10.1016/j.jacc.2017.11.025.

[19] Herman DS, Lam L, Taylor MR, Wang L, Teekakirikul P, Christodoulou D, et al. Truncations of titin causing dilated cardiomyopathy. N Engl J Med. 2012;366(7):619-28. doi: 10.1056/NEJMoa1110186.

[20] Kamisago M, Sharma SD, DePalma SR, Solomon S, Sharma P, McDonough B, et al. Mutations in sarcomere protein genes as a cause of dilated cardiomyopathy. N Engl J Med. 2000;343(23):1688-96. doi: 10.1056/NEJM200012073432304.

[21] Moller DV, Andersen PS, Hedley P, Ersboll MK, Bundgaard H, Moolman-Smook J, et al. The role of sarcomere gene mutations in patients with idiopathic dilated cardiomyopathy. Eur J Hum Genet. 2009;17(10):1241-9. doi: 10.1038/ejhg.2009.34.

[22] Lek M, Karczewski KJ, Minikel EV, Samocha KE, Banks E, Fennell T, et al. Analysis of protein-coding genetic variation in 60,706 humans. Nature. 2016;536(7616):285-91. doi: 10.1038/nature19057.

[23] Schafer S, de Marvao A, Adami E, Fiedler LR, Ng B, Khin E, et al. Titin-truncating variants affect heart function in disease cohorts and the general population. Nat Genet. 2017;49(1):46-53. doi: 10.1038/ng.3719.

[24] Roberts AM, Ware JS, Herman DS, Schafer S, Baksi J, Bick AG, et al. Integrated allelic, transcriptional, and phenomic dissection of the cardiac effects of titin truncations in

health and disease. Sci Transl Med. 2015;7(270):270ra6. doi: 10.1126/scitranslmed.3010134.

[25] Hinson JT, Chopra A, Nafissi N, Polacheck WJ, Benson CC, Swist S, et al. HEART DISEASE. Titin mutations in iPS cells define sarcomere insufficiency as a cause of dilated cardiomyopathy. Science. 2015;349(6251):982-6. doi: 10.1126/science.aaa5458.

[26] Bloemink M, Deacon J, Langer S, Vera C, Combs A, Leinwand L, et al. The hypertrophic cardiomyopathy myosin mutation R453C alters ATP binding and hydrolysis of human cardiac beta-myosin. J Biol Chem. 2014;289(8):5158-67. doi: 10.1074/jbc.M113.511204.

[27] Schmitt JP, Debold EP, Ahmad F, Armstrong A, Frederico A, Conner DA, et al. Cardiac myosin missense mutations cause dilated cardiomyopathy in mouse models and depress molecular motor function. Proc Natl Acad Sci U S A. 2006;103(39):14525-30. doi: 10.1073/pnas.0606383103.

[28] Ujfalusi Z, Vera CD, Mijailovich SM, Svicevic M, Yu EC, Kawana M, et al. Dilated cardiomyopathy myosin mutants have reduced force-generating capacity. J Biol Chem. 2018;293(23):9017-29. doi: 10.1074/jbc.RA118.001938.

[29] Olson TM, Kishimoto NY, Whitby FG, Michels VV. Mutations that alter the surface charge of alpha-tropomyosin are associated with dilated cardiomyopathy. J Mol Cell Cardiol. 2001;33(4):723-32. doi: 10.1006/jmcc.2000.1339.

[30] Thierfelder L, Watkins H, MacRae C, Lamas R, McKenna W, Vosberg HP, et al. Alpha-tropomyosin and cardiac troponin T mutations cause familial hypertrophic cardiomyopathy: a disease of the sarcomere. Cell. 1994;77(5):701-12. doi: 10.1016/0092-8674(94)90054-x.

[31] Gupte TM, Haque F, Gangadharan B, Sunitha MS, Mukherjee S, Anandhan S, et al. Mechanistic heterogeneity in contractile properties of alpha-tropomyosin (TPM1) mutants associated with inherited cardiomyopathies. J Biol Chem. 2015;290(11):7003-15. doi: 10.1074/jbc.M114.596676.

[32] Pankuweit S. Lamin A/C mutations in patients with dilated cardiomyopathy. Eur Heart J. 2018;39(10):861-3. doi: 10.1093/eurheartj/ehx650.

[33] Parks SB, Kushner JD, Nauman D, Burgess D, Ludwigsen S, Peterson A, et al. Lamin A/C mutation analysis in a cohort of 324 unrelated patients with idiopathic or familial dilated cardiomyopathy. Am Heart J. 2008;156(1):161-9. doi: 10.1016/j.ahj.2008.01.026.

[34] Laurini E, Martinelli V, Lanzicher T, Puzzi L, Borin D, Chen SN, et al. Biomechanical defects and rescue of cardiomyocytes expressing pathologic nuclear lamins. Cardiovasc Res. 2018;114(6):846-57. doi: 10.1093/cvr/cvy040.

[35] Muchir A, Wu W, Choi JC, Iwata S, Morrow J, Homma S, et al. Abnormal p38alpha mitogen-activated protein kinase signaling in dilated cardiomyopathy caused by lamin A/C gene mutation. Hum Mol Genet. 2012;21(19):4325-33. doi: 10.1093/hmg/dds265.

[36] Guo W, Schafer S, Greaser ML, Radke MH, Liss M, Govindarajan T, et al. RBM20, a gene for hereditary cardiomyopathy, regulates titin splicing. Nat Med. 2012;18(5):766-73. doi: 10.1038/nm.2693.

[37] Brauch KM, Karst ML, Herron KJ, de Andrade M, Pellikka PA,

Rodeheffer RJ, et al. Mutations in ribonucleic acid binding protein gene cause familial dilated cardiomyopathy. J Am Coll Cardiol. 2009;54(10):930-41. doi: 10.1016/j.jacc.2009.05.038.

[38] Li D, Morales A, Gonzalez-Quintana J, Norton N, Siegfried JD, Hofmeyer M, et al. Identification of novel mutations in RBM20 in patients with dilated cardiomyopathy. Clin Transl Sci. 2010;3(3):90-7. doi: 10.1111/j.1752-8062.2010.00198.x.

[39] van den Hoogenhof MMG, Beqqali A, Amin AS, van der Made I, Aufiero S, Khan MAF, et al. RBM20 Mutations Induce an Arrhythmogenic Dilated Cardiomyopathy Related to Disturbed Calcium Handling. Circulation. 2018;138(13):1330-42. doi: 10.1161/CIRCULATIONAHA.117.031947.

[40] Paulin D, Li Z. Desmin: a major intermediate filament protein essential for the structural integrity and function of muscle. Exp Cell Res. 2004;301(1):1-7. doi: 10.1016/j.yexcr.2004.08.004.

[41] Taylor MR, Slavov D, Ku L, Di Lenarda A, Sinagra G, Carniel E, et al. Prevalence of desmin mutations in dilated cardiomyopathy. Circulation. 2007;115(10):1244-51. doi: 10.1161/CIRCULATIONAHA.106.646778.

[42] Emery AE. Population frequencies of inherited neuromuscular diseases--a world survey. Neuromuscul Disord. 1991;1(1):19-29. doi: 10.1016/0960-8966(91)90039-u.

[43] Gao QQ, McNally EM. The Dystrophin Complex: Structure, Function, and Implications for Therapy. Compr Physiol. 2015;5(3):1223-39. doi: 10.1002/cphy.c140048.

[44] McNally EM. New approaches in the therapy of cardiomyopathy in muscular dystrophy. Annu Rev Med. 2007;58:75-88. doi: 10.1146/annurev.med.58.011706.144703.

[45] Arimura T, Ishikawa T, Nunoda S, Kawai S, Kimura A. Dilated cardiomyopathy-associated BAG3 mutations impair Z-disc assembly and enhance sensitivity to apoptosis in cardiomyocytes. Hum Mutat. 2011;32(12):1481-91. doi: 10.1002/humu.21603.

[46] Dominguez F, Cuenca S, Bilinska Z, Toro R, Villard E, Barriales-Villa R, et al. Dilated Cardiomyopathy Due to BLC2-Associated Athanogene 3 (BAG3) Mutations. J Am Coll Cardiol. 2018;72(20):2471-81. doi: 10.1016/j.jacc.2018.08.2181.

[47] Franaszczyk M, Bilinska ZT, Sobieszczanska-Malek M, Michalak E, Sleszycka J, Sioma A, et al. The BAG3 gene variants in Polish patients with dilated cardiomyopathy: four novel mutations and a genotype-phenotype correlation. J Transl Med. 2014;12:192. doi: 10.1186/1479-5876-12-192.

[48] Myers VD, Gerhard GS, McNamara DM, Tomar D, Madesh M, Kaniper S, et al. Association of Variants in BAG3 With Cardiomyopathy Outcomes in African American Individuals. JAMA Cardiol. 2018;3(10):929-38. doi: 10.1001/jamacardio.2018.2541.

[49] McNair WP, Ku L, Taylor MR, Fain PR, Dao D, Wolfel E, et al. SCN5A mutation associated with dilated cardiomyopathy, conduction disorder, and arrhythmia. Circulation. 2004;110(15):2163-7. doi: 10.1161/01.CIR.0000144458.58660.BB.

[50] Olson TM, Michels VV, Ballew JD, Reyna SP, Karst ML, Herron KJ, et al. Sodium channel mutations and susceptibility to heart failure and atrial fibrillation. JAMA. 2005;293(4):447-54. doi: 10.1001/jama.293.4.447.

[51] Mann SA, Castro ML, Ohanian M, Guo G, Zodgekar P, Sheu A, et al. R222Q SCN5A mutation is associated with

reversible ventricular ectopy and dilated cardiomyopathy. J Am Coll Cardiol. 2012;60(16):1566-73. doi: 10.1016/j.jacc.2012.05.050..

[52] Zakrzewska-Koperska J, FranaszczykM,BilinskaZ,TruszkowskaG, Karczmarz M, Szumowski L, et al. Rapid and effective response of the R222Q SCN5A to quinidine treatment in a patient with Purkinje-related ventricular arrhythmia and familial dilated cardiomyopathy: a case report. BMC Med Genet. 2018;19(1):94. doi: 10.1186/s12881-018-0599-4.

[53] Schmitt JP, Kamisago M, Asahi M, Li GH, Ahmad F, Mende U, et al. Dilated cardiomyopathy and heart failure caused by a mutation in phospholamban. Science. 2003;299(5611):1410-3. doi: 10.1126/science.1081578.

[54] Hof IE, van der Heijden JF, Kranias EG, Sanoudou D, de Boer RA, van Tintelen JP, et al. Prevalence and cardiac phenotype of patients with a phospholamban mutation. Neth Heart J. 2019;27(2):64-9. doi: 10.1007/s12471-018-1211-4.

[55] DeWitt MM, MacLeod HM, Soliven B, McNally EM. Phospholamban R14 deletion results in late-onset, mild, hereditary dilated cardiomyopathy. J Am Coll Cardiol. 2006;48(7):1396-8. doi: 10.1016/j.jacc.2006.07.016.

[56] Sylvius N, Duboscq-Bidot L, Bouchier C, Charron P, Benaiche A, Sebillon P, et al. Mutational analysis of the beta- and delta-sarcoglycan genes in a large number of patients with familial and sporadic dilated cardiomyopathy. Am J Med Genet A. 2003;120A(1):8-12. doi: 10.1002/ajmg.a.20003.

[57] Tsubata S, Bowles KR, Vatta M, Zintz C, Titus J, Muhonen L, et al. Mutations in the human delta-sarcoglycan gene in familial and sporadic dilated cardiomyopathy. J Clin Invest. 2000;106(5):655-62. doi: 10.1172/JCI9224.

[58] Schlame M, Kelley RI, Feigenbaum A, Towbin JA, Heerdt PM, Schieble T, et al. Phospholipid abnormalities in children with Barth syndrome. J Am Coll Cardiol. 2003;42(11):1994-9. doi: 10.1016/j.jacc.2003.06.015.

[59] Hsu P, Liu X, Zhang J, Wang HG, Ye JM, Shi Y. Cardiolipin remodeling by TAZ/tafazzin is selectively required for the initiation of mitophagy. Autophagy. 2015;11(4):643-52. doi: 10.1080/15548627.2015.1023984.

[60] Pasotti M, Klersy C, Pilotto A, Marziliano N, Rapezzi C, Serio A, et al. Long-term outcome and risk stratification in dilated cardiolaminopathies. J Am Coll Cardiol. 2008;52(15):1250-60. doi: 10.1016/j.jacc.2008.06.044.

[61] van Rijsingen IA, Arbustini E, Elliott PM, Mogensen J, Hermans-van Ast JF, van der Kooi AJ, et al. Risk factors for malignant ventricular arrhythmias in lamin a/c mutation carriers a European cohort study. J Am Coll Cardiol. 2012;59(5):493-500. doi: 10.1016/j.jacc.2011.08.078.

[62] Wahbi K, Ben Yaou R, Gandjbakhch E, Anselme F, Gossios T, Lakdawala NK, et al. Development and Validation of a New Risk Prediction Score for Life-Threatening Ventricular Tachyarrhythmias in Laminopathies. Circulation. 2019;140(4):293-302. doi: 10.1161/CIRCULATIONAHA.118.039410.

[63] Halliday BP, Cleland JGF, Goldberger JJ, Prasad SK. Personalizing Risk Stratification for Sudden Death in Dilated Cardiomyopathy: The Past, Present, and Future. Circulation. 2017;136(2):215-31. doi: 10.1161/CIRCULATIONAHA.116.027134.

[64] Chemello F, Bassel-Duby R, Olson EN. Correction of muscular dystrophies by CRISPR gene editing. J Clin Invest. 2020;130(6):2766-76. doi: 10.1172/JCI136873.

[65] Wang B, Li J, Xiao X. Adeno-associated virus vector carrying human minidystrophin genes effectively ameliorates muscular dystrophy in mdx mouse model. Proc Natl Acad Sci U S A. 2000;97(25):13714-9. doi: 10.1073/pnas.240335297.

[66] Fabb SA, Wells DJ, Serpente P, Dickson G. Adeno-associated virus vector gene transfer and sarcolemmal expression of a 144 kDa micro-dystrophin effectively restores the dystrophin-associated protein complex and inhibits myofibre degeneration in nude/mdx mice. Hum Mol Genet. 2002;11(7):733-41. doi: 10.1093/hmg/11.7.733.

[67] Gregorevic P, Allen JM, Minami E, Blankinship MJ, Haraguchi M, Meuse L, et al. rAAV6-microdystrophin preserves muscle function and extends lifespan in severely dystrophic mice. Nat Med. 2006;12(7):787-9. doi: 10.1038/nm1439.

[68] Ho PP, Lahey LJ, Mourkioti F, Kraft PE, Filareto A, Brandt M, et al. Engineered DNA plasmid reduces immunity to dystrophin while improving muscle force in a model of gene therapy of Duchenne dystrophy. Proc Natl Acad Sci U S A. 2018;115(39):E9182-E91. doi: 10.1073/pnas.1808648115.

[69] Konieczny P, Swiderski K, Chamberlain JS. Gene and cell-mediated therapies for muscular dystrophy. Muscle Nerve. 2013;47(5):649-63. doi: 10.1002/mus.23738.

[70] Mendell JR, Campbell K, Rodino-Klapac L, Sahenk Z, Shilling C, Lewis S, et al. Dystrophin immunity in Duchenne's muscular dystrophy. N Engl J Med. 2010;363(15):1429-37. doi: 10.1056/NEJMoa1000228.

[71] Aartsma-Rus A, Straub V, Hemmings R, Haas M, Schlosser-Weber G, Stoyanova-Beninska V, et al. Development of Exon Skipping Therapies for Duchenne Muscular Dystrophy: A Critical Review and a Perspective on the Outstanding Issues. Nucleic Acid Ther. 2017;27(5):251-9. doi: 10.1089/nat.2017.0682.

[72] Aartsma-Rus A, van Ommen GJ. Antisense-mediated exon skipping: a versatile tool with therapeutic and research applications. RNA. 2007;13(10):1609-24. doi: 10.1261/rna.653607.

[73] van Deutekom JC, Janson AA, Ginjaar IB, Frankhuizen WS, Aartsma-Rus A, Bremmer-Bout M, et al. Local dystrophin restoration with antisense oligonucleotide PRO051. N Engl J Med. 2007;357(26):2677-86. doi: 10.1056/NEJMoa073108.

[74] Sun C, Shen L, Zhang Z, Xie X. Therapeutic Strategies for Duchenne Muscular Dystrophy: An Update. Genes (Basel). 2020;11(8). doi: 10.3390/genes11080837.

[75] Verhaart IEC, Aartsma-Rus A. Therapeutic developments for Duchenne muscular dystrophy. Nat Rev Neurol. 2019;15(7):373-86. doi: 10.1038/s41582-019-0203-3.

[76] El Refaey M, Xu L, Gao Y, Canan BD, Adesanya TMA, Warner SC, et al. In Vivo Genome Editing Restores Dystrophin Expression and Cardiac Function in Dystrophic Mice. Circ Res. 2017;121(8):923-9. doi: 10.1161/CIRCRESAHA.117.310996.

[77] Xu L, Lau YS, Gao Y, Li H, Han R. Life-Long AAV-Mediated CRISPR Genome Editing in Dystrophic Heart Improves Cardiomyopathy without

Causing Serious Lesions in mdx Mice. Mol Ther. 2019;27(8):1407-14. doi: 10.1016/j.ymthe.2019.05.001.

[78] Hakim CH, Wasala NB, Nelson CE, Wasala LP, Yue Y, Louderman JA, et al. AAV CRISPR editing rescues cardiac and muscle function for 18 months in dystrophic mice. JCI Insight. 2018;3(23). doi: 10.1172/jci.insight.124297.

[79] Sicinski P, Geng Y, Ryder-Cook AS, Barnard EA, Darlison MG, Barnard PJ. The molecular basis of muscular dystrophy in the mdx mouse: a point mutation. Science. 1989;244(4912):1578-80. doi: 10.1126/science.2662404.

[80] Azibani F, Brull A, Arandel L, Beuvin M, Nelson I, Jollet A, et al. Gene Therapy via Trans-Splicing for LMNA-Related Congenital Muscular Dystrophy. Mol Ther Nucleic Acids. 2018;10:376-86. doi: 10.1016/j.omtn.2017.12.012.

[81] Bertrand AT, Renou L, Papadopoulos A, Beuvin M, Lacene E, Massart C, et al. DelK32-lamin A/C has abnormal location and induces incomplete tissue maturation and severe metabolic defects leading to premature death. Hum Mol Genet. 2012;21(5):1037-48. doi: 10.1093/hmg/ddr534.

[82] Repetti GG, Toepfer CN, Seidman JG, Seidman CE. Novel Therapies for Prevention and Early Treatment of Cardiomyopathies. Circ Res. 2019;124(11):1536-50. doi: 10.1161/CIRCRESAHA.119.313569.

[83] Wally V, Murauer EM, Bauer JW. Spliceosome-mediated trans-splicing: the therapeutic cut and paste. J Invest Dermatol. 2012;132(8):1959-66. doi: 10.1038/jid.2012.101.

[84] Lee YK, Lau YM, Cai ZJ, Lai WH, Wong LY, Tse HF, et al. Modeling Treatment Response for Lamin A/C Related Dilated Cardiomyopathy in Human Induced Pluripotent Stem Cells. J Am Heart Assoc. 2017;6(8). doi: 10.1161/JAHA.117.005677.

[85] Welch EM, Barton ER, Zhuo J, Tomizawa Y, Friesen WJ, Trifillis P, et al. PTC124 targets genetic disorders caused by nonsense mutations. Nature. 2007;447(7140):87-91. doi: 10.1038/nature05756.

[86] Gedicke-Hornung C, Behrens-Gawlik V, Reischmann S, Geertz B, Stimpel D, Weinberger F, et al. Rescue of cardiomyopathy through U7snRNA-mediated exon skipping in Mybpc3-targeted knock-in mice. EMBO Mol Med. 2013;5(7):1128-45. doi: 10.1002/emmm.201202168.

[87] Gramlich M, Pane LS, Zhou Q, Chen Z, Murgia M, Schotterl S, et al. Antisense-mediated exon skipping: a therapeutic strategy for titin-based dilated cardiomyopathy. EMBO Mol Med. 2015;7(5):562-76. doi: 10.15252/emmm.201505047.

[88] Kawada T, Sakamoto A, Nakazawa M, Urabe M, Masuda F, Hemmi C, et al. Morphological and physiological restorations of hereditary form of dilated cardiomyopathy by somatic gene therapy. Biochem Biophys Res Commun. 2001;284(2):431-5. doi: 10.1006/bbrc.2001.4962.

[89] Karakikes I, Stillitano F, Nonnenmacher M, Tzimas C, Sanoudou D, Termglinchan V, et al. Correction of human phospholamban R14del mutation associated with cardiomyopathy using targeted nucleases and combination therapy. Nat Commun. 2015;6:6955. doi: 10.1038/ncomms7955.

[90] Bass-Stringer S, Bernardo BC, May CN, Thomas CJ, Weeks KL, McMullen JR. Adeno-Associated Virus Gene Therapy: Translational Progress and Future Prospects in the Treatment of Heart Failure. Heart Lung Circ.

2018;27(11):1285-300. doi: 10.1016/j.hlc.2018.03.005.

[91] Calcedo R, Wilson JM. Humoral Immune Response to AAV. Front Immunol. 2013;4:341. doi: 10.3389/fimmu.2013.00341.

[92] Jessup M, Greenberg B, Mancini D, Cappola T, Pauly DF, Jaski B, et al. Calcium Upregulation by Percutaneous Administration of Gene Therapy in Cardiac Disease (CUPID): a phase 2 trial of intracoronary gene therapy of sarcoplasmic reticulum Ca2+-ATPase in patients with advanced heart failure. Circulation. 2011;124(3):304-13. doi: 10.1161/CIRCULATIONAHA.111.022889.

Chapter 8

Coronavirus Disease: Epidemiology, Aetiology, Pathophysiology and Involvement of the Cardiovascular System

David C. Gaze

Abstract

Since the emergence in China of coronavirus disease (COVID-19) in December 2019; the virus causing the pandemic has infected the human population in almost every country and territory on the globe. At the time of writing there are over 84 million confirmed cases of infection and over 1.8 million deaths globally. Rates of infection differ as does the number of severe cases and subsequent deaths between countries and continents. This is due in part to lockdown measures, social distancing and wearing of face coverings. It is also reflected by how healthcare systems record coronavirus deaths along with access to testing as well as tracking and tracing of infected individuals. Symptoms of COVID-19 include a novel persistent cough, fever and anosmia (loss of smell). In most cases, such symptoms are mild. A small proportion of those who become infected however, have a severe reaction to the disease affecting multiple organ systems and often require respiratory support in the intensive care setting. One such physiological system affected is the cardiovascular system. This is likely due to the increased number of ACE2 receptors in co-morbid cardiac pathologies. ACE2 receptors serve as the entry port for the coronavirus into human cells. Those individuals with underlying cardiovascular risk factors are therefore disproportionately at risk of COVID-19 infection. This chapter reviews the aetiology and epidemiology of the coronavirus infection; potential pathophysiological mechanisms of disease involving the cardiovascular system including the clinical utility of biomarkers, electrocardiography and echocardiography as well as autopsy cardiac pathology and histopathology.

Keywords: coronavirus disease, cardiovascular system, ACE2 receptors, pathophysiological mechanisms

1. Introduction

Coronavirus disease (COVID-19) is an emerging viral disease affecting humans. In December 2019, a small series of cases of a pneumonia-like illness presented to a hospital in Wuhan, Hubei province in China. The patients displayed bilateral pulmonary infiltrative lesions on chest x-ray. The disease was initially named 'viral pneumonia of unknown cause'. Many of those presenting with similar symptoms had visited or been closely associated with a local wholesale seafood market which also sold exotic species such as civets, snakes, rats and bats. The Chinese Centre for Disease Control and Prevention (China CDC) identified the virus as a novel coronavirus (nCoV) on 7th January 2020 and renamed the disease 'pneumonia caused by a novel coronavirus. Subsequently on 30th January 2020, the World Health Organisation (WHO) referred to the disease as 2019-nCoV. The *Coronaviridae* study group of the International Committee on Taxonomy of Viruses (ICTV) officially named the virus Severe Acute Respiratory Syndrome-Coronavirus-2 (SARS-CoV-2) on 11th February 2020. The WHO also announced a name change to *CO*rona*VI*rus *D*isease 2019 (COVID-19). The change reflected the greater reporting of a wide range of clinical presentations and multiple organ system involvement in severe cases of the disease. At the same time, it became apparent the disease was spreading significantly in Hubei Province due to an increase in numbers of cases with no identifiable association to the seafood market, demonstrating community (person-to-person) transmission.

The rate of escalation of COVID-19 infection is alarming. This is detailed in the following statistics (provided by many resources online via China CDC, news outlets and social media coverage). A retrospective epidemiological analysis by China CDC indicated there were 104 symptomatic cases by 31st December 2019. All cases were contained in Hubei province. Between 1st and 10th January 2020, this had risen to 566 cases showing symptoms in Hubei, with a further 87 cases in 19 other provinces. On January 20th 2020, 5 cases were reported in Beijing and 2 in Shanghai. Further analysis demonstrates that the number of cases of COVID-19 present in

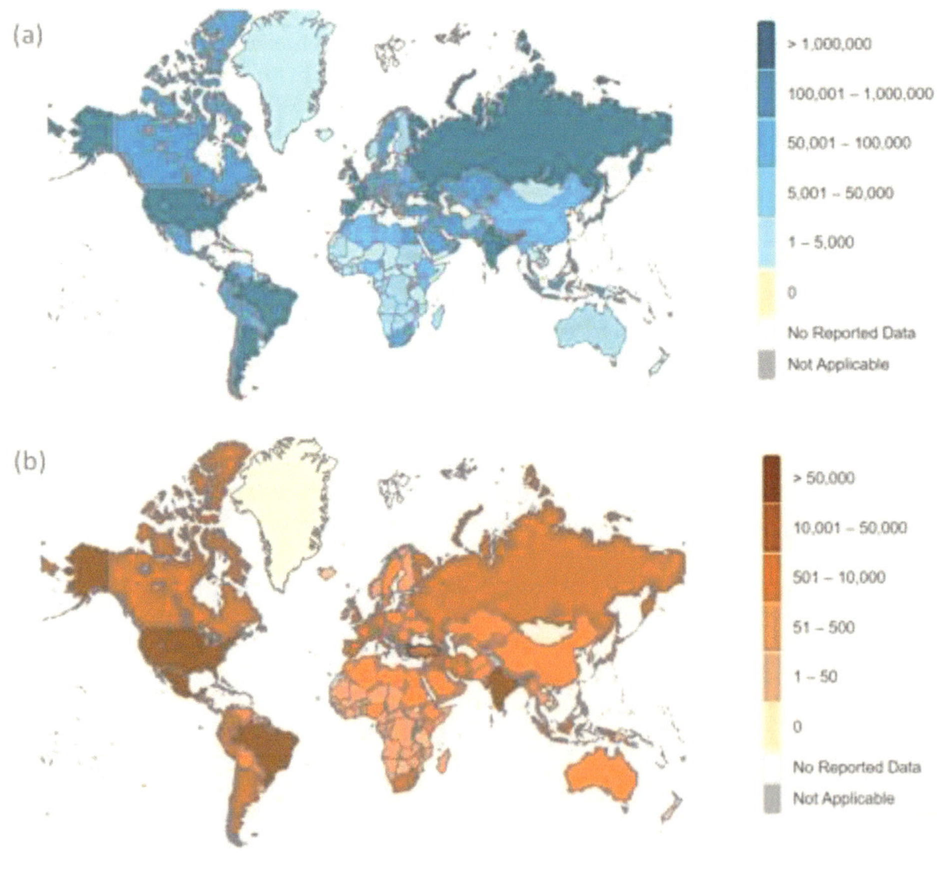

Figure 1.
Global epidemiology of COVID-19. (a) Confirmed cases of coronavirus and (b) deaths from coronavirus. (source WHO live situation dashboard www.covid19.who.int).

China by 31st January 2020 reached as staggering 32,642. 75% of these were in Hubei province. The incidence of the disease in mainland China had escalated to over 74,000 cases by 19th February 2020 along with 65 cases and 5 deaths in Hong Kong, 10 confirmed cases in Macao and 24 cases and one death in Taiwan.

From mid to late January countries other than China began reporting COVID-19 cases. The first non-mainland case was a Chinese national from Wuhan who travelled to Thailand and tested positive for COVID-19 on the 13th January 2020. The first reported case outside of Asia was announced on the 21st January 2020 in the United States of America (USA). At the end of February, the WHO declared the epidemic as a 'Public Health Emergency of International Concern' with evidence of infected cases in South Korea (2,337), Japan (210), Italy (650), Iran (245), Singapore (96) and USA (59). The cases in Japan are of note as they are associated with a contained infection on the Diamond Princess cruise ship. The ship departed Japan on 20th January 2020. Five days later a passenger developed a fever and tested positive on 1st February 2020 in Hong Kong. The ship returned to Japan and was placed in quarantine. By 12th February 492 passengers were tested of which 174 were positive for COVID-19. By 19th February 2020, the number of passengers infected rose to 621 and 705 nine days later. On 11th March 2020, at the daily briefing by the director general, Dr. Tedros Adhanom Ghebreyesus, the WHO declared COVID-19 as an offically recognised pandemic [1].

It is now a year since the initial outbreak in China. In this short time the WHO report via their live situation dashboard [2] to date (5th January 2021) 84,233,579 confirmed cases globally of which 1,843,293 individuals have died (**Figure 1**). What is shocking and apparent is the upward escalation of these figures on a daily basis, especially in the winter months in the Northern Hemisphere.

2. Novel SARS-CoV-2 variants

Late in 2020, two variants of the SARS-CoV-2 virus have been identified. The first was identified in September and sequenced in the United Kingdom [3]. The 'UK Kent variant' as it is commonly known has spread rapidly both in the UK and internationally. Since 26th December 2020, cases of the new UK Kent Variant have also been reported in other EU/EEA countries (Belgium, Denmark, Finland, France, Germany, Iceland, Ireland, Italy, the Netherlands, Norway, Portugal, Spain and Sweden) and globally (Australia, Canada, Hong Kong SAR, India, Israel, Japan, Jordan, Lebanon, South Korea, Switzerland, Singapore). The second variant originated in South Africa and is due to the mutation E484K; known as 501.V2. This variant was first detected in October 2020 and is associated with over 300 cases as of 26th December 2020. Both variants are highly transmissible, but data suggest they do not increase the severity of COVID-19 infection [4].

The first variant was identified following a surge in positive cases in the County of Kent in South East England and has spread extensively into London and beyond (**Figure 2**). The variant was named as variant under investigation (VUI) followed by year, month and number; thus, the designation given was VUI-202012/01 which was changed to variant of concern (VOC-202012/01). The variant is defined by 23 novel mutations. 13 of which are non-synonymous, 4 deletion and 6 synonymous. Of concern is nucleotide A23063T in the spike protein representing mutation N501Y. This mutation is located in the receptor-binding domain and is associated with increased binding affinity to ACE2; making viral entry into host cells easier than with the original strain, thus increasing transmissibility. Although more transmissible, recent data suggest this variant is less likely to cause severe infection and is likely to respond to the current vaccination programme [5].

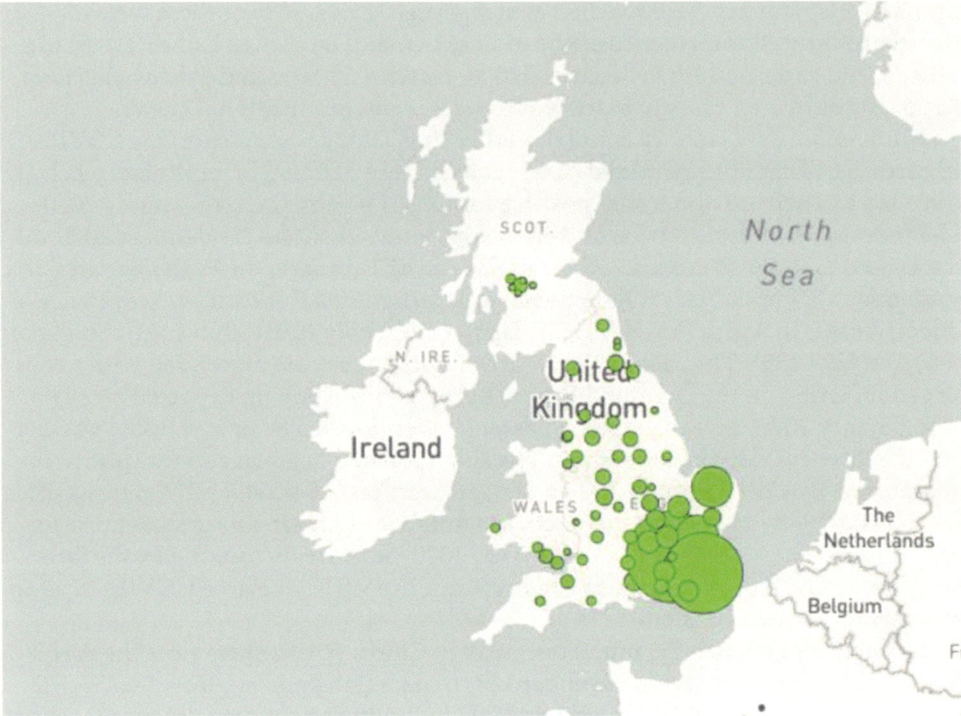

Figure 2.
Distribution of confirmed sequenced cases of VOC202012/01 as of 6th January 2021. [source: https://beta.microreact.org/project/vVnFfZG703qYUJ6bnDs3Jo-cog-uk-2020-12-20-sars-cov-2-in-the-uk].

3. Coronaviruses

3.1 Taxonomy and morphology

Coronaviruses are a large family of viruses found in animals such as camels, dogs, rats, cattle, mice, rats and bats; as well as several viruses known to infect humans. They were first discovered in 1968 and named *Coronaviridae* in 1975 by the ITCV. The viruses are positive-sense single stranded RNA viruses with 26 to 32 kb genomes and are classified into *Alpha, Beta, Gamma* and *Delta* genera (**Figure 3**). The viruses that infect mammals are *Alpha* and *Betacoronaviruses*. In humans, pathogenic coronaviruses include SARS-CoV, SARS-CoV-2, MERS-CoV, HCoV-HKU1, HCoV-229E, HCoV-NL63 HCoV-OC43. Most are inconspicuous and develop into common colds and mild-flu like symptoms, but recently since the emergence of SARS and MERS and now SARS-CoV-2, an increasing number of severe illnesses are developing associated with novel coronaviruses in humans.

Morphologically, the viral particle of coronaviruses are encased in a bilipid layer with three glycoproteins on the surface designated as membrane (M protein), envelope (E protein) and spike (S protein) proteins (**Figure 4a**). These give the virus the characteristic protrusions on the surface akin to a medieval European crown or *'corona'* hence the name coronavirus. An electron micrograph of viral particles isolated in alveolar tissue from the first infected case in the United States is shown in **Figure 4b**.

Utilising cryptoelecton tomography (Cryo-ET), Yao and colleagues determined the detailed molecular structure of the novel SARS-CoV-2 enveloped virus and elucidated the mechanism of packing the ~30 kb long single RNA into the 80 nm diameter luminal space [7].

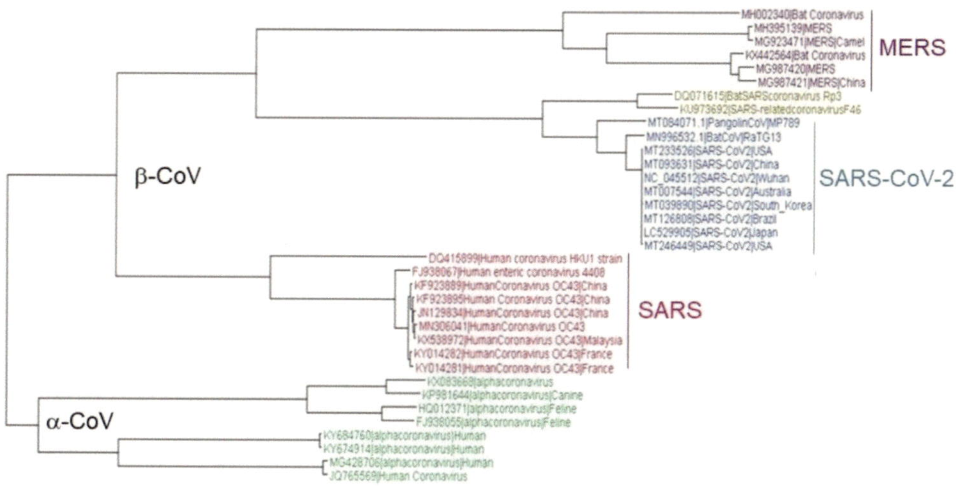

Figure 3.
Phylogenic tree of alpha and beta coronaviruses. MERS, Middle East respiratory syndrome; SARS, severe acute respiratory syndrome; SARS-COV-2, severe acute respiratory syndrome coronavirus 2.

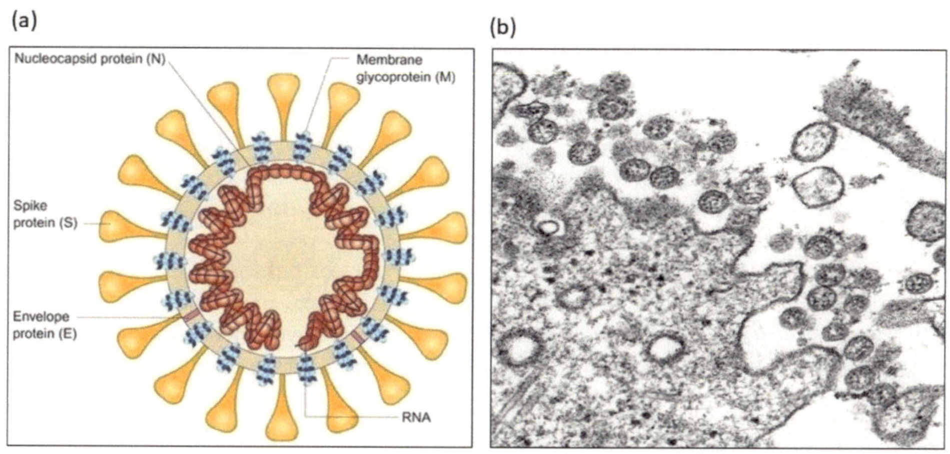

Figure 4.
(a) Schematic structure of a coronavirus particle [source: Peiris et al., [6]] (b) transmission electron microscopy image of an isolate from the first case of COVID-19 in the USA. The spherical extracellular viral particles contain cross-sections through the viral genome seen as black dots [source: cdc.gov].

3.2 Cellular entry of SARS-CoV-2

The SARS-CoV-2 virus enters human cells via interaction of the spike protein with the Angiotensin Converting Enzyme 2 protein (ACE2) [8]. ACE2 is integral to the renin-angiotensin-aldosterone (RAAS) system. Originally thought to have a systemic effect on maintenance of blood pressure and electrolyte balance, it has been found to be involved in inflammatory responses in many tissues including the cardiovascular system [9]. Activation of the RASS system has been associated with the development of hypertension, myocardial infarction, chronic heart failure, diabetes and inflammatory processes in lung tissue [10]. SARS-CoV-2 and ACE2 protein interaction is like the SARS-CoV virus responsible for the original SARS outbreak [11].

ACE2 is a metallopeptidase and is found in virtually all cell types. It is highly expressed on cell surfaces in lung alveolar epithelium, intestinal enterocytes as well as on vascular endothelial cells [12]. This is especially important in those individuals with underlying cardiovascular diseases as expression of ACE2 in the vasculature is altered [13]. This will be detailed further in the chapter under cardiovascular involvement. Following internalisation via vesicle entry, the ACE2 surface proteins are downregulated, potentiating the increasing physiological effects of angiotensin II (**Figure 5**) via proinflammatory mediators [14].

3.3 Routes of transmission of SARS-CoV-2

The major route of transmission in the human population is from person-to-person via respiratory droplets when infected individuals cough, sneeze and talk when in close contact with another person [15]. Susceptible individuals inhale droplets shed from an infected individual near one another. The risk of infection depends on the size of the particles and droplets, the extent of viral shedding from the infected individual, the force of expulsion of droplets from an infected individual, the proximity between infected and uninfected individuals as well as environmental factors such as air density, humidity and wind speed [16]. Aerosol transmission is an alternative route of infectivity; however, this has been subject to significant debate and scientific study.

Aerosol transmission occurs when proteins and pathogens float in the form of aerosols after droplets dry out. This may be possible with SARS-CoV-2 in enclosed areas if individuals are exposed to high levels of infected aerosol material such as in care home settings and hospital wards; thus, pose a risk to healthcare workers and others in close contact with infected individuals over a long period of time. Aerosol transmission is often successful with particles with a diameter of 5–10 μm and can be carried over a large distance, whereas droplets are often larger than 10 μm and fall from the air within 1 metre hence the global adoption of spacing between individuals of 1–2 metres [17].

Oral-faecal transmission is another potential route of person-to-person transmission [18]. SARS-CoV-2 has been detected in faecal material from known COVID-19 patients [15, 19]. This is unsurprising given the clinical gastrointestinal manifestations in some individuals. This poses as a rapid transmission route in

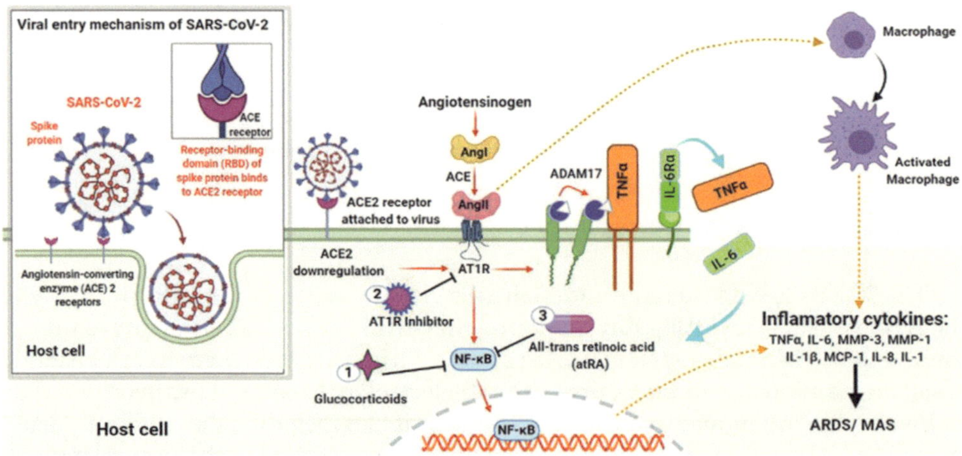

Figure 5.
Viral entry of SARS-CoV-2 in host cells via the ACE2 surface protein. Following entry ACE2 is downregulated resulting in upregulation of angiotensin II (Ang II) which via its AT1R receptor induces NF-kB signalling pathways to increase expression of inflammatory cytokines such as interleukins (IL-1, IL1β, IL-6), matrixmtalloproteinases (MMP-1, MMP-3) and tumour necrosis factor alpha (TNF-α). [source: Banu et al. [14]].

persons unable to maintain good hygiene such as neonates/infants, the infirm and the elderly with cognitive decline such as dementia. It is also a source of environmental viral transmission in developing countries with poor sanitation and no running clean water and soap for adequate hand washing. This has wider impact on those healthcare systems who provide screening of faecal material for colorectal cancer screening [20].

SARS-CoV-2 has not been detected in semen from individuals who have either recovered from or have active COVID-19 infections [21, 22], suggesting sexual transmission is very unlikely. Maternal-fetal transmission however has been described in a small number of clinical cases. A neonate born in Wuhan to a COVID-19 positive woman tested positive for COVID-19 in a nasopharyngeal swab taken 2 days after birth, however this does not confirm maternal-fetal transmission. Oher studies refute vertical intrauterine transmission from mother to child [23, 24] however a recent meta-analysis suggests vertical transmission is possible normally in the third trimester but the incidence is low at 2–3% [25]. This is in part due to the ACE2 receptor portal of SARS-CoV-2 entry into cells being expressed in low concentrations at the maternal-fetal barrier, limiting the route of vertical transmission.

4. General clinical presentation of COVID-19

With the emergence of the pandemic in earnest at the beginning of 2020, the medical and scientific literature has been flooded with case reports and small clinical series often on a regional (district/country) basis. In general, the clinical presentation of patients with SARS-CoV-2 is very similar to that of other coronavirus infections in humans. For the majority of those infected, individuals are either asymptomatic or have a mild fever, novel dry cough or anosmia (loss of smell).

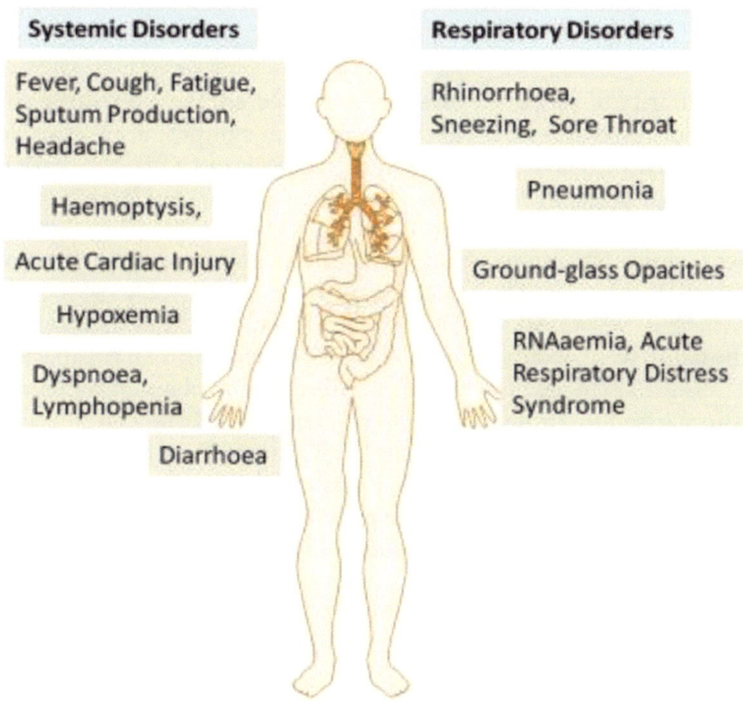

Figure 6.
Respiratory and systemic signs and symptoms associated with COVID-19 [source: Rothan and Byareddy [26]].

	Participants (n)	Value (%)	95% CI
Clinical Presentation			
Fever	15,921	78.8	76.2 to 81.3
Fatigue	13,680	32.2	28.0 to 36.6
Myalgia	10,728	21.3	18.1 to 24.9
Malaise	2,526	37.9	29.5 to 47.1
Respiratory symptoms			
Cough	12,782	53.9	50.0 to 57.7
Expectoration	6,072	7.5	5.7 to 9.6
Chest pain	3,512	9.0	6.2 to 13.1
Shortness of breath	11,205	18.9	15.7 to 22.8
Gastrointestinal symptoms			
Nausea	5,599	6.9	5.3 to 9.1
Vomiting	7,484	4.7	3.8 to 5.8
Diarrhoea	12,142	9.5	7.8 to 11.5
Prognosis			
Renal injury	77,679	3.6	1.2 to 10.1
Hepatic injury	77,331	7.9	2.6 to 21.7
Cardiac Injury	1,417	9.4	4.5 to 18.8
Mechanical ventilation	6,152	7.1	4.5 to 11.0
Mortality	52,808	5.6	4.2 to 7.5

Table 1.
Clinical characteristics and outcomes in COVID-19. Analysis of 281,461 confirmed cases. 95% CI, confidence interval. [source, data from Li et al. [27]].

In the small minority of those who are severely affected, the overriding clinical presentation is of respiratory distress however other symptoms are case-dependent.

The reported clinical characteristics and prognosis of COVID-19 patients varies greatly (**Figure 6**). A recent comprehensive meta-analysis has been performed of clinical characteristics, risk factors and outcomes by Li and colleagues [27]. This vast analysis includes 212 studies from 11 countries involving 281,461 laboratory confirmed COVID-19 cases. The mean age of patients was 46.7y (95%CI 42.8y to 50.6y) with 51.9 (95%CI 50.4 to 53.2) males. The mean time of illness onset to hospital admission was 5.5 days (95%CI 4.6 to 6.4 days) with an incubation period of 5.3 days (95%CI 4.5 to 5.9 days). Clinical presentation characteristics and outcome are summarised in **Table 1**. 79% of subjects were febrile and 53% developed a cough. Renal and hepatic injury occurred in 4% and 7% respectively but cardiac injury was higher at 9%. Overall mortality was reported to be 6% but this differed greatly by country. Mortality was significantly associated with age, male sex, the presence of hypertension or diabetes mellitus [27].

5. Chest imaging

Thoracic imaging is an important diagnostic tool in screening, early diagnosis and monitoring of patients with COVID-19. Although computed tomography (CT) is the gold standard, chest x-ray (CXR) is a cheap, readily available and a faster alternative. CXR lacks sensitivity for diagnosis in the early presentation of COVID-19 being 55% within two days, increasing to 79% at 11 days from onset of symptoms. Specificity decreased over time from 83–70% at ≤2d and > 11d respectively [28]. In approximately 60% of cases, CXR reveals interstitial and airspace opacities in an IA pattern. This increased over time from 51% at ≤2d vs. 73% at >11d [28]. Normal and mild severity CXR findings were the largest factor behind false-negative CXR and often associated with young age and some ethnic groups. In a real-world reader performance study by Cozzi and colleagues [29], experienced radiologist (>10 y experience) reported CXR with higher specificity than less experienced (<10 y experience) radiologists. Comparative CXR images from different respiratory diseases and a normal CXR are shown in **Figure 7**.

Computed tomography (CT) is the preferred radiological procedure for diagnosis. A Cochrane review of CT for diagnosis of COVID-19 found that in 84 studies with 8,279 participants; the pooled sensitivity for diagnosis was 86% (95%CI 90–95%) with a very low specificity of 18% (95%CI 4–56%) [31]. A retrospective study of chest CT findings in 121 symptomatic patients in 4 centres in China has been reported [32]. The classical findings were bilateral and peripheral ground-glass

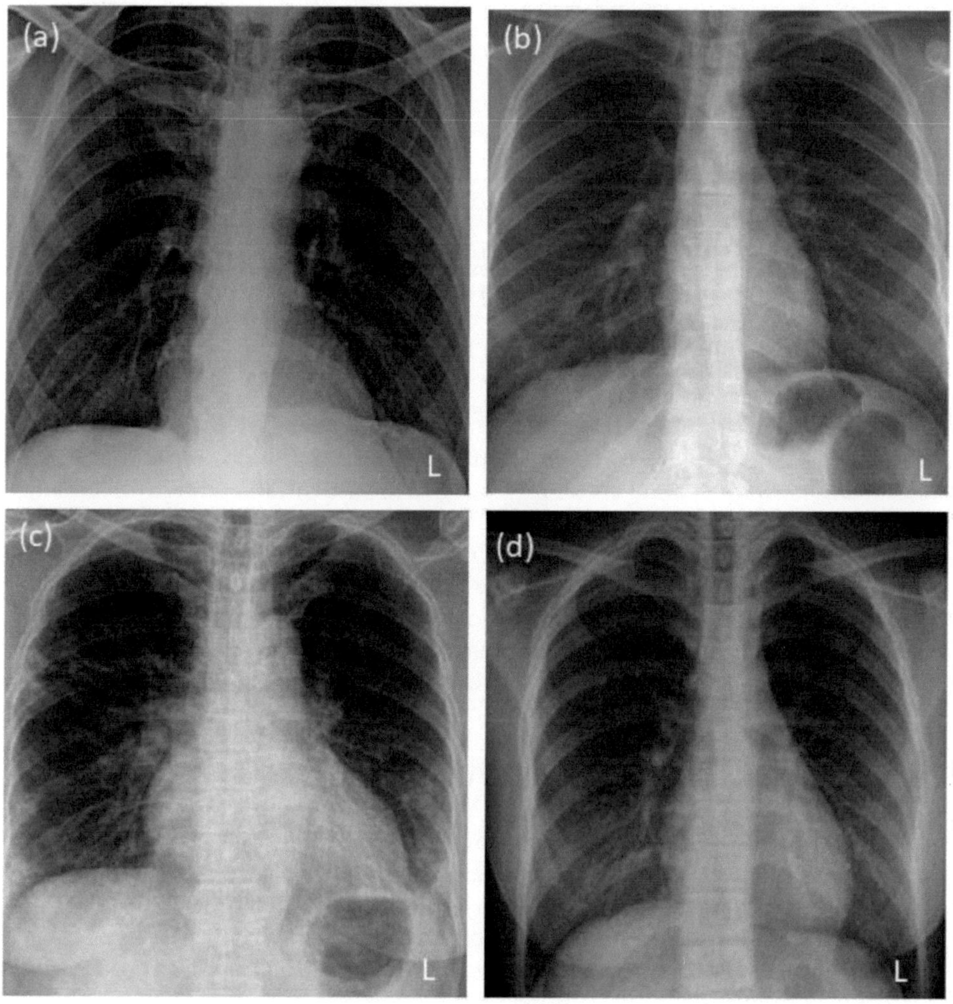

Figure 7.
Comparative chest X-ray findings in (a) normal CXR (b) SARS (c) MERS (d) COVID-19. [source: Images adapted from Pereira et al. [30]].

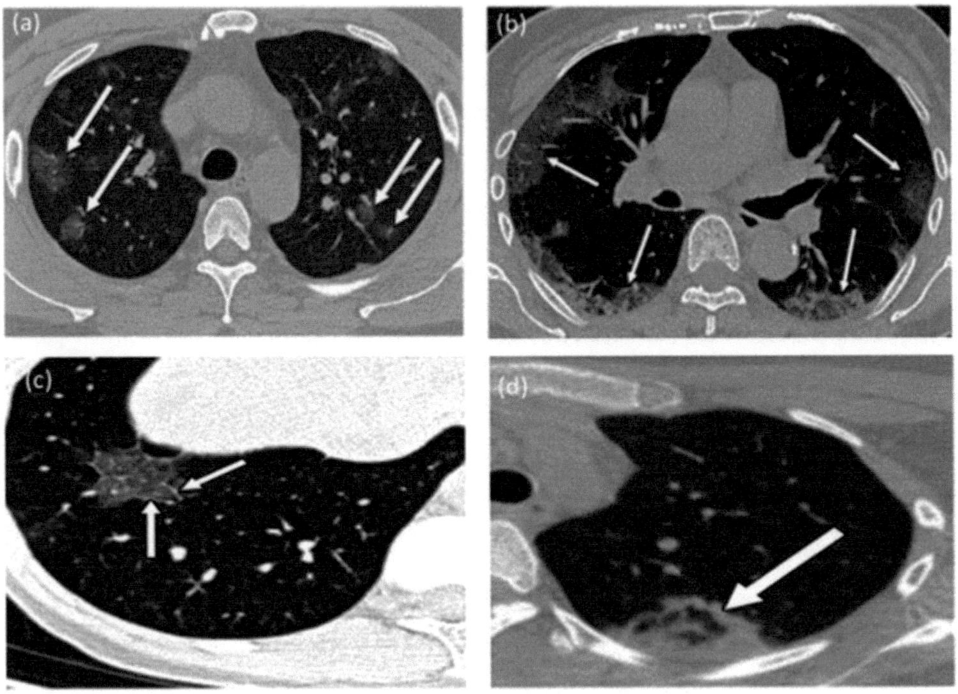

Figure 8.
Representative characteristic findings of COVID-19 infection on thoracic CT imaging: (a) axial CT image obtained without intravenous contrast. 36y male showing bilateral ground-glass opacities in upper lobes with rounded morphologies (arrows); (b) axial CT image. 65 y female, showing bilateral ground-glass and consolidative opacities with striking peripheral distribution (arrows); (c) axial CT image obtained without intravenous contrast material in a 43 y female, demonstrating crazy-paving pattern manifested by right lower lobe ground-glass opacification with interlobular septal thickening (arrows) with intralobular lines. (d) Axial CT image obtained in a 22y female, showing an area of faint ground-glass opacification in left upper lobe with a ring of denser consolidation or reverse halo sign (arrow). [source: Images modified from Bernheim et al. [32]].

consolidative opacity. 56% of subjects had normal CT images in the early phase (0 to 2 days) of the disease but more frequent in longer infections with consolidation, bilateral and peripheral and greater total lung involvement. Bilateral involvement occurred in 28%, 76% and 88% of early (0–2 days), intermediate (3–5 days) and late (6–12 days) infection times respectively. Further notable CT findings include linear opacity, crazy-paving patterns and reverse halo sign (**Figure 8**).

Following isolation and treatment, most COVID-19 patients stabilise and become well. Further CT imaging demonstrates regression of infection with absorbed lesions, and some cord-like shadows.

6. Gastrointestinal symptoms in COVID-19

Gastrointestinal (GI) symptoms are emerging in patients with COVID-19. This is due to the presence of the ACE2 receptor expressed in the GI tract [33, 34].

COVID-19 patients present with GI symptoms such as diarrhoea (10% of patients) with nausea and vomiting less common [35]. In a meta-analysis of 35 studies, 29 studies reported gastrointestinal symptoms in 6,064 COVID-19 patients with a pooled prevalence of gastrointestinal comorbidities of 4%. (95% CI 2 to 5%; range 0 to 15%; I^2 = 74%). The pooled prevalence of digestive symptoms was 15% (10 to 21%; range: 2 to 57%; I^2 = 96%) with nausea or vomiting, diarrhoea, and loss of appetite being the three most common [36].

7. Cardiovascular findings in COVID-19

In addition to respiratory and gastrointestinal symptoms, cardiovascular involvement is also common amongst patients with COVID-19. The symptoms are wide-ranging in manifestation and severity and are more common in the elderly and those hospitalised with the infection. Previous influenza epidemics have been associated with an increased prevalence of myocardial infarction, myocarditis and chronic/congestive heart failure [37]. Both SARS and MERS were associated with either bradycardia, tachycardia, cardiomegaly, diastolic impairments, cardiac arrest, cardiomegaly and acute cardiac failure [38–40].

Patients with cardiovascular risk factors or established cardiovascular disease disproportionately suffer with severe forms of the infection with worse clinical prognosis and outcome. In one of the earliest reports of clinical characteristics of COVID-19 from Wuhan China; 14% of 138 patients demonstrated baseline cardiovascular disease and 31% had hypertension [41]. Similar data has been reported in other population studies from Wuhan, China [42–44]; Italy [45, 46]; Iran [47], United Kingdom [48] and the USA [49] to varying cardiac involvement.

The pathophysiological mechanism of cardiac injury in COVID-19 infection are similar to those associated with other influenza pandemics and human coronavirus diseases (SARS and MERS). Although the pathophysiological mechanisms injury is not fully established in COVID-19 patients, it is likely that the elevation is related to (1) Systemic inflammatory involvement, cytokine storm mediated through T-cell and monocytes resulting in myocarditis. Often patients have concomitant elevations in C-reactive protein (CRP), eosinophil sedimentation rate (ESR) (2) Hypercoagulability.

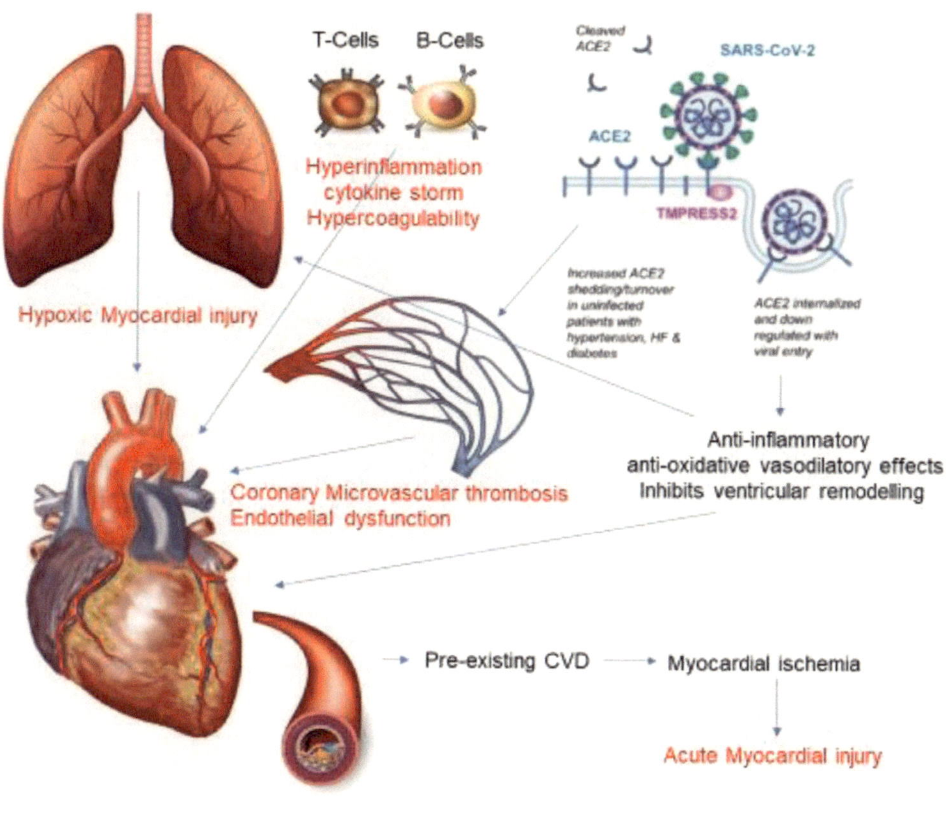

Figure 9.
Pathophysiological mechanisms of acute myocardial injury in COVID-19 infection.

Haematological differentials along with abnormal clotting factors and elevated D-dimer result in haemostasis and thrombosis as evident of coronary microvascular disease. (3) Endothelial injury causing diffuse disruption to the vasculature in several organs including the heart. (4) Down regulation of ACE2 expression in cardiomyocytes and loss of the protective signalling pathway (5) Inflammatory and stress response causing plaque rupture in those subjects with active coronary artery disease (**Figure 9**).

8. Biomarker evidence of myocardial injury in COVID-19

A significant proportion of patients requiring hospitalisation, intensive therapy and the need for mechanical ventilation demonstrate elevation of biomarkers of cardiac injury [42–44, 50–55], namely cardiac troponin T (cTnT); cardiac troponin I (cTnI) and the natriuretic peptides N-terminal pro-B-type natriuretic peptide (NTproBNP) and the active hormone b-type natriuretic peptide (BNP).

The evidence of cardiac injury in COVID-19 is wide ranging and its association with mortality differs between studies. Li and collages performed a meta-analysis of 28 studies involving 4,189 individuals with COVID-19. Elevated cardiac biomarkers (cTn, creatine kinase-MB, myoglobin and NTproBNP were associated with the severe forms of infection compared to subjects with mild forms of the disease (**Figure 10**). In addition, those with evidence of COVID-19

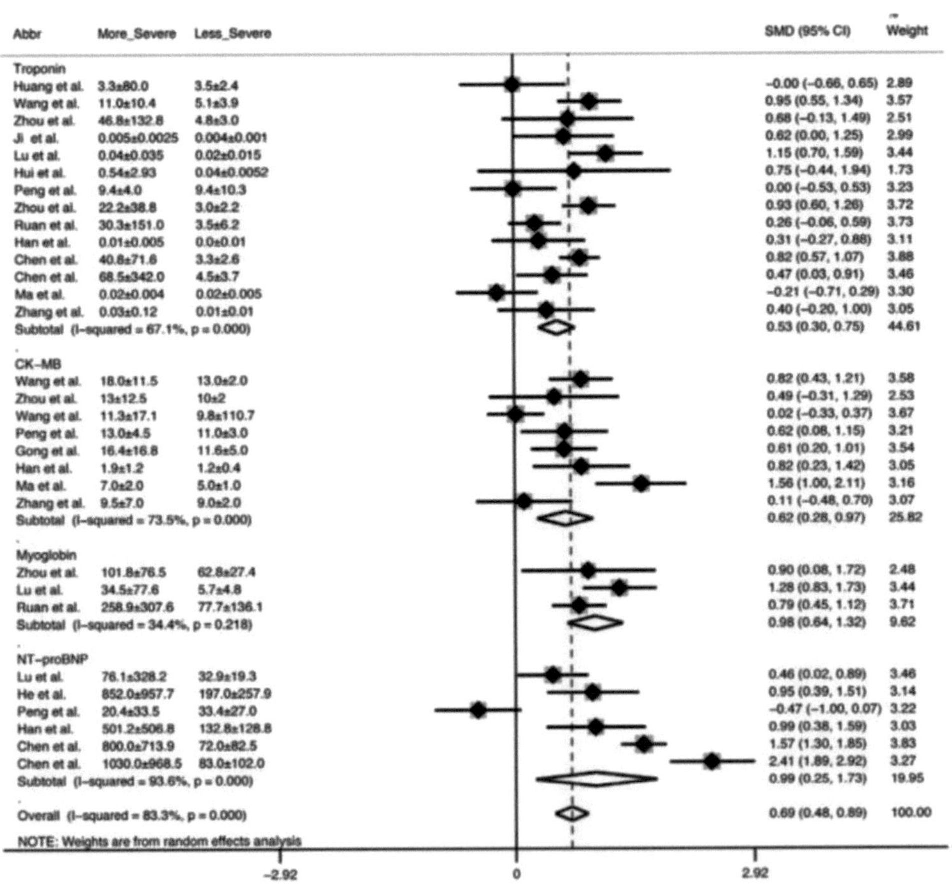

Figure 10.
Forest plot of cardiac biomarker standard mean difference between severe and less severe cases [source, Li et al. [53]].

related cardiac injury was more likely to die than those without (summary risk ratio 3.85 (95%CI 2.13 to 6.96, p = <0.001) [53].

With the emergence of cTn elevation in severe COVID-19 disease, attention turned to its prognostic value. A study of 416 COVID-19 patients by Shi and colleagues found elevated cTnI in 1 in 5 presenting patients, and positive cTn patients were more likely to require non-invasive ventilation and develop acute respiratory distress syndrome or acute kidney injury. In addition, the mortality rate was 10-fold higher in those patients with evidence of myocardial injury [43]. This is consistent with other studies.

Guo and colleagues reported 28% myocardial injury demonstrated by an elevated cTnT in 187 COVID-19 patients; with an in-hospital mortality of 60% and a higher incidence of mortality (69%) in those cTnT positive patients with underlying cardiovascular disease compared to 38% mortality in those without a cardiac history [55].

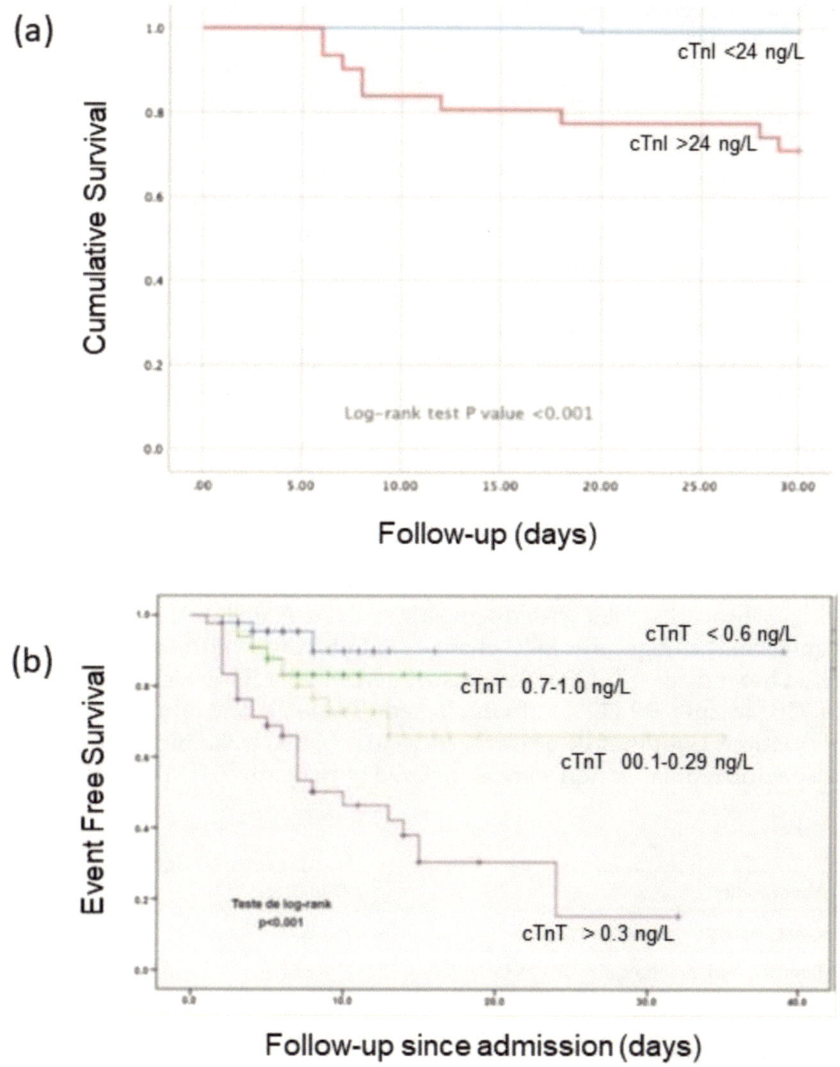

Figure 11.
Kaplan–Meier survival analysis of survival by (a) dichotomised cTnI over 40 days and by (b) cTnT quartiles over 30 days. [sources: Adapted from Cinar, et al. [61] and Almeida Jr. et al. [62] respectively].

Giustino and colleagues investigated 305 COVID-19 patients in 7 hospitals in New York City, USA and Milan, Italy. Patients exhibiting myocardial injury has elevated inflammatory markers, electrocardiographic abnormalities as well as transthoracic echocardiographic (TTE) evidence of left ventricular wall motion abnormalities, global left ventricular dysfunction, grade II or III left ventricular diastolic dysfunction, right ventricular dysfunction and pericardial effusion. In-hospital mortality was 32% in patients with myocardial damage and TT abnormalities, 19% with cTn positive myocardial injury only and 5% in those without evidence of cardiac involvement [56].

Lala and colleagues investigated the degree of myocardial injury in laboratory-confirmed cases of COVID-19 and correlated findings with outcome [57]. 36% of 2,736 patients had an elevated cTnI (>0.03 ng/mL).

Seven studies have investigated the prognostic value of elevated cTn in COVID-19. Five utilised cTnI [57–61], one cTnT [62] and one with combined cTnT and cTnI from different institutions [63]. In all cases, an elevated cTn (cTnI, **Figure 11a**; cTnT **Figure 11b**) was associated with poor outcome; be it in-hospital mortality, or combined endpoints of all-cause mortality and need for mechanical ventilation. Lala and colleagues [57] identified even minor elevations in cTnI (0.03 to 0.09 ng/ml) were associated with mortality (Hazard ratio 1.75; 95%CI = 1.37 to 2.24, $p < 0.001$). Those with greater cTnI concentrations above 0.09 ng/L conferred greater risk (Hazard ratio 3.03, 95% CI 2.42 to 3.80).

The underlying pathological mechanisms resulting in elevation in cTn in patients with COVID-19 have not been fully elucidated. The vast majority of reported cardiovascular complications in COVID-19 refer to acute cardiac injury, with an incidence of 8–22%. Other mechanisms (% incidence) include pulmonary thrombosis and arterial/venous thromboembolism (16–49%); chronic heart failure (52% in non-survivors, 12% in survivors); Acute coronary syndromes (44% with ST segment elevation myocardial infarction [STEMI]); arrhythmia (17% overall; 44% vs. 9% in severe and mild cases respectively). A few case reports have demonstrated myocarditis and pericardial disease [64].

9. Electrocardiographic and echocardiographic changes in COVID-19

The cardiac involvement in COVID-19 is diverse and as such varying different findings have been observed with diagnostic tools such as the electrocardiogram (ECG) and echocardiography. ECG changes in COVID-19 represent both left and right-sided heart disease [65] and are associated with a higher risk of mortality. In a study of 756 patients, 90 (12%) of which died (**Table 2**); one or more atrial premature contractions right bundle or intraventricular block, ischemic T-wave inversion and nonspecific repolarisation were associated with death [65]. These finding were

ECG Abnormality	Odds Ratio	95% CI
One or more atrial premature contraction	2.57	1.23 to 5.36
Right bundle branch or intraventricular block	2.61	1.32 to 5.18
Ischemic T-wave inversion	3.49	1.56 to 7.80
Nonspecific repolarisation	2.31	1.27 to 4.21

Table 2.
Odds ratio for ECG findings significantly associated with mortality. 95%CI, 95% confidence interval [source: McCullough et al. [65]].

further supported by De Vita and colleagues [66] who observed the ECG on admission was a helpful tool to identify COVID-19 patients with increased risk of death.

In a retrospective analysis of 319 severe and critically severe COVID-19 cases, Wang and colleagues observed 118 (37%) with normal ECG and 201 (63%) abnormal ECG traces. Differences were observed in ST-T changes, sinus tachycardia, atrial fibrillation, and atrial tachycardia between the group severity. Sinus tachycardia and atrial fibrillation were the independent risk factors of in-hospital death and ventilator use and could be used as an independent predictor of poor outcome [67].

A caveat to ECG induced changes is due to drug therapies given in severe COVID-19 infections. Drug-induced changes associated with chloroquine, hydroxychloroquine and azithromycin can result in a prolonged corrected QT (QTc), however such elongations do not induce arrhythmia-related death [68].

Echocardiographic findings demonstrate Left and right ventricular abnormalities in 39% and 33% of COVID-19 patients respectively [69]. severe ventricular dysfunction or tamponade is observed in approximately 15% of patients. In those without pre-existing cardiac disease the echocardiogram is abnormal in roughly half of COVID-19 patients with approximately 15% demonstrating severe disease. In a study of 90 hospitalised patients with severe (44, 49%) and non-severe (46, 51%) COVID-19; right ventricular (RV) and left ventricular (LV) functions were compared [70]. The RV and LV diameters were larger in severe patients compared to non-severe. Left ventricular ejection fraction (LVEF) were significantly ($p = <0.001$) lower (54.0% ±9.8%) in the severe-infections compared to the non-severe (61.9 ± 4.8%). Furthermore, pericardial effusions were observed in 23% of the severe patients with no observed cases in the non-severe patients.

In a study of 749 known COVID-19 positive patients undergoing transthoracic echocardiography (TTE), 38% were found to have LVEF ≤50% and 14% had moderately reduced right ventricular function. Stress-induced cardiomyopathy as evident by wall motion abnormalities were observed in four patients. A significant inverse relationship between cTnT and LVEF was observed ($P = -0.34$, $P = 0.006$). On the basis of the clinical TTE findings, therapeutic management was altered in 24% due to concern for a major cardiac even and in 14% where haemodynamic instability warranted TTE [71].

Both ECG and echocardiography are useful tools in the identification of left and right-sided cardiac dysfunction in COVID-19. Abnormalities are more frequent as infection severity increases and are often associated with poor prognosis.

10. Gross cardiac pathology and histopathology

A number of post-mortem (autopsy) studies have been performed on COVID-19 patients [72–79]. Four main pathological processes are generally observed: (a) Diffuse alveolar infiltration and damage with hyaline membrane formation, (b) thromboembolic disease in pulmonary and cardiac tissue and peripheral deep vein thrombosis, (c) hemophagocytes and (d) depletion of immune related cells [80, 81]. Gross cardiac examination (**Figure 12**) often reveals enlarged hearts [75, 76, 79] and the myocardium appears pale and flabby [76]. Thrombotic pathology is predominantly found in the lung, being present in 90% of cases; in 60% of hearts and 45% of kidneys [80].

In nine community deaths with suspected COVID-19 infections, Youd and colleagues did not observe any cases of myocarditis, however one case of bacterial bronchopneumonia had associated myocarditis. Contraction band necrosis was observed in a 86y Caucasian Male who had an underlying history of hypertension and cardiovascular disease. Cardiac amyloidosis was evident in one case [79].

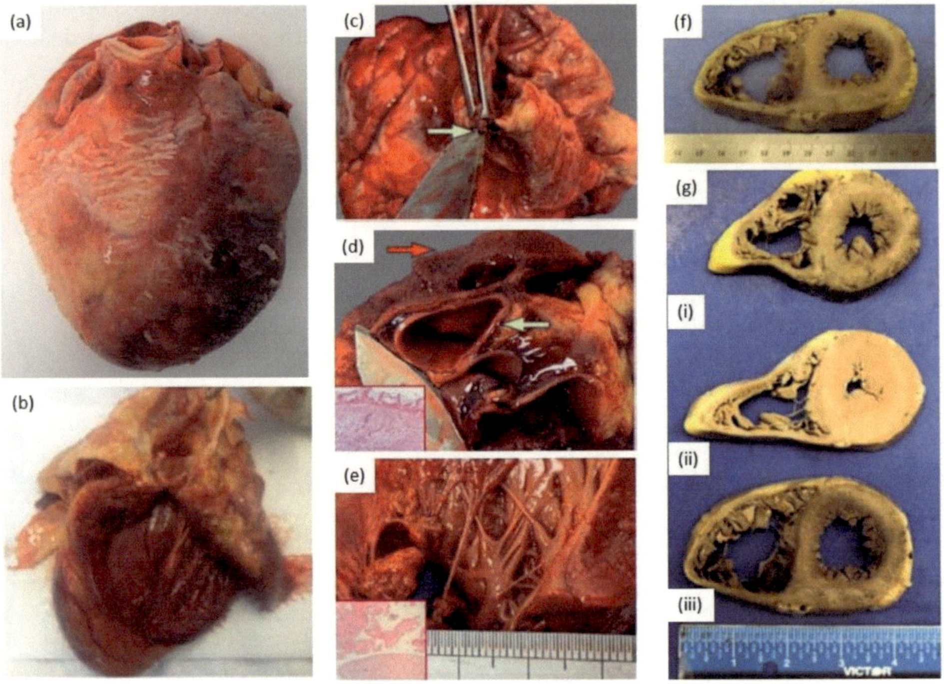

Figure 12.
Gross macroscopic cardiac pathology in COVID-19. (a) Fibrinous myocarditis; (b) cardiac hypertrophy with pale flabby myocardium; (c) macroscopic right coronary artery thrombosis (green arrow); (d) contained aortic dissection (green arrow) and fibrinous pericarditis (red arrow and H&E histology inset) in a 22y male; (e) gross marantic endocarditis with associated H&E histology inset; (f) extreme right ventricular dilatation with intraventricular septum straightening in a formalin fixed heart; (g) transverse sections demonstrating extensive right ventricular dilation of (i) 2.9:1.7 cm, (ii) 4.0:0.9 cm, (iii) 3.6:3.4 cm. [sources: Adapted from Youd et al. [79], Hanley et al. [80], Fox et al. [82, 83]].

An Italian study of 22 autopsies (18 with comorbid conditions, 4 without) demonstrated significant pulmonary and cardiovascular pathologies. All 22 deaths were reported as cardiorespiratory failure [76]. Cardiovascular pathologies are reported in **Table 3**.

A systematic review of histopathological findings by physiological system have identified cardiovascular findings such as focal lymphocytic inflammation, acute cardiomyocyte necrosis, presence of inflammatory cells and apoptotic bodies [74].

A multicentre study of 21 autopsy examinations by Basso and colleagues [73] examined cardiac tissue. Lymphocytic myocarditis was present in 3 (14%) cases, two of which were CD4 predominant T-cells, and one CD8 prominent. 86% of cases demonstrated interstitial macrophage infiltration. Mild pericarditis was evident in 4 cases. Common histological findings from cardiac tissue are presented in **Figure 13**.

Although the underlying mechanisms of cardiac involvement in COVID-19 infection remain to be fully elucidated, cardiac fibrosis occurs in tandem with local and systemic inflammatory responses [84]. Whilst these mechanisms are designed to facilitate healing following tissue damage, an excess of the inflammatory response along with the development of fibrotic tissue are pathological drivers for global organ damage. Overt inflammation and fibrosis in the heart can result in abnormal cardiac remodelling potentiating the development of acute and chronic heart failure. Anti-inflammatory and anti-fibrotic therapies are in general unsuccessful in improving damaged cardiac tissue function. With respect to COVID-19,

Histopathological findings	COVID-19 deaths with comorbid conditions (n = 18) (%)	COVID-19 deaths without comorbid conditions (n = 4) (%)
Myocarditis	9 (50.0)	3 (75.0)
Vasculitis	5 (27.8	3 (75.0)
Inflammatory infiltrate	13 (72.3)	3 (75.0)
Focal necrosis	6 (33.4)	2 (50.0)
Pericarditis	9 (50.0)	4 (100)
Vascular fibrosis	4 (22.3)	2 (50.0)

Table 3.
Cardiovascular histopathological findings in COVID-19 cadavers with and without comorbid conditions [source: Falasca et al. [76]].

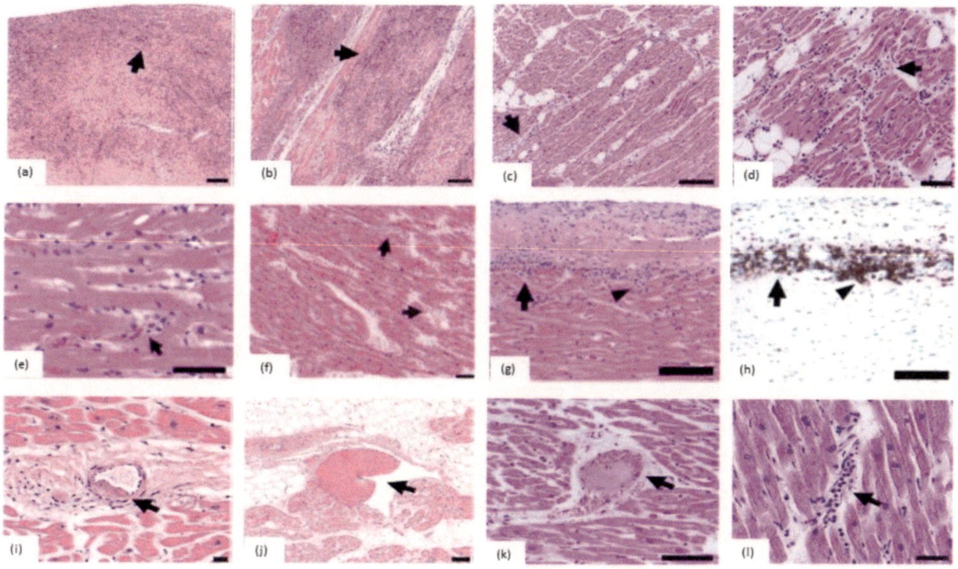

Figure 13.
(a and b) Myocarditis. Biventricular multifocal and diffuse lymphocytic myocarditis (arrows) with extensive myocyte injury and previously undiagnosed cardiac amyloidosis (H&E) x50 in an 86y male; (c and d) Biventricular multifocal lymphocytic myocarditis (arrows) with myocyte injury (H&E x100). Atrial fibrillation developed 2 d before death, 64y male; (e) Increased interstitial macrophage H&E x400) in a 60y male; (f) Increased macrophage cells within the myocardial interstitum (H&E x100) in a 73y female; (g) Focal lymphocytic pericarditis (arrows, H&E, x400) comprised of (h) CD8+ lymphocytes associated with focal myocardial inflammation in the absence of myocyte injury (arrowhead, CD8 immunostaining x400); (I and j) Small vessel changes. Microthrombus in a small myocardial artery (a, arrow H&E x100) and organised venous thrombosis (b, arrow H&E x100) in a 70y male; (k) Thrombus in a small myocardial vein (arrow, H&E x200) in a 71y male; (l) Leucocyte aggregates of eosinophils and mononuclear cells in capillaries and small veins (arrow, H&E x400) in a 64y male.[Source: Adapted from Basso et al., [73]].

further work is required to identify potential therapeutic targets of regulation and moderation of cardiac fibroblast function and thus reduce the burden of inflammatory-responsive fibrotic-based heart failure.

11. Conclusion

The novel Coronavirus disease, COVID-19 that emerged just over one year ago has caused substantial disruption to everyday life for every human on the planet. In the ensuing year, science and medicine have fought a race against time to understand the aetiology and pathogenicity of the disease. The overriding signs and symptoms supported by diagnostic testing indicates diffuse alveolar infiltration with vascular thromboembolic involvement in pulmonary, cardiac and renal tissue. Cardiac electrocardiography, echocardiography and cardiac biomarker testing are vital in the identification and management of patients with COVID-19 and concomitant cardiovascular involvement. Pathological findings at autopsy aid in the understanding of the pathophysiology of cardiovascular involvement in the disease. With the development of vaccines and mass vaccination programmes for the vulnerable along with herd immunity in the young, the global population will survive this novel pandemic but to significant cost both socially, economically and emotionally.

Author details

David C. Gaze
School of Life Sciences, University of Westminster, London, United Kingdom

*Address all correspondence to: d.gaze@westminster.ac.uk

References

[1] Cucinotta D, Vanelli M. WHO Declares COVID-19 a Pandemic. Acta Biomed. 2020 03 19,;91(1):157-60.

[2] WHO Coronavirus Disease (COVID-19) Dashboard [Internet]. []. Available from: www.covid19.who.int.

[3] Wise J. Covid-19: New coronavirus variant is identified in UK. BMJ. 2020 December 16;371:m4857.

[4] European Centre for Disease Prevention and Control. Risk related to spread of new SARS-CoV-2 variants of concern in the EU/EEA. 2020 29 December.

[5] Conti P, Caraffa A, Gallenga CE, Kritas SK, Frydas I, Younes A, et al. The British variant of the new coronavirus-19 (Sars-Cov-2) should not create a vaccine problem. J Biol Regul Homeost Agents. 2021 February 24;35(1):3.

[6] Peiris JSM, Yuen KY, Osterhaus ADME, Stöhr K. The severe acute respiratory syndrome. The New England journal of medicine. 2003 Dec 18,;349(25):2431-2441.

[7] Yao H, Song Y, Chen Y, Wu N, Xu J, Sun C, et al. Molecular architecture of the SARS-CoV-2 virus. Cell. 2020 October 29,;183(3):730,738.e13.

[8] Wang Q, Zhang Y, Wu L, Niu S, Song C, Zhang Z, et al. Structural and Functional Basis of SARS-CoV-2 Entry by Using Human ACE2. Cell (Cambridge). 2020 May 14,;181(4):894,904.e9.

[9] Balakumar P, Jagadeesh G. A century old renin-angiotensin system still grows with endless possibilities: AT1 receptor signaling cascades in cardiovascular physiopathology. Cell Signal. 2014 Oct;26(10):2147-2160.

[10] Gonzalez NC, Allen J, Schmidt EJ, Casillan AJ, Orth T, Wood JG. Role of the renin-angiotensin system in the systemic microvascular inflammation of alveolar hypoxia. Am J Physiol Heart Circ Physiol. 2007 May 01;292(5):2285.

[11] Lin C, Huang Y. Does the direct renin inhibitor have a role to play in attenuating severity of the outbreak coronavirus disease 2019 (COVID-19)?: Therapeutic Advances in Endocrinology and Metabolism. 2020 April 16,.

[12] Hamming I, Timens W, Bulthuis ML, Lely AT, Navis G, van Goor H. Tissue distribution of ACE2 protein, the functional receptor for SARS coronavirus. A first step in understanding SARS pathogenesis. J Pathol. 2004 June 01;203(2):631-637.

[13] Bos JM, Hebl VB, Oberg AL, Sun Z, Herman DS, Teekakirikul P, et al. Marked up-regulation of ACE2 in hearts of patients with obstructive hypertrophic cardiomyopathy: Implications for SARS-CoV-2-mediated COVID-19. Mayo Clin Proc. 2020 July 01;95(7):1354-1368.

[14] Banu N, Panikar SS, Leal LR, Leal AR. Protective role of ACE2 and its downregulation in SARS-CoV-2 infection leading to macrophage activation syndrome: Therapeutic implications. Life sciences (1973). 2020 Sep 1,;256:117905.

[15] Li H, Wang Y, Ji M, Pei F, Zhao Q, Zhou Y, et al. Transmission Routes Analysis of SARS-CoV-2: A Systematic Review and Case Report. Front Cell Dev Biol. 2020 -7-10;8.

[16] Fennelly KP. Particle sizes of infectious aerosols: Implications for infection control. The lancet respiratory medicine. 2020 Sep;8(9):914-924.

[17] Jones NR, Qureshi ZU, Temple RJ, Larwood JPJ, Greenhalgh T, Bourouiba L. Two metres or one: what is the evidence

for physical distancing in covid-19? BMJ. 2020 08 25,;370:m3223.

[18] Hindson J. COVID-19: Faecal–oral transmission? Nature reviews. Gastroenterology & hepatology. 2020 Mar 25,;17(5):259.

[19] Xu Y, Li X, Zhu B, Liang H, Fang C, Gong Y, et al. Characteristics of pediatric SARS-CoV-2 infection and potential evidence for persistent fecal viral shedding. Nature medicine. 2020 Mar 13,;26(4):502-505.

[20] Benton SC, Fraser CG. Faecal immunochemical tests in the COVID-19 pandemic; safety-netting of patients with symptoms and low faecal haemoglobin concentration – Can a repeat test be used? Ann Clin Biochem. 2020 October 5,:0004563220967569.

[21] Kayaaslan B, Korukluoglu G, Hasanoglu I, Kalem A, Eser F, Akinci E, et al. Investigation of SARS-CoV-2 in semen of patients in the acute stage of COVID-19 infection. Urologia internationalis. 2020 Sep;104(9-10): 678-683.

[22] Holtmann N, Edimiris P, Andree M, Doehmen C, Baston-Buest D, Adams O, et al. Assessment of SARS-CoV-2 in human semen—a cohort study. Fertil Steril. 2020 -8;114(2):233-8.

[23] Schwartz DA. An Analysis of 38 Pregnant Women With COVID-19, Their Newborn Infants, and Maternal-Fetal Transmission of SARS-CoV-2: Maternal Coronavirus Infections and Pregnancy Outcomes. Arch Pathol Lab Med. 2020 /07/01;144(7):799-805.

[24] Schwartz DA, Dhaliwal A. Infections in Pregnancy With COVID-19 and Other Respiratory RNA Virus Diseases Are Rarely, If Ever, Transmitted to the Fetus: Experiences With Coronaviruses, Parainfluenza, Metapneumovirus Respiratory Syncytial Virus, and Influenza. Arch Pathol Lab Med. 2020 /08/01;144(8):920-8.

[25] Kotlyar AM, Grechukhina O, Chen A, Popkhadze S, Grimshaw A, Tal O, et al. Vertical transmission of coronavirus disease 2019: a systematic review and meta-analysis. Am J Obstet Gynecol. 2020 -7-31.

[26] Rothan HA, Byrareedy SN. The epidemiology and pathogenesis of coronavirus disease (COVID-19) outbreak. Journal of Autoimmunity. 2020 May;109:102433.

[27] Li J, Huang DQ, Zou B, Yang H, Hui WZ, Rui F, et al. Epidemiology of COVID-19: A systematic review and meta-analysis of clinical characteristics, risk factors, and outcomes. Journal of Medical Virology;n/a(n/a).

[28] Stephanie S, Shum T, Cleveland H, Challa SR, Herring A, Jacobson FL, et al. Determinants of Chest X-Ray Sensitivity for COVID- 19: A Multi-Institutional Study in the United States. Radiology: Cardiothoracic Imaging. 2020 September 24,;2(5):e200337.

[29] Cozzi A, Schiaffino S, Arpaia F, Della Pepa G, Tritella S, Bertolotti P, et al. Chest x-ray in the COVID-19 pandemic: Radiologists' real-world reader performance. European journal of radiology. 2020 Nov;132:109272.

[30] Pereira RM, Bertolini D, Teixeira LO, Silla CN, Costa YMG. COVID-19 identification in chest X-ray images on flat and hierarchical classification scenarios. Computer methods and programs in biomedicine. 2020 Oct;194:105532.

[31] Salameh J, Leeflang MM, Hooft L, Islam N, McGrath TA, Pol CB, et al. Thoracic imaging tests for the diagnosis of COVID-19. Cochrane Database of Systematic Reviews. 2020(9).

[32] Bernheim A, Mei X, Huang M, Yang Y, Fayad ZA, Zhang N, et al. Chest CT findings in coronavirus Disease-19 (COVID-19): Relationship to duration of

infection. Radiology. 2020 Feb 20,;295(3):200463.

[33] Harmer D, Gilbert M, Borman R, Clark KL. Quantitative mRNA expression profiling of ACE 2, a novel homologue of angiotensin converting enzyme. FEBS Letters. 2002 December 4,;532(1):107-110.

[34] Yan R, Zhang Y, Li Y, Xia L, Guo Y, Zhou Q. Structural basis for the recognition of SARS-CoV-2 by full-length human ACE2. Science. 2020 March 27;367(6485):1444-1448.

[35] Yang L, Tu L. Implications of gastrointestinal manifestations of COVID-19. The Lancet Gastroenterology & Hepatology. 2020 /07/01;5(7):629-30.

[36] Mao R, Qiu Y, He J, Tan J, Li X, Liang J, et al. Manifestations and prognosis of gastrointestinal and liver involvement in patients with COVID-19: A systematic review and meta-analysis. The lancet. Gastroenterology & hepatology. 2020 Jul;5(7):667-678.

[37] Nguyen JL, Yang W, Ito K, Matte TD, Shaman J, Kinney PL. Seasonal Influenza Infections and Cardiovascular Disease Mortality. JAMA Cardiol. 2016 06 01,;1(3):274-81.

[38] Alhogbani T. Acute myocarditis associated with novel middle east respiratory syndrome coronavirus. Ann Saudi Med. 2016 Jan-Feb;36(1):78-80.

[39] Corrales-Medina VF, Suh KN, Rose G, Chirinos JA, Doucette S, Cameron DW, et al. Cardiac complications in patients with community-acquired pneumonia: A systematic review and meta-analysis of observational studies. PLoS Med. 2011 Jun;8(6):e1001048.

[40] Yu C, Wong RS, Wu EB, Kong S, Wong J, Yip GW, et al. Cardiovascular complications of severe acute respiratory syndrome. Postgrad Med J. 2006 Feb;82(964):140-144.

[41] Wang D, Hu B, Hu C, Zhu F, Liu X, Zhang J, et al. Clinical Characteristics of 138 Hospitalized Patients With 2019 Novel Coronavirus–Infected Pneumonia in Wuhan, China. JAMA. 2020 -3-17; 323(11):1061-9.

[42] Huang C, Wang Y, Li X, Ren L, Zhao J, Hu Y, et al. Clinical features of patients infected with 2019 novel coronavirus in Wuhan, China. Lancet. 2020 02 15,;395(10223):497-506.

[43] Shi S, Qin M, Shen B, Cai Y, Liu T, Yang F, et al. Association of Cardiac Injury With Mortality in Hospitalized Patients With COVID-19 in Wuhan, China. JAMA Cardiol. 2020 07 01,;5(7):802-10.

[44] Zhou F, Yu T, Du R, Fan G, Liu Y, Liu Z, et al. Clinical course and risk factors for mortality of adult inpatients with COVID-19 in Wuhan, China: a retrospective cohort study. Lancet. 2020 03 28,;395(10229):1054-62.

[45] Lombardi CM, Carubelli V, Iorio A, Inciardi RM, Bellasi A, Canale C, et al. Association of Troponin Levels with Mortality in Italian patients hospitalized with coronavirus disease 2019: Results of a multicenter study. JAMA Cardiol. 2020 August 26.

[46] Grasselli G, Zangrillo A, Zanella A, Antonelli M, Cabrini L, Castelli A, et al. Baseline Characteristics and Outcomes of 1591 Patients Infected With SARS-CoV-2 Admitted to ICUs of the Lombardy Region, Italy. JAMA. 2020 04 28,;323(16):1574-81.

[47] Akbariqomi M, Hosseini MS, Rashidiani J, Sedighian H, Biganeh H, Heidari R, et al. Clinical characteristics and outcome of hospitalized COVID-19 patients with diabetes: A single-center, retrospective study in Iran. Diabetes research and clinical practice. 2020 Nov;169:108467.

[48] Docherty AB, Harrison EM, Green CA, Hardwick HE, Pius R,

Norman L, et al. Features of 20 133 UK patients in hospital with covid-19 using the ISARIC WHO clinical characterisation protocol: Prospective observational cohort study. BMJ. 2020;369:m1985.

[49] Goyal P, Choi JJ, Pinheiro LC, Schenck EJ, Chen R, Jabri A, et al. Clinical characteristics of Covid-19 in new York City. New England Journal of Medicine. 2020 June 11,;382(24):2372-2374.

[50] Bavishi C, Bonow RO, Trivedi V, Abbott JD, Messerli FH, Bhatt DL. Acute myocardial injury in patients hospitalized with COVID-19 infection: A review. Progress in Cardiovascular Diseases. 2020 June 6,.

[51] Chen T, Wu D, Chen H, Yan W, Yang D, Chen G, et al. Clinical characteristics of 113 deceased patients with coronavirus disease 2019: retrospective study. BMJ. 2020 03 26,;368:m1091.

[52] Gaze DC. Clinical utility of cardiac troponin measurement in COVID-19 infection. Ann Clin Biochem. 2020 May 01;57(3):202-205.

[53] Li J, Han T, Woodward M, Anderson CS, Zhou H, Chen Y, et al. The impact of 2019 novel coronavirus on heart injury: A Systematic review and Meta-analysis. Prog Cardiovasc Dis. 2020 Jul - Aug;63(4):518-24.

[54] Lippi G, Lavie CJ, Sanchis-Gomar F. Cardiac troponin I in patients with coronavirus disease 2019 (COVID-19): Evidence from a meta-analysis. Prog Cardiovasc Dis. 2020 June 01;63(3):390-391.

[55] Guo T, Fan Y, Chen M, Wu X, Zhang L, He T, et al. Cardiovascular Implications of Fatal Outcomes of Patients With Coronavirus Disease 2019 (COVID-19). JAMA Cardiol. 2020 07 01,;5(7):811-8.

[56] Giustino G, Croft LB, Stefanini GG, Bragato R, Silbiger JJ, Vicenzi M, et al. Characterization of myocardial injury in patients with COVID-19. J Am Coll Cardiol. 2020 November 03;76(18):2043-2055.

[57] Lala A, Johnson KW, Januzzi JL, Russak AJ, Paranjpe I, Richter F, et al. Prevalence and Impact of Myocardial Injury in Patients Hospitalized With COVID-19 Infection. J Am Coll Cardiol. 2020 -08-04;76(5):533-46.

[58] Al Abbasi B, Torres P, Ramos-Tuarez F, Dewaswala N, Abdallah A, Chen K, et al. Cardiac troponin-I and COVID-19: A prognostic tool for In-hospital mortality. Cardiol Res. 2020 December 01;11(6):398-404.

[59] Shah P, Doshi R, Chenna A, Owens R, Cobb A, Ivey H, et al. Prognostic value of elevated cardiac troponin I in hospitalized Covid-19 patients. Am J Cardiol. 2020 August 28.

[60] Cordeanu EM, Duthil N, Severac F, Lambach H, Tousch J, Jambert L, et al. Prognostic value of troponin elevation in COVID-19 hospitalized patients. J Clin Med. 2020 December 17;9(12):10.3390/jcm9124078.

[61] Cinar T, Hayiroglu MI, Cicek V, Kilic S, Asal S, Dogan S, et al. Prognostic significance of cardiac troponin level in Covid-19 patients without known cardiovascular risk factors. Am J Emerg Med. 2020 December 18.

[62] Almeida Junior, G L G, Braga F, Jorge JK, Nobre GF, Kalichsztein M, Faria PMP, et al. Prognostic value of troponin-T and B-type natriuretic peptide in patients hospitalized for COVID-19. Arq Bras Cardiol. 2020 October 01;115(4):660-666.

[63] Schiavone M, Gasperetti A, Mancone M, Kaplan AV, Gobbi C, Mascioli G, et al. Redefining the prognostic value of high-sensitivity

troponin in COVID-19 patients: The importance of concomitant coronary artery disease. J Clin Med. 2020 October 12;9(10):10.3390/jcm9103263.

[64] Imazio M, Klingel K, Kindermann I, Brucato A, De Rosa FG, Adler Y, et al. COVID-19 pandemic and troponin: Indirect myocardial injury, myocardial inflammation or myocarditis? Heart. 2020 August 01;106(15):1127-1131.

[65] McCullough SA, Goyal P, Krishnan U, Choi JJ, Safford Mokika M, Okin Peter M. Electrocardiographic findings in coronavirus Disease-19: Insights on mortality and underlying myocardial processes. Journal of cardiac failure. 2020 Jul;26(7):626-632.

[66] De Vita A, Ravenna SE, Covino M, Lanza O, Franceschi F, Crea F, et al. Electrocardiographic Findings and Clinical Outcome in Patients with COVID-19 or Other Acute Infectious Respiratory Diseases. J Clin Med. 2020 -11-12;9(11).

[67] Wang Y, Chen L, Wang J, He X, Huang F, Chen J, et al. Electrocardiogram analysis of patients with different types of COVID-19. Annals of Noninvasive Electrocardiology. 2020;25(6):e12806.

[68] Mehraeen E, Seyed Alinaghi SA, Nowroozi A, Dadras O, Alilou S, Shobeiri P, et al. A systematic review of ECG findings in patients with COVID-19. Indian Heart J. 2020 December 01;72(6):500-507.

[69] Dweck MR, Bularga A, Hahn RT, Bing R, Lee KK, Chapman AR, et al. Global evaluation of echocardiography in patients with COVID-19. European Heart Journal - Cardiovascular Imaging. 2020 September 1,;21(9):949-58.

[70] Barman HA, Atici A, Tekin EA, Baycan OF, Alici G, Meric BK, et al. Echocardiographic features of patients with COVID-19 infection: A cross-sectional study. Int J Cardiovasc Imaging. 2020 October 08.

[71] Jain SS, Liu Q, Raikhelkar J, Fried J, Elias P, Poterucha TJ, et al. Indications for and Findings on Transthoracic Echocardiography in COVID-19. J Am Soc Echocardiogr. 2020 -10;33(10): 1278-84.

[72] Barton LM, Duval EJ, Stroberg E, Ghosh S, Mukhopadhyay S. COVID-19 Autopsies, Oklahoma, USA. Am J Clin Pathol. 2020 May 05;153(6):725-733.

[73] Basso C, Leone O, Rizzo S, De Gaspari M, van der Wal, A C, Aubry MC, et al. Pathological features of COVID-19-associated myocardial injury: A multicentre cardiovascular pathology study. Eur Heart J. 2020 October 14;41(39):3827-3835.

[74] Deshmukh V, Motwani R, Kumar A, Kumari C, Raza K. Histopathological observations in COVID-19: A systematic review. J Clin Pathol. 2020 August 18.

[75] Elsoukkary SS, Mostyka M, Dillard A, Berman DR, Ma LX, Chadburn A, et al. Autopsy findings in 32 patients with COVID-19: A single-institution experience. Pathobiology. 2020 September 17:1-13.

[76] Falasca L, Nardacci R, Colombo D, Lalle E, Di Caro A, Nicastri E, et al. Postmortem findings in Italian patients with COVID-19: A descriptive full autopsy study of cases with and without comorbidities. J Infect Dis. 2020 November 09;222(11):1807-1815.

[77] Sperhake J. Autopsies of COVID-19 deceased? Absolutely! Leg Med (Tokyo). 2020 -11;47:101769.

[78] Xu Z, Shi L, Wang Y, Zhang J, Huang L, Zhang C, et al. Pathological findings of COVID-19 associated with acute respiratory distress syndrome. Lancet Respir Med. 2020 April 01;8(4):420-422.

[79] Youd E, Moore L. COVID-19 autopsy in people who died in community settings: The first series. J Clin Pathol. 2020 December 01;73(12):840-844.

[80] Hanley B, Naresh KN, Roufosse C, Nicholson AG, Weir J, Cooke GS, et al. Histopathological findings and viral tropism in UK patients with severe fatal COVID-19: A post-mortem study. The Lancet Microbe. 2020 Oct;1(6):e245-e253.

[81] Maiese A, Manetti AC, La Russa R, Di Paolo M, Turillazzi E, Frati P, et al. Autopsy findings in COVID-19-related deaths: A literature review. Forensic Sci Med Pathol. 2020 October 07.

[82] Fox SE, Akmatbekov A, Harbert JL, Li G, Quincy Brown J, Vander Heide RS. Pulmonary and cardiac pathology in African American patients with COVID-19: An autopsy series from New Orleans. Lancet Respir Med. 2020 July 01;8(7):681-686.

[83] Fox SE, Li G, Akmatbekov A, Harbert JL, Lameira FS, Brown JQ, et al. Unexpected features of cardiac pathology in COVID-19 infection. Circulation. 2020 September 15;142(11):1123-1125.

[84] Smolgovsky S, Ibeh U, Tamayo TP, Alcaide P. Adding insult to injury - Inflammation at the heart of cardiac fibrosis. Cell Signal. 2021 -01;77:109828.

Chapter 9

The Function of Seven Transmembrane Receptors in the Cardiovascular System and Their Role in the Development of Cardiomyopathy

Valentina Kubale, Ewelina Prozorowska, Kristýna Glocová, Lucy Slater and Catrin Sian Rutland

Abstract

The G-protein-coupled receptors (GPCRs, also called seven-transmembrane receptor, 7TMRs, or heptahelical receptor) are a conserved family of seven transmembrane receptors which are essential not only in the healthy heart and blood vessels but also in for treatment and therapy of cardiovascular disease and failure. Heart failure is a global leading cause of morbidity and death and as such understanding 7TMRs, their functions, structures and potential for therapy is essential. This review will investigate the roles of the receptors in the healthy functioning cardiovascular system, and in cardiac disorders with an emphasis in cardiomyopathy. It will also explore the role of autoimmunity and autoantibodies against the G-protein-coupled receptors in cardiomyopathy.

Keywords: angiotensin, adrenoreceptors, cardiomyopathy, heart disease, endothelin-1, muscarinic receptors, vascular

1. Introduction

The 7 transmembrane receptors (7TMRs) also known as G-protein coupled receptors (GPCRs) constitute the largest family of plasma membrane receptors. The superfamily of 7TMRs includes receptors for hormones, neurotransmitters and ion channels, and is critical to mediate physiological and cellular processes [1, 2].

Composed of seven transmembrane hydrophobic alpha (α) helices joined by three intracellular and three extracellular loop structures, a cytoplasmic carboxyl terminus and an extracellular amino terminus (**Figure 1**), 7TMRs signal by stimulating heterotrimeric G proteins following the presentation of an agonist to the receptor [3]. Agonist binding at the 7TMR extracellular region initiates the formation of a G protein. Guanosine diphosphate (GDP) is released from the G protein in exchange for guanosine triphosphate (GTP). The GTP bound α subunit disassociates from the βγ dimer, both of which activate several effectors such as adenylyl cyclase, phospholipases and ion channels [3]. The Gα subunit can be categorised in

IntechOpen

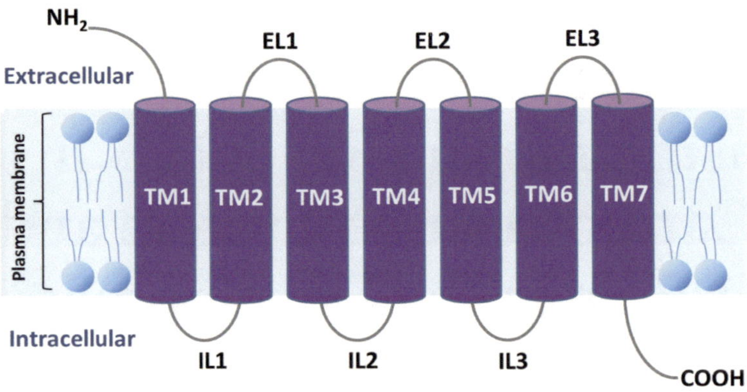

Figure 1.
General structure of a seven transmembrane receptor (7TMR)/G protein coupled receptor (GPCR). Extracellular loops 1–3 (EL1–3) and intracellular loops (IL1–3) connecting the 7 transmembrane helices (TM1–7). NH_2–N-terminal chain and COOH–C-terminal chain.

to sub groups $G\alpha_s$, $G\alpha_i$, $G\alpha_{q/11}$ and $G\alpha_{12/13}$ [3]. The Gα subunits and the Gβγ dimer deriving from the heterotrimeric G protein can combine with downstream effector molecules such as adenylyl cyclase or phospholipase C to control cellular signalling pathways involving secondary messengers [3]. Examples of secondary messengers include cyclic adenosine monophosphate (cAMP), inositol-1,4,5-trisphosphate (IP_3) and diacylglycerol (DAG) which elicit cellular and physiological responses [4].

2. Cardiovascular effects of 7TMRs and therapeutic drug targets

7TMRs are the target for a large proportion of therapeutic drugs, currently encompassing more than 30% of prescription medications [5] which directly or indirectly alter cellular signalling mechanisms.

2.1 Adrenoreceptors (β-adrenergic receptors)

Adrenergic receptors (ARs; also known as adrenoreceptors) are a class of 7TMRs located in the heart and vasculature and are responsible for relaying sympathetic nervous system (SNS) messages into cardiovascular reactions [1]. The neurotransmitters norepinephrine (NE) and epinephrine (Epi), which originate from the SNS, exert their effects on cardiac cells and tissues by binding to adrenoreceptors [6]. A number of adrenoreceptor subgroups are present in the mammalian heart, including three α_1-ARs, three α_2-ARs and three β-ARs (β_1, β_2 and β_3) [6].

β-Adrenergic receptors (β-ARs) are the most important and one of the most frequently studied receptors belonging to the family of G-protein coupled receptors [7]. There are three subtypes of β-ARs: β_1, β_2 and β_3, activation of which regulates important cardiovascular functions [7, 8]. The β1-ARs are characterised mainly for the heart, β_2-ARs for blood vessels and β_3-ARs for adipose tissue [9]. Within the vasculature the predominant subtype is β_2-AR, which is 65–70% homologous to β1- and β_3-ARs [8]. The agonists that bind with all three subtypes of β-ARs are the hormones adrenaline and noradrenaline, which help regulate cardiovascular and pulmonary function [10, 11].

Human genes encoding the β_2-ARs are without introns and have been mapped to chromosome 5q31–32 [12]. The β-ARs consist of 413 amino acid residues, approximately 46.5 kDa [8]. There are three domains of β_2-ARs: The extracellular domain, the transmembrane domain responsible for the ligands binding and the intracellular domain, which interacts with G protein and kinases such as β-ARK [13]. β_2-ARs occur mainly in the lungs, where their presence has been shown in airway smooth muscle (30,000–40,000 per cell), epithelial and endothelial cells, type II cells and mast cells [8]. Moreover β_2-ARs are in heart, kidney and blood vessels—mainly arterioles [8, 14].

As in the other G-receptors the signalling pathway of β_2-ARs, which bind with a hormone ligand includes three basic steps: Receptor binding, G protein activation and effector system activation. β_2-ARs may occur in two forms, activated and inactivated [6]. The binding of β-ARs agonist with β2-receptor activates the pathway in which Gs coupled proteins are involved. The stimulation of G proteins causes guanosine triphosphate (GTP) to bind to the α-subunit (Gsα) that activates it. The G-subunits dissociate, and α-subunits stimulate adenylate cyclase (AC) to formation of cyclic adenosine 3′,5′-monophosphate (cAMP). It is stated that cAMP acts as a catalyst for the process of activation of protein kinase A (PKA) and due to that it is involved in control of muscle tone. On the other hand cAMP inhibits the release of cytosolic calcium ion (Ca^{2+}) in the smooth muscle cells, which leads to vascular relaxation (vasodilation) [8, 15].

Although the β_2-ARs activated by β_2-ARs agonists mostly influence the blood vessels (mainly arterioles and coronary arteries), they can also act in the heart and kidney. In the atrial and ventricular myocardium, stimulation of β_2-ARs leads to increase in cardiac muscle contractility or relaxation, whilst in the kidneys it stimulates the release of renin, what it turn influences activation of the renin-angiotensin-aldosterone system [1, 8].

The primary role of the β-ARs in the heart is to coordinate the heart rate and contractility in response to the SNS neurotransmitters [6]. β_1-AR is the most abundant subtype accounting for 75–80% in a healthy myocardium [6]. Around 15–18% of cardiomyocyte β-ARs are β_2-AR whilst the remaining 2–3% of β-AR density is composed of β_3-ARs [6]. Activation of β_1-ARs and to a smaller degree β_2-ARs, leads to an increase in cardiac contractility and an accelerated cardiac rate. Stimulation of the two predominate β-ARs also increases impulse transmission via the atrioventricular node [6]. The activation of cardiomyocyte β_1- and β_2-ARs also leads to a significant increase in free intracellular Ca^{2+} concentration [6]. Calcium is a secondary messenger in many biological systems. In cardiomyocytes, calcium affects ion channels which regulate ionic currents, impacting upon action potentials and muscle contractility [16]. B_3-AR appears to illicit an opposite effect on cardiac function to that induced by β_1- and β_2-ARs in that it acts to prevent cardiac hyperstimulation from NE and Epi (**Table 1**) [6].

Constant elevation of catecholamines leading to β-AR signalling changes results in overstimulation of cardiac function [1]. Reducing the β-AR activity is vital to alleviate the risk of long-term cardiac tissue damage such as cardiomyopathy. Propanolol was discovered to be a β-AR antagonist in 1964, a so called β-blocker. Alprenolol and Practolol β-blockers have also been used for the management of heart failure [1]. β-Blockers function to overcome the harmful effects of norepinephrine which overstimulate the β_1-AR, leading to a reduction in cardiac workload [1]. The most recently used β-blockers bisoprolol and carvedilol target both β_1- and β_2-ARs produce a survival benefit for heart failure patients [1]. In rats β_2-AR agonists (fenoterol and zinterol) were shown to reduce progression of left ventricular modelling in dilated cardiomyopathy in addition to decreasing myocardial cell death [17]. In a later study the same group determined that in a rat model of dilated ischemic cardiomyopathy, Metoprolol, a β_1-AR blocker, action is enhanced when given in combination with the β_2-AR agonist fenoterol [18].

Action	β_1-AR	β_2-AR	B_3-AR
Heart muscle contraction		Yes	Yes
Increases cardiac output	Yes	Yes	
Increases heart rate in SA node	Yes	Yes	
Increases atrial contractility	Yes	Yes	
Increases contractility and automaticity of ventricular muscle	Yes	Yes	
Dilates muscular blood vessels		Yes	Yes
Increases perfusion in blood vessels		Yes	
Metabolism/lipolysis/thermogenesis			Yes
Prevent cardiac hyperstimulation			Yes

Table 1.
Actions of β-adrenergic receptors.

The β_2-ARs have also been directed implicated in patients with ischaemic cardiomyopathy. A Gln27Glu polymorphism of β_2-AR was discovered in a study investigating 155 people with heart failure of ischaemic aetiology with impaired Left Ventricular Ejection Fraction ≤35% [19]. Three allele categories were discovered, the most common genotype in heart failure was Gln27Gln, and the least common was Glu27Glu, whilst Gln27Glu was not significantly different between heart failure and control subjects. The study concluded that the Glu allele was associated with lower myocardial infarction rate and highlighted that patient response to β-blockade therapy may be altered [19]. Likewise β_1-AR (Ser49Gly, Arg389Gly) and β2-AR (Arg16Gly, Gln27Glu, Thr164Ile) polymorphisms did not alter in a Polish cohort study of patients with idiopathic dilated cardiomyopathy [20]. It is of interest that in patients with Takotsubo cardiomyopathy, β-AR polymorphisms (β_1-AR (Gly389Arg) and β_2-AR (Arg16Gly and Gln27Glu)) were significantly different to controls but similar to patients with ST-elevation myocardial infarction [21]. Work combining beta-blockers with ACE-inhibitors/angiotensin receptor blockers over the years using meta-analysis data has shown reduced recurrence of the disorder [22].

A murine model depleting levels of β_2-ARs also resulted in diabetic cardiomyopathy in vivo and reduced β_2-ARs in cardiomyocytes grown under in hyperglycemic conditions [23]. Conversely, overexpression of β_2-ARs (by 300 fold) in mice showed that over time severe cardiomyopathy was observed, resulting in interstitial fibrosis, loss of myocytes and myocyte hypertrophy. In the majority of the 81% of mice that died within 15 months, heart failure was observed [24]. These results were similar to other transgenic overexpression mouse lines. The authors hypothesised that a number of mechanisms from activation of growth or transcriptional factors, cross-talk with other pathways, necrosis or apoptosis of cardiac myocytes and/or high heart rates limiting energy supply.

The human heart also possesses α_1 adrenoreceptors (α_1-AR) although in a smaller quantity to the β-ARs [25]. The α_1-ARs are expressed in the heart, both the $\alpha 1_A$-and $\alpha 1_B$-AR subtypes are expressed in human myocytes, and have been shown to regulate contractility [26, 27]. The α_1-ARs combine with the $G_{q/11}$ family of G proteins, in turn activating phospholipase C. The secondary messenger IP_3 binds to receptors on the membrane of the sarcoplasmic reticulum, triggering the release of intracellular Ca^{2+} [6]. The raised Ca^{2+} level leads an increase in vasoconstriction [6]. The coupling of α_1-ARs to the $G_{q/11}$ family of G proteins also produces DAG and subsequent protein kinase C [6].

In heart failure the α_1-ARs may offer a protective benefit to maintain cardiac inotropy, preventing cardiomyocyte apoptosis and maladaptive cardiac remodelling [6]. Although a small study, loss of β_1-AR and no change in β_2-AR levels in end-stage dilated cardiomyopathy patients was observed alongside a loss of α_{1A}-ARs [28]. Although the role of β_1-AR in heart failure has long been described, this interaction between the α-ARs was novel as the few previous studies had shown no change or increases in α-ARs binding but these were different types of heart failure. In addition a total of 26 proteins of interest were also identified in the cardiomyopathy patients, some of which have been linked to G-protein coupled receptor signalling and desensitisation [28]. Prostatic binding protein levels decreased whereas increases in ANP32A and clathrin were noted. Also of interest are Takotsubo cardiomyopathy (also known as stress cardiomyopathy) patients. This condition is often reversible, and two studies have shown that several β_1-AR and α2c-AR polymorphisms were not implicated in Takotsubo cardiomyopathy [29, 30].

2.2 Angiotensin II type 1 and 2 receptors

Angiotensin II (AngII) is an important protein in the renin-angiotensin system (RAS). In the bloodstream renin converts angiotensinogen (derived from liver) into angiotensin I, which in turn is transformed into AngII by angiotensin converting enzyme (ACE) [14, 31, 32]. AngII can be also secreted in some local tissues including within the brain, heart, arteries and kidney [32].

The Angiotensin II type 1 and 2 receptors (AT_1 and AT_2 receptors) belong to the wide family of G-protein coupled receptors (GPCRs), members of which have seven transmembrane spanning domains and is the biggest member of the human genome [31, 33]. The distinction and classification of AT_1 and AT_2 receptors is based on their varied affinity for different non-peptide antagonists [34]. Moreover the AT_1 and AT_2 receptors differ between each other in their number of amino acids, tissue-specific expression and mechanisms of signal transferring [13]. Both of these receptors occur in all mammals and bind a peptide hormone angiotensin II (AngII), which is the most important effector in the RAS [32].

The main role of angiotensin becomes apparent in the cardiovascular and endocrine systems where it regulates blood pressure and hydro-electrolytic homeostasis [32, 33]. It is stated that the main physiological functions of AngII (vasoconstriction, aldosterone secretion, renal regulations cellular dedifferentiation and proliferation) are mediated mostly by the AT_1 subtype of angiotensin receptor [14, 31, 33–36]. In humans, the genes encoding AT_1 receptors are mapped on chromosome 3q21–3q25 [37]. The AT_1 receptors consist of 359 amino acids, with a molecular weight of 41 kDa, and their amino sequence reveals 20–35% homology with other GPCRs [31].

In adult mammals, AT_1 receptors are mainly expressed in kidney (glomeruli, proximal tubules, vasculature, medullary interstitial cells), adrenal glands (cortex, medulla), heart (myocardium, ganglia, conduction system), brain (circumventricular organs, thalamus, basal ganglia, cerebellar cortex, medulla oblongata) and vasculature (smooth muscles, adventitia) [32, 38]. Rats and mice can have two isoforms of the Angiotensin II 1 receptor: AT_{1A} and AT_{1B} with amino acid sequence convergence seen at 94% [14, 31, 33, 34]. AT_{1A} receptors are present predominantly in vascular smooth muscle, liver, lung and kidney whilst AT_{1B} receptors occur mainly in the adrenal gland and anterior pituitary [31, 34, 38]. The rodent AT_{1A} and AT_{1B} receptor genes are situated on chromosomes 17 and 2 respectively [38].

The activity of angiotensin II through AT_1 receptors should be considered in physiological and pathophysiological conditions. The physiological signalling pathway involves the renin-angiotensin-aldosteron system and leads to changes in blood pressure primarily through vasoconstriction of arteries and arterioles, secretion of aldosterone from adrenal gland and sodium reabsorption by via the kidney tubules [32]. Ang II mediates vasoconstriction through the IP3/DAG pathway, which uses Gq/11 protein-coupled receptors. Gq/11 activates phospholipase C (PLC), which hydrolyses phosphatidylinositol 4,5-bisphosphate (PIP2) and produces diacyl glycerol (DAG) and inositol trisphosphate (IP3). IP3 causes an increase in intracellular calcium whilst DAG activates protein kinases C [31]. The increased concentration of calcium (Ca^{2+} ions) within vascular smooth muscle cells leads to vasoconstriction which results in an increase in blood pressure or may causing a localised reduction in blood flow in some specific tissues [32, 36]. AngII acting through the AT_1 receptors located in the zona glomerulosa of the adrenal gland stimulates the release of aldosterone [32]. Aldosterone then acts on the distal convoluted tubules and the cortical collecting ducts in kidney, firstly causing sodium (Na^+) retention, leading to increased peripheral resistance and secondly causing resorption of water from urine which also increases extracellular fluid volume. Both of these mechanisms lead to an elevation in arterial pressure [32].

Considering the pathological conditions, the activity of AngII through AT_1 receptors may induce the proliferation of vascular smooth muscle cells which in turn promotes myocyte hypertrophy and causes vascular fibrosis. Proliferation of smooth muscle cells is also involved in the initial stages of atherosclerotic plaques formation in arteries [32]. AngII binding to AT_1 receptors also activate the multiple intracellular signalling pathway that promotes atherosclerosis. The pathway includes oxidative stress, inflammation, endothelial dysfunction, tissue remodelling, proliferation fibrosis, thrombosis and autostimulation. Moreover AngII may participate in the process of atherosclerosis lesion formation as it stimulates the release of endothelin-1 (ET-1) from the endothelial cells [32]. In addition to inducing proliferation and atherosclerotic plaques formation, AngII may have an effect on the developing/developed plaques. Atherosclerotic plaque stability and disruption is in turn associated with matrix metalloproteinase (MMP) enzymes, the production of which can be stimulated by AngII [32]. The MMPs are inhibited by tissue inhibitors of metalloproteinases (TIMPs) and disruption of the balance between MMPs and TIMPs may lead to cardiovascular diseases [37, 39]. Moreover, in pathological states, the activation of AT_1 receptor by AngII may cause vascular remodelling and growth by expression of autocrine growth factors (including fibroblast growth factor and platelet-derived growth factor) in vascular smooth muscle cells [32, 40].

The activation of AT_2 receptors by AngII has an opposite effect to AT_1 receptors. It means that the functions of AngII mediated by AT_2 receptors are vasodilation, natriuresis and inhibition of cellular growth and proliferation [14]. Genes encoding AT_2 receptors are localised on chromosome Xq22-q2 [13, 31]. The molecular weight of AT_2 receptors is approximately 41 kDa and they consist of 363 amino acids [13, 41].

AT_2 receptor expression has been localised in both foetal and adult tissues. In foetuses, expression of AT_2 receptors is intense, especially in a cardiovascular system [13]. In adult mammals the expression of AT_2 receptor is still observed in heart (mainly in myocardium) and renal blood vessels but is significantly lower than before birth [13, 38]. Expression of AT_2 receptors has been also noted in the adrenal gland (cortex and medulla), brain (thalamus, cerebellar cortex), mesenteric and uterine arteries [38, 42].

It is stated that the AT_2 receptor acts to stabilise blood pressure by controlling vascular tone by vasodilation [13]. In this action the AT_2 receptor together with other GPCR family B2 receptors for bradykinin form a stable functional heterodimer, which causes the increase of nitric oxide (NO) and stimulating cyclic guanosine monophosphate (cGMP) synthesis. The cGMP contributes to relaxation of smooth muscles, which in large veins, large arteries, and smaller arterioles leads to vasodilation and causes decreased blood pressure. It has also been suggested that activation of AT_2 receptors by AngII may inhibit arterial and myocardial hypertrophy and fibrosis in the ageing heart and vasculature.

Therefore AngII exerts its influence via the activation of the Angiotensin II type I receptor (AT_1R), a 7TMR located in vascular smooth muscle as well as in the kidneys, brain and adrenal glands in an effort to maintain sodium/water homeostasis and moderate vasoconstriction [1]. AT_1R acts to control arterial pressure, blood volume and to encourage growth and proliferation through the activation of cellular signalling mechanisms [15]. The AT_1R is a $G_{q/11}$ coupled receptor [25]. Stimulation by AngII leads to the activation of phospholipase C-β and the release of DAG and IP_3, followed by the activation of protein kinase C and movement of intracellular calcium [3]. AT_1Rs are upregulated in cardiac tissue in response to hypertrophic triggers, encouraging unfavourable cardiac remodelling in heart failure [9]. These complex roles have resulted in a number of angiotensin receptor blockers (ARBs) and angiotensin converting enzyme (ACE) inhibitors to be developed and used as cardiovascular treatments. ARBs and ACE inhibitors have demonstrated a reduction in deleterious left ventricular remodelling, such as hypertrophy and myocardial stiffness which as associated with heart failure [6]. ACE inhibitors alongside antagonists of the AT_1R, the -sartans, have become one of the main pharmaceutical treatments for hypertension and cardiovascular disease [1]. Commonly used ARBs include Losartan, Valsartan and Candesartan [43]. ARBs function to interfere with the renin-angiotensin system by preventing the binding of AngII to AT_1R. This inhibition of AngII result in vascular smooth muscle relaxation, a reduction in cellular hypertrophy, and a decrease in plasma volume resulting from an increase in salt and water excretion [43].

A number of advances in terms of cardiomyopathy and ANGII and its receptors have been made in the last few years. In terms of cardiomyopathy, the AngII receptor inhibitor LCZ696 has been shown to inhibit extracellular signal-regulated kinase (ERK), resulting in increased survival in pregnancy-associated cardiomyopathy mice. The authors indicated that by reducing cardiac hypertrophy, fibrosis and apoptosis it could act as a potential treatment for this cardiomyopathy [44]. Another study showed that this angiotensin receptor-neprilysin inhibitor reduced inflammation, oxidative stress and apoptosis in vitro and in vivo [45]. It has also been stated that in end-stage hypertrophic cardiomyopathy, the modern Angiotensin receptor neprilysin inhibitor treatments are both safe and effective [46]. Angiotensin-converting enzyme 2 (ACE2) has also showed therapeutic potential when looking at doxorubicin-induced cardiomyopathy rat models [47]. The enzyme reduced apoptosis, inflammatory responses, and oxidative stress and reduced mortality and myocardial fibrosis whilst improving ventricular remodelling and cardiac function. They also showed activation of the AMPK and PI3K-AKT pathways, inhibition of the ERK pathway, and decreased TGF-β1 [47]. Sulforaphane, which activates nuclear factor erythroid 2-related factor 2 (Nrf2), has also been shown to present angiotensin II-induced cardiomyopathy via Akt/GSK-3ß/Fyn -mediated Nrf2 activation [48].

Aldehyde dehydrogenase 2 (ALDH2) has also been shown to protect against alcoholic cardiomyopathy [49]. By decreasing angiotensinogen and AngII this cardioprotective enzyme inhibited local RAS in mice by inhibiting the p38 MAPK/CREB pathway. In another form of cardiomyopathy, hypertrophic, ACE inhibitors angiotensin-receptor blockers have been used to try and regulate the renin-angiotensin-aldosterone system [50]. This has resulted in patients having a lower risk of developing atrial fibrillation which is associated with hypertrophic cardiomyopathy.

Much work has looked into polymorphisms in the angiotensin-converting enzyme gene itself in relation to hypertrophic cardiomyopathy risk; however, the studies have sometimes shown conflicting results. A systematic review and meta-analysis indicated that the ACE insertion/deletion (I/D of 287 base pairs in intron 16) polymorphism was probably a risk for hypertrophic cardiomyopathy [51]. People with the DD genotype have increased levels of ACE and angiotensin II and therefore more hypertrophy and fibrosis, as seen in other situations where their levels increase. Although many of the 1 in 500 people affected by hypertrophic cardiomyopathy have mutations in the genes coding for sarcomeric proteins, polymorphisms in the components of the RAS are implicated. ACE DD has also been associated with dilated cardiomyopathy patients, angiotensin receptor type 11166CC genotypes with both hypertrophic and dilated cardiomyopathy and the 235TT genotype of angiotensinogen (M235T) is associated with hypertrophic, dilated and restrictive cardiomyopathy [52].

Overstimulation of AngII has also been reported in dilated cardiomyopathy [53] and AT1R overexpression resulted in female mice being more affected (especially in terms of heart failure and increased mortality) than males [53]. In particular, ventricular hypertrophy and dilation and changes in Ca^{2+} activity and homeostasis were observed, and these reflect that clinical observations that dilated cardiomyopathy can be exacerbated in women in comparison to men. This can also be linked to oestrogen which increases angiotensinogen and decreased renin, ACE and AT1R expression but of course following menopause these effects are lost [54].

Much has been investigated in relation to the use of ACE inhibitors in patients with ischemic cardiomyopathy. Much work has been carried out in patients with an ejection fraction of less than 40% with these enzymes working well. More recently attention has turned to those with an ejection fraction of more than 40% who were studied less. In patients with 40–50% ejection fraction, the ACE inhibitors were seen to reduce the risk of mortality, nonfatal myocardial infarction and stroke by 21% [55].

2.3 Endothelin-1 (ET-1) receptor

There are three different forms of 21-amino acid peptides, which belong to the endothelin peptide family: ET-1, ET-2, and ET-3 [56]. They vary in biological function and may affect blood vessels as well as other tissues both within and outside of the cardiovascular system [56]. The predominant form of endothelin peptide is an isopeptide ET-1 with potent vasoconstrictor and proliferative properties [57]. ET-1 is synthetized by endothelial cells, airway smooth muscles cells, cardiomyocytes, macrophages, leukocytes and mesangial cells [57].

There are two subtypes of receptors which are mediated by endothelin, known as Endothelin Type A receptor (ET_A) and type B (ET_B) [57]. Although mediated by the same peptide agonist, activity of these two subtypes is usually opposite, as the ET_A receptor promotes vasoconstriction, growth, and inflammation whilst ET_B receptors may cause both vasoconstriction and vasodilation and also increases in sodium excretion and inhibition of growth and inflammation [57–59].

The potential to bind with ET_A receptors is the same for ET-1 and ET-2 endothelin but lower for ET-3 endothelin, whilst the potential binding rate with ET_B receptors is equal for every form of endothelin [57, 58]. In people the genes responsible for expression of the ET_A receptors are situated on chromosome 4q31.22-q31.23, whilst genes encoding ET_B receptors are mapped onto chromosome 13q22.3 [60]. The molecular weight of the ET_A and ET_B receptors are 48 and 50 kDa respectively [61, 62]. The human 427 amino acid long ET_A receptors and 442 amino acid long ET_B receptors are approximately 64% homologous [58]. The homology of ET_A and ET_B receptors in humans and other mammalian species is between 88% and 97% [58].

ET_A receptors are expressed predominantly in the heart (coronary vasculature and cardiomyocytes), lungs (pulmonary artery), kidney (renal artery, afferent and efferent arteriole, cortical vasculature, mesangial cells), brain (cerebral vasculature) and adrenal gland. ET_B receptors also occur in the heart (coronary vasculature and cardiomyocytes), lungs (pulmonary artery), kidney (renal artery, afferent and efferent arteriole, medullar vasculature), brain (cerebral vasculature) and adrenal gland [63].

The ET_A receptors mediated by ET-1 endothelin in vascular smooth muscle cells promoting vasoconstriction, hypertension, hypertrophy, fibrosis and inflammatory changes, including atherosclerosis and due to that has activity similar to the AT_1 receptors mediated by AngII [63]. The vasoconstrictive pathway of ET_A receptors includes: Coupling to phospholipase C (PLC) via GTP-binding protein, phospholipase C activation, phosphatidyl inositol hydrolysis, inositol 1,4,5 triphosphate (IP3) generation and 1,2-diacylglycerol (DCG) accumulation. Inositol triphosphate is a signalling molecule that leads to mobilisation of Ca^{2+} from intra- and extra-cellular sources resulting in long-lasting vasoconstriction [56, 64].

The ET_B receptors mediated by ET-1 endothelin in the vascular endothelium are involved in the clearance of ET-1 and stimulate vasodilation due to the nitric oxide and cyclooxygenase metabolites production, which also exert vasorelaxant effects on the underlying smooth muscle. Moreover, the ET_B receptors have a natriuretic action causing sodium and water resorption from the distal tubules and collecting ducts in the kidney. The ET_B receptors, which occur in smooth muscle cells, additionally act as vasoconstrictors [57, 63, 64].

In the last few years research into endothelin has progressed the information known about links to cardiomyopathies. Some of the early published studies showed that ET-1 and its receptor either played a causative role in hypertrophic cardiomyopathy, idiopathic dilated cardiomyopathy and uremic cardiomyopathy or could be a marker [65–68]. Indeed work in cats has even reflected the increased ET-1 levels in cases of hypertrophic, dilated, restrictive and unclassified cardiomyopathy [69]. More work has now been carried out into other cardiomyopathies and the potential mechanisms of action. Much like ACE2, the endothelin receptor blocker bosentan has been shown to inhibit doxorubicin-induced cardiomyopathy in a rodent model [70]. This study looked at the receptor blocker as elevated levels of ET-1 were discovered in doxorubicin treated patients. The in vitro studies indicated that activation of the epidermal growth factor (EGF) receptor and the MEK1/2-ERK1/2 cascade were possible mechanisms of action [70]. A good review looking at endothelin-1 and atrial cardiomyopathy, published in 2019 brings together the information in this area. The work over the years has indicated that endothlin-1 plays an active role affecting Ca^{2+} levels, via the ET-1-superoxide-MMP9 cascade and via apoptosis, resulting in both electrical and anatomical remodelling [71].

Not only is endothelin-1 a potential therapeutic route but it also shows promise in predicting patient outcomes. A recent study investigating new-onset atrial fibrillation in patients with obstructive hypertrophic cardiomyopathy has shown that elevated pre-operative levels may indicate increased likelihood of atrial fibrillation [72]. Big endothelin-1, the precursor of endothelin-1 has also been shown to be useful when predicting prognosis for hypertrophic cardiomyopathy patients and the authors have suggested that it should be added to marker panels [73, 74]. Endothelin

1 has also been implicated as a modifier in dilated cardiomyopathy. With variations including the rare G > A and a C > T at c.90 seen in dilated cardiomyopathy patients and *EDN1* polymorphisms linked to increased risk of the disorder, likely by altered the stability of the protein [75]. A model of diabetic cardiomyopathy in rats also showed that plasma endothelin-2 levels were higher that controls and that overexpression of the protein results in a more severe phenotype [76].

2.4 Muscarinic receptors

Cardiac function is controlled by the SNS and parasympathetic nervous system (PNS). Parasympathetic vagal nerves are distributed throughout all areas of the heart, particularly in the ventricles [77]. Cardiac muscarinic receptors are activated by acetylcholine, having been stimulated by vagal nerve activation. The muscarinic acetylcholine receptors (M-ChR) are glycoproteins belonging to the 7TMR superfamily [77]. The M_2 subtype of M-ChR are the most prevalent group within the mammalian heart and their function is opposed to the β-ARs in that they cause a reduction in myocardium contractility and a lower cardiac rate [10]. M-ChR exert their influence on the myocardium via the $G\alpha_1$-coupled receptors which inhibit adenylyl cyclase whilst the Gβγ dimer impedes the activity of potassium channels in the sinoatrial node [1]. M-ChR can also exert an effect over Ca^{2+} channels [77] affecting cardiac contractility.

Heart failure patients demonstrate an increase in M_2 muscarinic receptor density, with activated M_2 receptors encouraging an inotropic response [9]. One study using serum from a patient showed that when autoantibodies to the muscarinic receptors and β-ARs were activated it resulted in cardiomyopathy and atrial tachyarrhythmias [78]. Along a similar line, autoantibodies against β1-ARs have been shown to cause sudden death in idiopathic dilated cardiomyopathy patients [79]. Antibodies to β-ARs have been discovered in people with idiopathic dilated cardiomyopathy, even leading to the suggestion of a form of 'adrenergic cardiomyopathy' [80]. In addition autoantibodies against muscarinic receptors have also been noted in cases of peripartum cardiomyopathy [81], dilated cardiomyopathy [82–85], and M2-muscarinic acetylcholine receptor autoantibodies have been implicated in playing a role in atrial fibrillation in dilated cardiomyopathy patients [86] Similar increases were not observed in patients with Takotsubo cardiomyopathy [87] or in rats with cirrhotic cardiomyopathy [88]. Autoantibodies against cardiomyocytes, β_1- or β_2-ARs or M_2 muscarinic receptors were not noted in 20 people with Takotsubo cardiomyopathy in comparison to healthy controls, or in rats with cirrhotic cardiomyopathy.

3. Conclusions

The superfamily of 7TMRs includes receptors for hormones, neurotransmitters and ion channels, and are critical to mediate physiological and cellular processes [1, 2]. This chapter has investigated adrenoreceptors (both α- and β-adrenergic receptors) and the components of the renin-angiotensin system (RAS) especially AngII, ACE and the AT1 and AT2 receptors. The chapter has also looked at endothelin-1 (ET-1) and its receptor, and precursor Big endothelin-1 and finally the muscarinic receptors. By looking at their numerous effects in both healthy and diseased vasculature and cardiac disorders, especially cardiomyopathies, it can be seen that there are wide ranging effects. Developing these 7TMRs as markers of disease, for prognosis, diagnosis and therapeutic treatments is becoming more important as their many roles as being uncovered in the cardiovascular system.

Acknowledgements

The authors would like to thank their institutions for funding them. Ewelina Prozorowska, Kristýna Glocová, and Lucy Slater were undertaking research internships with Catrin Sian Rutland at The University of Nottingham, UK. Kristýna Glocová had her internship funded by The European Association of Veterinary Anatomists (EAVA), Young Research Career Development Award; therefore, Kristýna and Catrin would like to thank the EAVA. The ORCID ID of Catrin Rutland is https://orcid.org/0000-0002-2009-4898.

Conflicts of interest

The authors declare no conflicts of interest.

Author details

Valentina Kubale[1], Ewelina Prozorowska[2,4], Kristýna Glocová[3,4], Lucy Slater[4] and Catrin Sian Rutland[4*]

1 Veterinary Faculty, Institute for Preclinical Sciences, University of Ljubljana, Ljubljana, Slovenia

2 Department of Histology and Embryology, Poznań University of Life Sciences, Poznań, Poland

3 University of Veterinary and Pharmaceutical Sciences Brno, Brno, Czech Republic

4 School of Veterinary Medicine and Science, Medical Faculty, University of Nottingham, Nottingham, UK

*Address all correspondence to: catrin.rutland@nottingham.ac.uk

References

[1] Foster SR, Roura E, Molenaar P, Thomas WG. G protein-coupled receptors in cardiac biology: Old and new receptors. Biophysical Reviews. 2015;7(1):77-89

[2] Pierce KL, Premont RT, Lefkowitz RJ. Seven-transmembrane receptors. Nature Reviews. Molecular Cell Biology. 2002;**3**(9):639-650

[3] Nieto Gutierrez A, McDonald PH. GPCRs: Emerging anti-cancer drug targets. Cellular Signalling. 2018;**41**:65-74

[4] Rockman HA, Koch WJ, Lefkowitz RJ. Seven-transmembrane-spanning receptors and heart function. Nature. 2002;**415**(6868):206-212

[5] Shenoy SK. Seven-transmembrane receptors and ubiquitination. Circulation Research. 2007;**100**(8):1142-1154

[6] Siryk-Bathgate A, Dabul S, Lymperopoulos A. Current and future G protein-coupled receptor signaling targets for heart failure therapy. Drug Design, Development and Therapy. 2013;**7**:1209-1222

[7] Sigg DD, Hezi-Yamit A. Cardiac and Vascular Receptors and Signal Transduction. Handbook of Cardiac Anatomy, Physiology and Devices. New York, USA: Humana Press; 2009. pp. 191-218

[8] Johnson M. Molecular mechanisms of beta(2)-adrenergic receptor function, response, and regulation. The Journal of Allergy and Clinical Immunology. 2006;**117**(1):18-24

[9] Wang J, Gareri C, Rockman HA. G-protein-coupled receptors in heart disease. Circulation Research. 2018;**123**(6):716-735

[10] Myslivecek J, Trojan S. Regulation of adrenoceptors and muscarinic receptors in the heart. General Physiology and Biophysics. 2003;**22**(1):3-14

[11] Rosenbaum DM, Cherezov V, Hanson MA, Rasmussen SGF, Thian FS, Kobilka TS, et al. GPCR engineering yields high-resolution structural insights into beta(2)-adrenergic receptor function. Science. 2007;**318**(5854):1266-1273

[12] Johnson JA, Terra SG. Beta-adrenergic receptor polymorphisms: Cardiovascular disease associations and pharmacogenetics. Pharmaceutical Research. 2002;**19**(12):1779-1787

[13] Li Y, Li XH, Yuan H. Angiotensin II type-2 receptor-specific effects on the cardiovascular system. Cardiovascular Diagnosis and Therapy. 2012;**2**(1):56-62

[14] Carey RM, Padia SH. Angiotensin AT2 receptors: Control of renal sodium excretion and blood pressure. Trends in Endocrinology and Metabolism. 2008;**19**(3):84-87

[15] Ainscough JF, Drinkhill MJ, Sedo A, Turner NA, Brooke DA, Balmforth AJ, et al. Angiotensin II type-1 receptor activation in the adult heart causes blood pressure-independent hypertrophy and cardiac dysfunction. Cardiovascular Research. 2009;**81**(3):592-600

[16] Bers DM. Calcium cycling and signaling in cardiac myocytes. Annual Review of Physiology. 2008;**70**:23-49

[17] Ahmet I, Lakatta EG, Talan MI. Complimentary effects of chronic pharmacologic manipulation of beta-adrenergic receptor (beta AR) subtype signaling in rodent dilated ischemic cardiomyopathy. Circulation. 2003;**108**(17):95

[18] Ahmet I, Lakatta EG, Talan MI. Pharmacological stimulation of beta2-adrenergic receptors (beta2AR) enhances therapeutic effectiveness of beta1AR blockade in rodent dilated ischemic cardiomyopathy. Heart Failure Reviews. 2005;**10**(4):289-296

[19] Metaxa S, Missouris C, Mavrogianni D, Miliou A, Oikonomou E, Toli E, et al. Polymorphism Gln27Glu of beta2 adrenergic receptors in patients with ischaemic cardiomyopathy. Current Vascular Pharmacology. 2018;**16**(6):618-623

[20] Paczkowska A, Szperl M, Malek L, Mazurkiewicz L, Skora E, Grzybowski J, et al. Polymorphisms of the beta-1 and beta-2 adrenergic receptors in Polish patients with idiopathic dilated cardiomyopathy. Kardiologia Polska. 2009;**67**(3):235-241

[21] Vriz O, Minisini R, Zito C, Boccato E, Fimiani F, Pirisi M, et al. Can apical ballooning cardiomyopathy and anterior STEMI be differentiated based on beta1 and beta2-adrenergic receptors polymorphisms? International Journal of Cardiology. 2015;**199**:189-192

[22] Brunetti ND, Santoro F, De Gennaro L, Correale M, Gaglione A, Di Biase M, et al. Combined therapy with beta-blockers and ACE-inhibitors/angiotensin receptor blockers and recurrence of takotsubo (stress) cardiomyopathy: A meta-regression study. International Journal of Cardiology. 2017;**230**:281-283

[23] Mishra PK, Givvimani S, Metreveli N, Tyagi SC. Attenuation of beta2-adrenergic receptors and homocysteine metabolic enzymes cause diabetic cardiomyopathy. Biochemical and Biophysical Research Communications. 2010;**401**(2):175-181

[24] Du XJ, Gao XM, Wang B, Jennings GL, Woodcock EA, Dart AM. Age-dependent cardiomyopathy and heart failure phenotype in mice overexpressing beta(2)-adrenergic receptors in the heart. Cardiovascular Research. 2000;**48**(3):448-454

[25] Capote LA, Mendez Perez R, Lymperopoulos A. GPCR signaling and cardiac function. European Journal of Pharmacology. 2015;**763**(Pt B):143-148

[26] Skomedal T, Borthne K, Aass H, Geiran O, Osnes JB. Comparison between alpha-1 adrenoceptor-mediated and beta adrenoceptor-mediated inotropic components elicited by norepinephrine in failing human ventricular muscle. The Journal of Pharmacology and Experimental Therapeutics. 1997;**280**(2):721-729

[27] Jensen BC, Swigart PM, De Marco T, Hoopes C, Simpson PC. Alpha 1-adrenergic receptor subtypes in nonfailing and failing human myocardium. Circulation: Heart Failure. 2009;**2**(6):654-663

[28] Shi T, Moravec CS, Perez DM. Novel proteins associated with human dilated cardiomyopathy: Selective reduction in alpha(1A)-adrenergic receptors and increased desensitization proteins. Journal of Receptor and Signal Transduction Research. 2013;**33**(2):96-106

[29] Handy AD, Prasad A, Olson TM. Investigating genetic variation of adrenergic receptors in familial stress cardiomyopathy (apical ballooning syndrome). Journal of Cardiology. 2009;**54**(3):516-517

[30] Sharkey SW, Maron BJ, Nelson P, Parpart M, Maron MS, Bristow MR. Adrenergic receptor polymorphisms in patients with stress (tako-tsubo) cardiomyopathy. Journal of Cardiology. 2009;**53**(1):53-57

[31] Guo DF, Sun YL, Hamet P, Inagami T. The angiotensin II type

1 receptor and receptor-associated proteins. Cell Research. 2001;**11**(3):165-180

[32] Naik P, Murumkar P, Giridhar R, Yadav MR. Angiotensin II receptor type 1 (AT1) selective nonpeptidic antagonists—A perspective. Bioorganic & Medicinal Chemistry. 2010;**18**(24):8418-8456

[33] Petrel C, Clauser E. Angiotensin II AT(1) receptor constitutive activation: From molecular mechanisms to pathophysiology. Molecular and Cellular Endocrinology. 2009;**302**(2):176-184

[34] Audoly LP, Oliverio MI, Coffman TM. Insights into the functions of type 1 (AT(1)) angiotensin II receptors provided by gene targeting. Trends in Endocrinology and Metabolism. 2000;**11**(7):263-269

[35] Unal H, Karnik SS. Constitutive activity in the angiotensin II type 1 receptor: Discovery and applications. Advances in Pharmacology. 2014;**70**:155-174

[36] Kawai T, Forrester SJ, O'Brien S, Baggett A, Rizzo V, Eguchi S. AT1 receptor signaling pathways in the cardiovascular system. Pharmacological Research. 2017;**125**(Pt A):4-13

[37] Liu P, Sun M, Sader S. Matrix metalloproteinases in cardiovascular disease. The Canadian Journal of Cardiology. 2006;**22**(Suppl B):25B-30B

[38] Allen AM, Zhuo J, Mendelsohn FA. Localization and function of angiotensin AT1 receptors. American Journal of Hypertension. 2000;**13**(1 Pt 2):31S-38S

[39] Hassoun PM, Mouthon L, Barbera JA, Eddahibi S, Flores SC, Grimminger F, et al. Inflammation, growth factors, and pulmonary vascular remodeling. Journal of the American College of Cardiology. 2009;**54** (1 Suppl):S10-S19

[40] Rubenstein DA, Yin W. Platelet-activation mechanisms and vascular remodeling. Comprehensive Physiology. 2018;**8**(3):1117-1156

[41] Kambayashi Y, Bardhan S, Takahashi K, Tsuzuki S, Inui H, Hamakubo T, et al. Molecular cloning of a novel angiotensin II receptor isoform involved in phosphotyrosine phosphatase inhibition. The Journal of Biological Chemistry. 1993;**268**(33):24543-24546

[42] Hannan RE, Widdop RE. Vascular angiotensin II actions mediated by angiotensin II type 2 receptors. Current Hypertension Reports. 2004;**6**(2):117-123

[43] Israili ZH. Clinical pharmacokinetics of angiotensin II (AT1) receptor blockers in hypertension. Journal of Human Hypertension. 2000;**14** (Suppl 1):S73-S86

[44] Wang Y, Guo Z, Gao Y, Liang P, Shan Y, He J. Angiotensin II receptor blocker LCZ696 attenuates cardiac remodeling through the inhibition of the ERK signaling pathway in mice with pregnancy-associated cardiomyopathy. Cell & Bioscience. 2019;**9**:86

[45] Ge Q, Zhao L, Ren XM, Ye P, Hu ZY. Feature article: LCZ696, an angiotensin receptor-neprilysin inhibitor, ameliorates diabetic cardiomyopathy by inhibiting inflammation, oxidative stress and apoptosis. Experimental Biology and Medicine (Maywood, N.J.). 2019;**244**(12):1028-1039

[46] Rubis P, Wisniowska-Smialek S, Holcman K, Lesniak-Sobelga A, Kostkiewicz M, Podolec P. Angiotensin receptor neprilysin inhibitor treatment is safe and potentially efficacious in endstage hypertrophic cardiomyopathy. Polish Archives of Internal Medicine. 2017;**127**(3):216-218

[47] Ma H, Kong J, Wang YL, Li JL, Hei NH, Cao XR, et al. Angiotensin-converting enzyme 2 overexpression protects against doxorubicin-induced cardiomyopathy by multiple mechanisms in rats. Oncotarget. 2017;**8**(15):24548-24563

[48] Xin Y, Bai Y, Jiang X, Zhou S, Wang Y, Wintergerst KA, et al. Sulforaphane prevents angiotensin II-induced cardiomyopathy by activation of Nrf2 via stimulating the Akt/GSK-3ss/Fyn pathway. Redox Biology. 2018;**15**:405-417

[49] Liu B, Zhang R, Wei S, Yuan Q, Xue M, Hao P, et al. ALDH2 protects against alcoholic cardiomyopathy through a mechanism involving the p38 MAPK/CREB pathway and local renin-angiotensin system inhibition in cardiomyocytes. International Journal of Cardiology. 2018;**257**:150-159

[50] Huang CY, Yang YH, Lin LY, Tsai CT, Hwang JJ, Chen PC, et al. Renin-angiotensin-aldosterone blockade reduces atrial fibrillation in hypertrophic cardiomyopathy. Heart. 2018;**104**(15):1276-1283

[51] Yuan Y, Meng L, Zhou Y, Lu N. Genetic polymorphism of angiotensin-converting enzyme and hypertrophic cardiomyopathy risk: A systematic review and meta-analysis. Medicine (Baltimore). 2017;**96**(48):e8639

[52] Rani B, Kumar A, Bahl A, Sharma R, Prasad R, Khullar M. Renin-angiotensin system gene polymorphisms as potential modifiers of hypertrophic and dilated cardiomyopathy phenotypes. Molecular and Cellular Biochemistry. 2017;**427**(1-2):1-11

[53] Mathieu S, El Khoury N, Rivard K, Paradis P, Nemer M, Fiset C. Angiotensin II overstimulation leads to an increased susceptibility to dilated cardiomyopathy and higher mortality in female mice. Scientific Reports. 2018;**8**(1):952

[54] Fischer R, Dechend R, Gapelyuk A, Shagdarsuren E, Gruner K, Gruner A, et al. Angiotensin II-induced sudden arrhythmic death and electrical remodeling. American Journal of Physiology. Heart and Circulatory Physiology. 2007;**293**(2):H1242-H1253

[55] Alzahrani T, Tiu J, Panjrath G, Solomon A. The effect of angiotensin-converting enzyme inhibitors on clinical outcomes in patients with ischemic cardiomyopathy and midrange ejection fraction: A post hoc subgroup analysis from the PEACE trial. Therapeutic Advances in Cardiovascular Disease. 2018;**12**(12):351-359

[56] Luscher TF, Barton M. Endothelins and endothelin receptor antagonists—Therapeutic considerations for a novel class of cardiovascular drugs. Circulation. 2000;**102**(19):2434-2440

[57] Ergul A. Endothelin-1 and endothelin receptor antagonists as potential cardiovascular therapeutic agents. Pharmacotherapy. 2002;**22**(1):54-65

[58] Schneider MP, Boesen EI, Pollock DM. Contrasting actions of endothelin ET(A) and ET(B) receptors in cardiovascular disease. Annual Review of Pharmacology. 2007;**47**:731-759

[59] Roig JC, Fink J, Burchfield DJ. Pharmacologic Adjuncts. I. Assisted Ventilation of the Neonate. 5th ed. London, UK: Elsevier Health Sciences; 2016. pp. 347-370

[60] Braasch I, Volff JN, Schartl M. The endothelin system: Evolution of vertebrate-specific ligand-receptor interactions by three rounds of genome duplication. Molecular Biology and Evolution. 2009;**26**(4):783-799

[61] Mazzuca MQ, Khalil RA. Vascular endothelin receptor type B: Structure, function and dysregulation in vascular

disease. Biochemical Pharmacology. 2012;**84**(2):147-162

[62] Hayzer DJ, Rose PM, Lynch JS, Webb ML, Kienzle BK, Liu ECK, et al. Cloning and expression of a human endothelin receptor—Subtype-A. The American Journal of the Medical Sciences. 1992;**304**(4):231-238

[63] Dhaun N, Webb DJ. Endothelins in cardiovascular biology and therapeutics. Nature Reviews. Cardiology. 2019;**16**(8):491-502

[64] Miyauchi T, Sakai S. Endothelin and the heart in health and diseases. Peptides. 2019;**111**:77-88

[65] Hasegawa K, Fujiwara H, Koshiji M, Inada T, Ohtani S, Doyama K, et al. Endothelin-1 and its receptor in hypertrophic cardiomyopathy. Hypertension. 1996;**27**(2):259-264

[66] Hiroe M, Hirata Y, Fujita N, Umezawa S, Ito H, Tsujino M, et al. Plasma endothelin-1 levels in idiopathic dilated cardiomyopathy. The American Journal of Cardiology. 1991;**68**(10):1114-1115

[67] Wolf SC, Gaschler F, Brehm S, Klaussner M, Amann K, Risler T, et al. Endothelin-receptor antagonists in uremic cardiomyopathy. Journal of Cardiovascular Pharmacology. 2000;**36**(5 Suppl 1):S348-S350

[68] Kiowski W. The endothelin-type-A receptor in dilated cardiomyopathy: Another key player? European Heart Journal. 2001;**22**(20):1849-1851

[69] Prosek R, Sisson DD, Oyama MA, Biondo AW, Solter PE. Measurements of plasma endothelin immunoreactivity in healthy cats and cats with cardiomyopathy. Journal of Veterinary Internal Medicine. 2004;**18**(6):826-830

[70] Bien S, Riad A, Ritter CA, Gratz M, Olshausen F, Westermann D, et al. The endothelin receptor blocker bosentan inhibits doxorubicin-induced cardiomyopathy. Cancer Research. 2007;**67**(21):10428-10435

[71] Matsubara TJ, Fujiu K. Endothelin-1 and atrial cardiomyopathy. International Heart Journal. 2019;**60**(2):238-240

[72] Song C, Wang S, Guo Y, Zheng X, Lu J, Fang X, et al. Plasma big endothelin-1 predicts new-onset atrial fibrillation after surgical septal myectomy in patients with hypertrophic cardiomyopathy. BMC Cardiovascular Disorders. 2019;**19**(1):122

[73] Wang Y, Tang Y, Zou Y, Wang D, Zhu L, Tian T, et al. Plasma level of big endothelin-1 predicts the prognosis in patients with hypertrophic cardiomyopathy. International Journal of Cardiology. 2017;**243**:283-289

[74] Schwebe M, Ameling S, Hammer E, Monzel JV, Bonitz K, Budde S, et al. Protective effects of endothelin receptor A and B inhibitors against doxorubicin-induced cardiomyopathy. Biochemical Pharmacology. 2015;**94**(2):109-129

[75] Matsa LS, Sagurthi SR, Ananthapur V, Nalla S, Nallari P. Endothelin 1 gene as a modifier in dilated cardiomyopathy. Gene. 2014;**548**(2):256-262

[76] Liefeldt L, Rylski B, Walcher F, Manhart J, Kron S, Rosenke YW, et al. Effects of transgenic endothelin-2 overexpression on diabetic cardiomyopathy in rats. European Journal of Clinical Investigation. 2010;**40**(3):203-210

[77] Dhein S, van Koppen CJ, Brodde OE. Muscarinic receptors in the mammalian heart. Pharmacological Research. 2001;**44**(3):161-182

[78] Yu X, Patterson E, Stavrakis S, Huang S, De Aos I, Hamlett S, et al. Development of cardiomyopathy and

atrial tachyarrhythmias associated with activating autoantibodies to beta-adrenergic and muscarinic receptors. Journal of the American Society of Hypertension. 2009;**3**(2):133-140

[79] Iwata M, Yoshikawa T, Baba A, Anzai T, Mitamura H, Ogawa S. Autoantibodies against the second extracellular loop of beta1-adrenergic receptors predict ventricular tachycardia and sudden death in patients with idiopathic dilated cardiomyopathy. Journal of the American College of Cardiology. 2001;**37**(2):418-424

[80] Rosenbaum MB, Chiale PA, Schejtman D, Levin M, Elizari MV. Antibodies to beta-adrenergic receptors disclosing agonist-like properties in idiopathic dilated cardiomyopathy and Chagas' heart disease. Journal of Cardiovascular Electrophysiology. 1994;**5**(4):367-375

[81] Ma G, Wang Y, Hou D, Liu J, Zhang J, Xu L, et al. Association of autoantibodies against the M2-muscarinic receptor with long-term outcomes in peripartum cardiomyopathy patients: A 5-year prospective study. Journal of Cardiology. 2019;**74**(3):251-257

[82] Martinez CG, Zamith-Miranda D, da Silva MG, Ribeiro KC, Brandao IT, Silva CL, et al. P2x7 purinergic signaling in dilated cardiomyopathy induced by auto-immunity against muscarinic M2 receptors: Autoantibody levels, heart functionality and cytokine expression. Scientific Reports. 2015;**5**:16940

[83] Wallukat G, Fu HM, Matsui S, Hjalmarson A, Fu ML. Autoantibodies against M2 muscarinic receptors in patients with cardiomyopathy display non-desensitized agonist-like effects. Life Sciences. 1999;**64**(6-7):465-469

[84] Le Guludec D, Cohen-Solal A, Delforge J, Delahaye N, Syrota A, Merlet P. Increased myocardial muscarinic receptor density in idiopathic dilated cardiomyopathy: An in vivo PET study. Circulation. 1997;**96**(10):3416-3422

[85] Fu ML. Anti-M2 muscarinic receptor autoantibodies and idiopathic dilated cardiomyopathy. International Journal of Cardiology. 1996;**54**(2):127-135

[86] Baba A, Yoshikawa T, Fukuda Y, Sugiyama T, Shimada M, Akaishi M, et al. Autoantibodies against M2-muscarinic acetylcholine receptors: New upstream targets in atrial fibrillation in patients with dilated cardiomyopathy. European Heart Journal. 2004;**25**(13):1108-1115

[87] Juenemann M, Nef H, Mollmann H, Singh P, Troidl C, Schramm P, Kaps M, Gerriets T, Blaes F, Tschernatsch M. No evidence for humoral autoimmunity against cardiomyocytes, adrenergic or muscarinic receptors in patients with tako-tsubo cardiomyopathy. Immunobiology 2019;224(2):220-2

[88] Jaue DN, Ma Z, Lee SS. Cardiac muscarinic receptor function in rats with cirrhotic cardiomyopathy. Hepatology. 1997;**25**(6):1361-1365

Section 2

Cardiorenal Pathology

Chapter 10

Hemodialysis Vascular Access with Central Venous Disease

Hemant J. Mehta

Abstract

Vascular access (VA) for hemodialysis (HD) is the lifeline of a patient. Arteriovenous fistula (AVF) is the gold standard of VA, but there are challenging situations when providing long-term VA becomes challenging, in the presence of central vein stenosis (CVS), which is common in patients on hemodialysis, but its exact prevalence is not known. It would be ideal to have proper venous mapping with imaging modality to be able to plan central venous access. This prior venous mapping will help to plan the target vein and delineate venous path to be able to place HD catheter in the best position or resolve the VA-related problems. However, digital subtraction angiography remains the gold standard of the procedure, during which the target vein is accessed via ultrasound guidance, and subsequent passage of wire is done under fluoroscopic guidance. Venous angiography and, if indicated, angioplasty are performed. For complete chronically occluded thrombotic veins, recanalization needs to be attempted. Stenting is reserved for a select group of patients. There are advances in endovascular techniques to deal with CVS, and it needs a multidisciplinary team approach to tackle the complex issues of VA-related central venous disease (CVD).

Keywords: hemodialysis vascular access, central venous disease, central venous stenosis, central vein angioplasty, central vein stenting, complete thrombotic occlusion of central veins

1. Introduction

Long-term hemodialysis (HD) is dependent on reliable vascular access (VA), which is the lifeline of a patient. We have come a long way in the chronic HD treatment due to advances in VA. Starting from Scribbner's shunt to single-lumen HD catheters in the femoral vessels to double-lumen non-tunneled non-cuff HD catheters, to tunneled cuff catheters (TCC), and to early stick arteriovenous grafts; all for urgent start HD. Over the years, we also moved the catheters from subclavian veins (SCV) to internal jugular veins (IJV), for VA in the upper part of the body, basically for access draining to the superior vena cava (SVC). Unfortunately, the non-cuffed HD catheters became a tool to continue HD for a prolonged period (a practice very commonly encountered in the part of the world where the author is working, mainly due to nonavailability of VA expertise) in the absence of matured arteriovenous fistula (AVF) or graft. This led to injury to the vessel wall, leading to thrombosis and central vein occlusion and compromised VA for HD due to central venous stenosis (CVS). Even the TCCs are associated with CVS. Two major factors implicated in development of CVS are venous trauma resulting from cannulation of central veins and hemodynamic stress secondary to high flow due to access site AVF, causing central venous disease (CVD).

AVF is the gold standard of VA. Ideally, all patients starting HD should have AVF in place, but that is not possible. In 2015, 80% of patients were using a catheter at HD initiation, a rate that has changed only marginally since 2005, and at 90 days after the initiation of HD, 68.5% of patients were still using catheters [1, 2]. Late referral by nephrologists to surgeons has been an underappreciated cause of initiation of HD with central catheters. [3]. There are situations when a patient has multiple AVF failures, in the upper limbs. It then becomes a challenging situation to provide dialysis to these patients with a reliable access. The problem is further compounded in patients with prior central vein HD catheters, resulting in CVD. CVS is considered to be common in patients on hemodialysis, but its exact prevalence is not known. The CVS may have occurred due to insertion of central catheters, PICC, or pacemaker leads. Due to direct contact of these devices with the wall of the central veins, and the constant movement, both lateral (like a pendulum) and cephalocaudal direction associated with breathing and the cardiac cycle cause endothelial injury. Pathological examinations of central veins obtained at autopsy have shown that even short-term catheters are associated with foci of local intimal injury with endothelial denudation and adherent thrombus [4].

In patients with AVF, development of CVS is partly related to turbulent blood flow and neointimal hyperplasia (NIH). Infection related to prior catheter insertion may also be responsible for CVS. Extrinsic compression, either musculoskeletal or arterial, can be contributing to CVS.

However, in an otherwise healthy person, the CVS hardly, if ever, causes problems. The problem comes to light when an AVF or graft is placed on the ipsilateral side where there is presence of CVS. It also gets recognized when a fresh attempt is made to insert cuffed or non-cuffed tunnel catheter in the central vein. We should realize that CVS leading to CVD is difficult to treat and often resistant to treatment. In CVD, VA for HD sometimes need to be abandoned, or in serious cases, the patient's life may be threatened. Therefore, one should strive for the ideal situation of catheter avoidance and central vein preservation and remember that prevention is ideal and better than cure.

2. Clinical case study

This is a 52-year-old diabetic female, who was on regular hemodialysis 3 times a week with right internal jugular vein (IJV) TCC as her vascular access for 7 months and a non-maturing left brachiocephalic vein AVF. She presented with progressively increasing orthopnea of 1-week duration and was presumed to have coronary artery disease. She was referred to our hospital cardiology department for coronary angiography (CAG), who subsequently asked nephrology services to give her a post CAG dialysis. Her CAG was normal. When on dialysis and on attempting to ultrafilter her, she had intradialytic hypotension, with persistent and increasing breathlessness. She was examined by a consultant and a clinical diagnosis of CVS was made. The patient was clinically not in fluid overload state. HD was terminated, and her blood pressure and symptoms settled. The next day, she underwent contrast-enhanced tomography of central vein, which proved stenosis at the cavo-atrial junction, at the site of the tip of the dialysis catheter. She was subjected to central vein angioplasty and her symptoms resolved (**Figure 1**) (author's personal work).

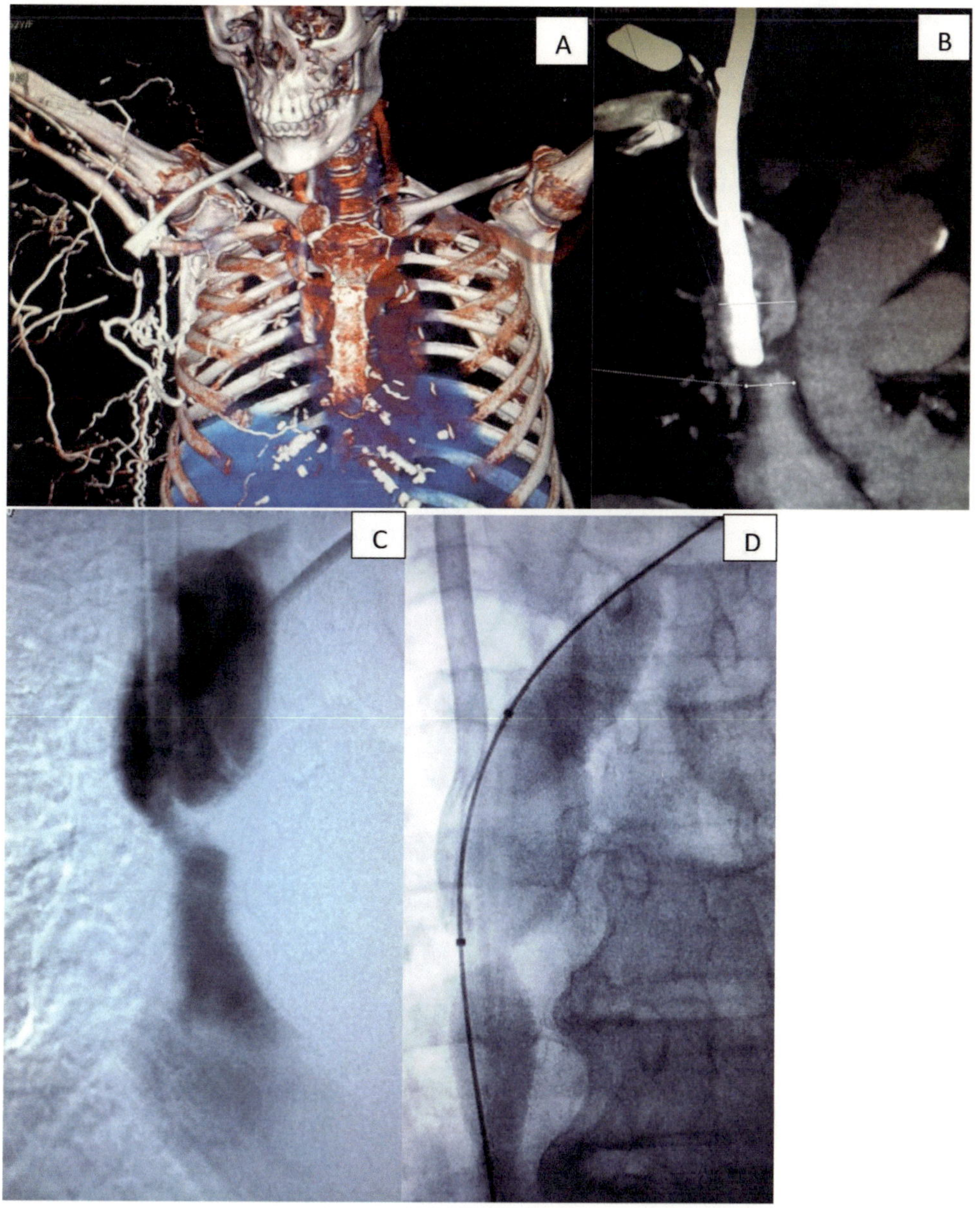

Figure 1.
CT scan and angiography images: (a) 3D reconstructed image showing clots around the TCC tip and also multiple collateral veins in the thoracic cage, suggestive of CTO; (b) stenosis at cavo-atrial junction at the site of TCC tip; (c) findings of (b) on CT scan are confirmed on angiography; and (d) angioplasty of the CVS with TCC in situ.

3. What are central veins?

In the neck, SVC, bilateral brachiocephalic vein (BCV), IJV, external jugular vein (EJV), and SCVs would constitute the central veins for upper limb access, whereas femoral, common iliac, and external iliac veins and the infrarenal inferior vena cava could constitute the lower limb central veins.

4. Preservation of central veins

Since CVS precludes to a creation of successful VA for long-term HD, it is essential to spread the awareness about preservation of central veins. It is a common practice to preserve peripheral veins (especially in nondominant hand) in a patient with chronic kidney disease (CKD, G III or higher). This is known to residents, fellows, nursing staff, etc. However, the concept of preservation of central veins in CKD is not widespread. CKD patients do get repeated central catheters at pre-HD stage due to medical problems, or PICC line, or the cardiologists requiring to put cardiac rhythm devices. There needs to be a dialog with cardiology colleagues to try and avoid insertion of SCV leads in CKD patients who are going to need HD in future. They can be requested to go for epicardial lead pacemakers (**Figure 2**) (author's personal work). Also, stiff non-cuffed HD catheters should not be kept in situ in jugular veins for more than 15 days. Even if patient has acute kidney injury and likely to need prolonged HD beyond 15 days, it is essential to change them to TCC, which has lesser chances of CVS than non-cuffed catheters. SCV catheterization should not be performed in CKD patients, although it still occurs frequently. Many intensivists prefer SCVs for central line insertion, and they should be convinced to avoid it in CKD patients.

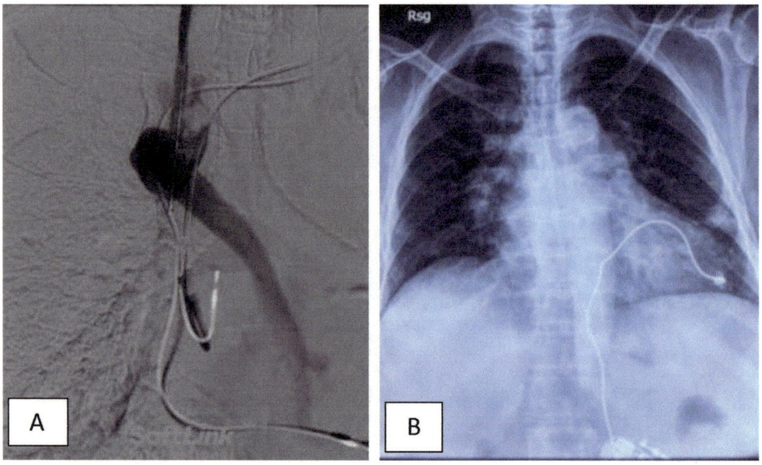

Figure 2.
(A) Pacemaker lead, with TCC. Pull back angiograph shows SVC occlusion and filling of azygous vein. (B) Pacemaker with epicardial leads in a patient with CKD GIIIb due to DKD.

5. Pathophysiology

CVS can be either related or unrelated to current or previous catheters. Catheter-associated CVS are related to type of catheter, i.e., stiff non-tunneled or softer tunneled catheter, duration, number of catheters in the same site, vein site, and tip position are all related to CVS. The material of catheter can be responsible for platelet aggregation and thrombosis. This can lead to episodes of catheter-related bloodstream infections (CRBSI). Also, the blood turbulence produced due to tip design can be responsible for CVS. Traditionally, catheters inserted in SCVs are known to cause CVS, as the SCV is located between the clavicle and first rib. However, left IJV or EJV catheters passing through the left brachiocephalic veins are responsible for left BCV stenosis. In the left BCV, stenosis occurs at two points, at the junction of the left IJV to the left SCV and junction of the left BCV to the right BCV continuing as the SVC. So, the stenosis occurs at the contact points of catheters with vessel wall in this situation. Also, left BCV is situated between aorta and sternum and can contribute to stenosis. Right IJV catheters were not considered to cause CVS; however, prolong catheters in the right IJV, passing through the right BCV, can also cause right BCV CVS. Catheter tips in the SVC or SVC-right atrium junction are also known to cause thrombosis and/or CVS at the tip position site, (as illustrated in the clinical case above). Catheters on the ipsilateral side of cardiac rhythm device lines or ipsilateral AVF are also known to cause CVS. In the later situation, it is due to turbulent blood flow at high flow generated by AVF. This is more prominently seen in cephalic arch with proximal brachiocephalic AVF and rarely with distal radio-cephalic AVF.

6. Asymptomatic CVS

Patients with prior history of central catheters or pacemaker leads may have CVS but are usually asymptomatic. The CVS comes to notice only when a VA is placed on ipsilateral side of CVS or a patient undergoes imaging for some other indications. Even in the presence of VA, asymptomatic CVS (<50%) are sometimes detected during other radiological procedures. These are usually found in cephalic arch or brachiocephalic veins. If these lesions are asymptomatic, one need not do intervention, even if stenosis is >50%. These require only observation for development of any symptoms or signs. This is because central veins are more elastic and prone to recoil after angioplasty. Also, the intimal damage to the veins caused by angioplasty balloon (cracking and fissuring of the vessel intima) may accelerate further stenosis, due to aggregation of thrombocytes and occurrence of thrombi leading to intimal hyperplasia and fibrosis at the site of the original stenosis [5, 6].

Prophylactic treatment of a stenosis that fulfills the anatomic criteria (>50% diameter reduction) but is not associated with a hemodynamic, functional, or clinical abnormality is not warranted and should not be performed. This is especially important for central venous lesions [7]. Two studies in one cohort were performed to address the issue of likelihood of developing CVS. Among 2811 patients, central venous stenosis was diagnosed in 120 (4.3%), at a median dialysis vintage of 2.9 (interquartile range, 1.8–4.6) years. Among a subset of 500 patients, all with a history of catheter use, 34 (6.8%) developed central venous stenosis, at a rate of 2.2 per 100 patient-years. The incidence of central venous stenosis was higher with a larger number of previous catheters [relative risk (RR), 2.2; 95% confidence interval (95% CI), 1.6–2.9]and pacemaker insertion (RR, 3.9; 95% CI, 1.7–8.9) and was lower with older age (RR, 0.7 per decade; 95% CI, 0.6–0.8) [8].

7. Diagnosis of CVS in symptomatic patients

The diagnosis of CVS is made from clinical and imaging findings. Most patients will have a history of previous central venous catheter placement and will present with ipsilateral arm, breast, face, or neck swelling. Many patients will have evidence of AV access dysfunction, with decreased access flows, increased venous pressures during dialysis, and a history of excessive bleeding from the puncture site after removal of needle. CVS leading to venous hypertension (VH) in the ipsilateral extremity and chest wall is a frequently encountered problem affecting 17 to 40% patients on HD. On physical examination, there may be numerous dilated collaterals in the neck or chest and arm edema or dilated tortuous draining veins of fistula on the side of the CVS. In the cases of bilateral innominate vein or SVC stenosis or occlusion, patients may present with SVC syndrome. CVS can often be diagnosed by duplex ultrasound, with an absence of normal respiratory variation in the diameter of central veins and polyphasic atrial waves. It is difficult to visualize the central veins with duplex ultrasound in obese and muscular patients [9]. The author has seen patients with severe CVS presenting with not only ipsilateral limb edema but hemifacial swelling, diminished vision, and hearing loss on the right side and throbbing headache. We have also encountered a patient in whom there was no prior history of any catheters or lines but had narrowed fibrosed right IJV. This was detected at the time of insertion of TCC for initiation of chronic dialysis. In this particular patient, right EJV was patent (indirect evidence that the right IJV was blocked for a long time, but patient was asymptomatic). We had a patient with right upper limb oedema and history of multiple right IJV non-cuffed catheters for dialysis but never had any SCV catheters. During angiography, right SCV was found to be thrombosed. As per the European Best Practice Guidelines on VA [10], if symptomatic CVS is suspected, digital subtraction angiography (DSA) of the access and the complete venous outflow tract should be performed. In certain cases, ultrasonography with Doppler, computerized tomography (CT) of central veins or magnetic resonance imaging (MRI) plain study with time of flight (TOF) technique (**Figure 3**) may be deployed prior to DSA for venous mapping.

The main regions of central vein which are affected are the right BCV or SCV, right IJV, left BCV or SCV, and left IJV or SVC. The problem of cephalic arch stenosis in proximal brachiocephalic AVF (prevalence ~30%) or sometimes due to radio-cephalic AVF should also be kept in mind. Percutaneous transluminal angioplasty (PTA) with balloon dilatation is the primary basis for endovascular therapy. However, balloon dilation should be performed only if there is a clinical indication such as arm or face swelling. Several studies have reported that balloon dilation for a narrowed lesion found incidentally on angiogram and without symptoms accelerates lesion growth [11–13].

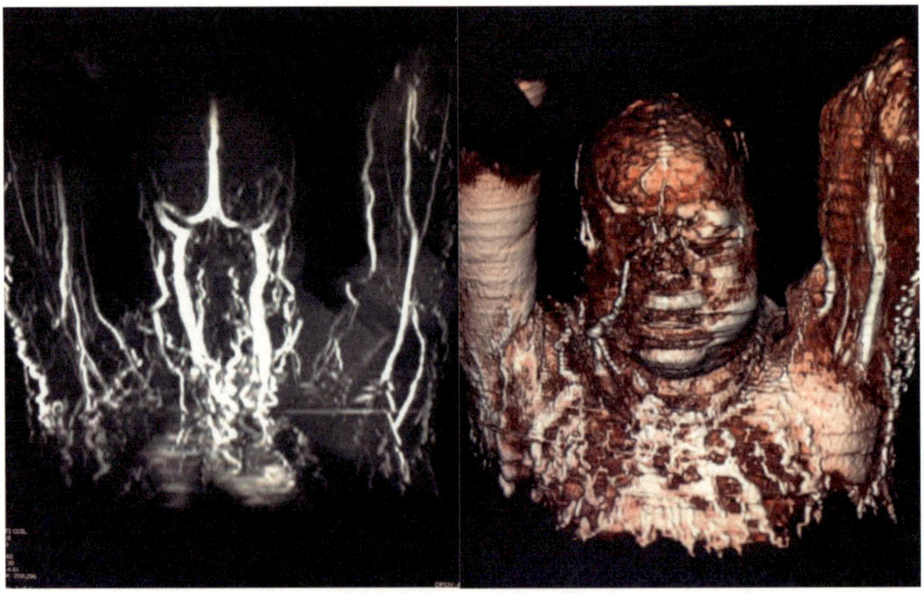

Figure 3.
MRI using TOF protocol, without contrast, to have venous mapping prior to intervention, in a patient who was grossly edematous and had no veins available to perform CT venography. It showed multiple levels of CVS, including bilateral IJVs, EJVs, and bilateral BCVs.

A major problem with lesions in the central veins is that many are elastic. It has been postulated that there are actually two types of lesions based upon their response to angioplasty, elastic and inelastic [14].

It is reasonable to perform PTA for central venous lesion if this intervention is required to maintain stable dialysis therapy. However, the presence of large fresh thrombus at the lesion site represents a contraindication to PTA unless the thrombus can first be removed by thrombectomy or another method. The left brachiocephalic lesions can be due to not only compressive stenosis but also organic stenosis. In particular, the left brachiocephalic vein may be compressed between the sternum and the right brachiocephalic artery [15].

8. CVD and similar conditions

The lesions can be partial but significant (>60% stenosis, for intervention purpose, however, venography demonstrating more than 50% stenosis of the subclavian, brachiocephalic vein, and superior vena cava in the upper extremity or the iliac vein or inferior vena cava in the lower extremity is considered central venous occlusion) or complete thrombotic occlusion [or chronic total occlusion (CTO)]. In addition, patients with TCC present with catheter malfunction and may have catheter-related sheath (CRS) (old term: fibrin sheath), with or without clot at the catheter tip (called catheter-related atrial thrombus, CRAT).

9. Options for patients with CVS needing VA

They can change to peritoneal dialysis if feasible. One can plan for thigh AVF or graft. But if both these are not the options, one is left with exploring central venous access with angioplasty and insertion of HD catheters, with TCC or Hemodialysis Reliable Outflow (HeRO®) device. For the purpose of this chapter, we would focus on upper limb CVS. Not to forget the fact that in the presence of SVC stenosis, no AVF or upper limb grafts will be feasible if the SVC stenosis is tight and has a chance for recurrence in spite of SVC angioplasty with or without stent. With improved dialysis survival, there are increasing numbers of patients who have exhausted definitive access options due to central venous stenosis and are maintaining dialysis on a central venous catheter. The HeRO allows an alternative by providing a definitive access solution [16].

10. The procedure: approaching and crossing stenosis

The approach to central vein could be from femoral veins, internal jugular veins, and brachial or cephalic veins. One needs to have thorough history, clinical examination, and Doppler study to arrive at a conclusion about suspected site of CVS. When these are unable to point the site of likely lesion, one may perform contrast-enhanced computer tomography (CT) venogram. The problem with CT venography is the need to inject iodinated contrast. This can be a problem in HD patients at times, who have no peripheral access to inject contrast. In such cases, magnetic resonance (MR) venography without gadolinium, using time-of-flight protocol, may yield equally good results and help plan the procedure. Gadolinium should be avoided in patients with eGFR of <30 ml/min due to risk of nephrogenic systemic fibrosis.

Once the procedure of angiography is decided, one needs to be ready with proper hardware, including various types of wires (0.35 and 0.14 regular and double length wires, hydrophilic wires, and stiff wires), various types of diagnostic and guiding catheters, larger-size high-pressure balloons, stents, or stent grafts. One may need large length vascular sheaths to provide stability to the catheter and guide wire, especially when femoral venous access is used.

10.1 How are the target lesion approached?

The indications to perform central vein angioplasty are either the patient is symptomatic with functioning vascular access in the upper limb, or the patient has had multiple vascular access failures in upper limb, and no reliable long-term vascular access is available. In such cases, the aim of central vein angioplasty is to create a passage to insert central dialysis catheter, which can be either TCC or hybrid graft if a reliable arterial inflow is available.

If the target lesion is right brachiocephalic vein or SVC, the right IJV is punctured, lesion attempted to be crossed with 0.014′ hydrophilic wire. If that is not successful, the right femoral vein is punctured and the lesion approached. The combination of this approach from either side helps take simultaneous angiographic shoots to define site and extent of lesion in terms of its length and diameter. We have encountered several cases, in which the thinnest of wires, sometimes even the coronary wires, or CTO wires (chronic thrombotic occlusion) fail to cross the lesion. In such cases, recanalization is attempted, which is described as sharp needle recanalization. When traditional endovascular methods fail, experienced interventionalists may utilize sharp or radiofrequency (RF)-assisted recanalization techniques. Sharp recanalization techniques require the use of the back end of a wire, 20- to 22-gauge (15–20 cm) percutaneous or transseptal needles, or transjugular intrahepatic portosystemic shunt needles [17]. In the absence of any other alternatives, we have been doing it with a long Chiba needle. One has to have simultaneous projections in anterior-posterior and lateral views to be sure that the puncture is in the proper venous plain and perforation is avoided. There is no true vessel wall, and a stent is placed to reconstitute the vessel wall if this is being done for upper extremity vascular access preservation. Otherwise, a catheter is inserted after balloon angioplasty of target lesion and creating enough venous diameters to allow smooth passage of the dialysis catheter. Recently, a new device called Surfacer® Inside-Out® access catheter system is available. The Surfacer Device offers a new approach for repeated venous access in patients with thoracic central venous occlusion (TCVOs) that enables the avoidance of left-sided catheter placement in individuals awaiting creation or maturation of permanent AV access or in patients who have exhausted all thoracic venous access options [18]. The author has no personal experience of using it; however, it is meant to restore and preserve access in the chronically occluded veins. Its advantages include restoration and sustenance of access, reliable and repeatable central venous access to the right IJV, preserving viability of secondary central veins, and optimization of the placement and maturation of permanent AV access.

TCVO [19], the authors divided TCVO as type 1, defined as any unilateral obstruction affecting either the internal jugular or subclavian vein. Type 2 includes all cases with ipsilateral occlusion of the brachiocephalic vein or ipsilateral obstruction of both internal jugular and subclavian veins. In TCVO type 3, both brachiocephalic veins are obstructed. Type 4 is characterized by central obstruction of the SVC. Thirty-six patients with TCVO treated in Vienna, Austria; Oxford, England; or Cologne, Germany, who required hemodialysis access between July 2016 and June 2018, with TCVO and history of multiple CVCs and AVF, were referred to the participating centers for vascular access. Thirty-two (89%) patients were eligible for the inside-out approach (IOA) approach. Thirty-nine treatments were performed, with seven patients undergoing the IOA procedure for the second time more than 3 months after initial CVC placement. Dialysis access was established successfully in 38 of 39 (97%) implementations of the IOA procedure. Median intervention time was 43 minutes. No complications occurred. This appears to be a promising method, although this was an observational study and no comparison was made to any other methods.

If CVS is bypassed, and adequate inflow with axillary artery is available, the HeRO® device can be implanted, which will avoid the need for external TCC and minimize risk of CRBSI.

a. If the target lesion is in the subclavian vein or cephalic arch or left brachiocephalic vein, approach from arm cephalic, basilic, or rarely brachial vein is required, usually combined with femoral vein approach. In cases of tight CTO, to provide adequate support and stability to the procedure of angioplasty, the wire from the arm vein is passed all the way down to the femoral vein and snared out. The hydrophilic wire is then changed over to a stiff wire, and the procedure of angioplasty is completed.

b. If attempting to put femoral vein or inferior vena cava (IVC) TCC and dealing with iliac vein or IVC stenosis, approach will be from the femoral vein, and again recanalization is attempted with thin wire or sharp needle.

PTA with balloon dilatation is the primary basis for endovascular therapy. If symptoms are present, PTA is performed; however, patency is poor, so repeat procedures are often required. If it is a first PTA and there is no elastic recoil of the vein on table, one should not consider stenting. Recent studies using intravascular ultrasound (IVUS) for CVS showed that, although the lesion was sufficiently enlarged on angiography after PTA, IVUS demonstrated insufficient dilation or extrusion by the balloon catheter [20]. In such cases, repeat angioplasty with larger-size and higher-pressure balloons can be tried, keeping in mind the risk of central venous rupture. Insertion of stents in such situation can be tried. However, numerous studies showed failure of stent use, especially in HD VA, because of neointimal hyperplasia within the stent, leading to a lower patency rate than that of PTA [21, 22].

The stent graft (SG) is a structure that applies graft material to the inside or outside of the stent to create a physical barrier to NIH. Various studies and author's experience have been that even the SGs do not provide long-term venous patency. There have been reports of using drug-coated balloons for CVS; however, at present, the benefit seems limited.

Stenting for TCVO is appropriate in the following situations, provided there are associated hemodynamic or clinical abnormalities: acute elastic recoil (>50%) following PTA and recurrent stenosis within a 3-month period of PTA. If balloon angioplasty achieves insufficient dilation (e.g., severe recoil) or leads to dissection or acute occlusion of the affected vein, bailout stenting is performed. [15]. Balloon angioplasty is a basic treatment for central venous lesion, but stent implantation is sometimes required. The self-expandable or balloon-expandable stent is chosen by the lesion location and characteristics. The lesion in SCV is generally treated by self-expandable stent, and right BCV is treated by balloon-expandable stent. The organic lesion of innominate vein with plaque is treated by self-expandable stent. Note that the innominate venous stenosis is sometimes caused by compression between the right brachiocephalic artery and the sternum and this lesion is treated by balloon-expandable stent because the radial force of balloon-expandable stent is stronger than self-expandable stent. It is important to understand the indication and stent selection for central venous PTA [15].

It is also important to remember to choose a proper-sized stent. This is sometimes not possible to judge from the angiographic images, and what appears to be adequate angioplasty could be inadequate in terms of adequate vein diameter. IVUS is sometimes useful to guide the choice of proper balloon or stent size, as what appears to be an adequately treated vein could be having significant underlying stenosis, which is not possible to realize on conventional two-dimensional angiography. IVUS is an invasive modality that provides cross-sectional imaging of the veins but without the need for ionizing radiation or contrast administration. In addition to being a diagnostic tool that is easy and repeatable, it aids treatment decision-making. Though IVUS may be better suited than traditional venography to identify intraluminal narrowing and pre-/post-intervention outcomes, additional study is warranted to better characterize the value of IVUS in the VA-related CVS patient population. In a patient with CVS and prior allergy to iodinated contrast, angiography was performed using 1 cc of contrast, CVS confirmed, and the rest of the procedure of angioplasty and confirmation of adequate result was completed using IVUS (personal communication, Dr. Daniel Patel, Interventional Nephrologist, Volusia-Flagler Vascular Centre, Daytona Beach, Florida, USA).

If CRS is the cause for catheter malfunction, the same can be confirmed during catheter exchange procedure by doing pullback angiography prior to full removal of TCC. There can be only CRS, which can be tackled by balloon angioplasty and fibrin sheath disruption. Rarely (and in the authors' own experience), the CRS can be snared out. However, the CRS can be associated with CRAT. And it can become tricky to perform angioplasty, as the risk of pulmonary thromboembolism due to large CRAT, attached to TCC tip, is high. Sometimes, CRAT is attached to the wall of the right atrium. In such a case, if TCC is functioning well, the patient can be anticoagulated and kept under close observation. For a large CRAT or infected CRAT, attached to TCC tip, and where it is risky and not advisable to remove the CRAT, AngioVac thrombectomy device can be used. If these patients are poor candidates for conventional therapy of thrombolytics or surgical thromboembolectomy because of bleeding, failure of thrombolytics, or hemodynamic instability, they may benefit from percutaneous mechanical thrombectomy by AngioVac, which is proved to be effective for complete evacuation in most patients [23].

Surgical options may be considered for CVS, when the stenosis persists, and there are no alternative avenues to provide long-term reliable VA. One must assess the AVF for flow velocity, as this may be the cause of CVD. In such cases, inflow reduction either surgically or percutaneously can be performed. Another surgical option is unusual bypass including reconstruction surgery and claviculectomy or first rib resection if there is thoracic outlet syndrome. If an experienced vascular surgeon is available, the bypass surgery can be performed using graft (PTFE) from the brachial artery to ipsilateral or contralateral internal jugular veins or axillary or femoral veins. Direct connection to SVC or right atrium have also been attempted. One must remember that such surgeries are complicated and carries its own risks and complications.

There are occasions when there is coexistence of CVS and stenosis in the draining vein, either juxta-anastomotic or away from the site of anastomosis. In such situation, one must attempt and achieve patency of CVS lesion. Failure to do so can lead to severe swelling of the ipsilateral arm. The best way to relieve symptomatic CVS is closure of AVF. But it is not possible in patients, who have the last surviving access and shortage of vascular estate.

But, sometimes, there are more than one possible approach to a problem, and the opinion varies as per the specialist handling the case. For example, refer to **Figure 4**, a middle-aged lady on hemodialysis with CVS who had undergone angioplasty with stenting and resolution of right upper limb painful edema. She

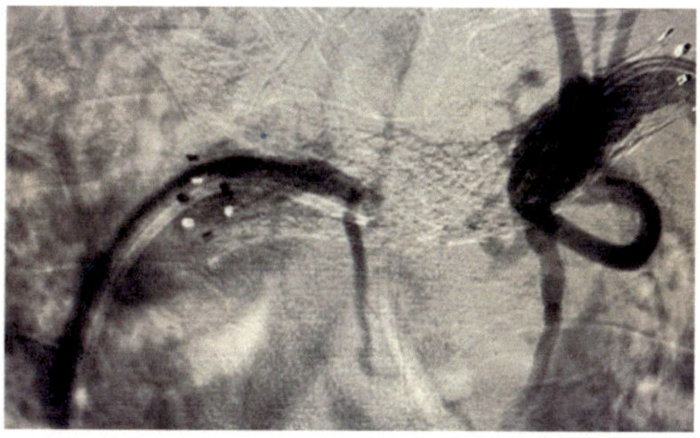

Figure 4.
Right SCV in-stent thrombosis.

presented with the same symptoms 6 months later. The angiography image shows in-stent stenosis. It was difficult to negotiate the stenosis. Various opinions were sought. The interventional nephrologist found that it was the high-flow fistula (flow volume 2600 ml/min, very high) which was responsible for her symptoms, and the patient should undergo flow reduction procedure. The interventional radiologist said that attempt to do in-stent angioplasty, followed by stent placement within the stent, should be the first option. The vascular access surgeon said that the stenosis is due to external compression and the patient should undergo middle 1/3rd claviculectomy to relieve her symptoms.

11. Cardiovascular consequences of AVF

Sometimes very-high-flow AVFs can lead to VH, progressive aneurysmal dilatation of vein with skin ulceration, hemodialysis access-induced distal ischemia, and high-output heart failure with or without pulmonary hypertension. AVFs have effects on cardiac functions related to the increase in preload and cardiac output (CO). It is difficult to define cardiovascular consequences due to AVF in a precise manner. This is due to the fact that patients requiring long-term hemodialysis tend to have volume overload due to water and salt retention. There could also be pressure load due to arterial sclerosis and hypertension and increased CO secondary to chronic anemia. In addition, many hemodialysis patients have significant pre-existing myocardial, valvular, or coronary heart disease, as the vascular calcification due to CKD-MBD (chronic kidney disease—mineral and bone disorder). Congestive heart failure (CHF) is highly prevalent among patients with ESRD. Approximately 35–40% of patients with ESRD have an established CHF diagnosis at initiation of hemodialysis. Worsening in cardiac functions soon after AVF creation has also been observed favoring a causative effect of the AVF on certain cardiac functions [24].

12. Conclusion

CVD is a common occurrence in HD patients, either due to mechanical or hemodynamic factors. It could be related to catheters or AVF. It can be symptomatic or asymptomatic. Interventions will be required in symptomatic patients and in those who have VA malfunction. There are various options, and one needs to choose the modality based on the patient's need. The outcomes cannot be predicted as each vein behaves differently. Proper knowledge of anatomical lesion, pathophysiology of the lesion, patient needs, and expertise available will determine the intervention modality and outcomes. There is a need for multidisciplinary approach to tackle the situation. We, at our institute, work with a motto which is slightly modified from the old proverb, and we proudly say that "if there's a will and a vein, there's a way." Prevention of CVS by catheter avoidance is an ideal situation; however CVD due to hemodynamic issues not related to catheters cannot be avoided, and VA surveillance is the best way for early diagnosis and management of such lesions.

Acknowledgements

The author acknowledges the support of department of interventional radiology, cardiac catheterization lab, and its staff. Special thanks go to Dr. Gireesh Warawadekar, interventional radiologist and past president of the Indian Society of Interventional Radiology, and Dr. Nikhil Karnik, interventional radiologist. Special thanks to all the fellows, clinical associates, and junior consultants in the department of nephrology, Lilavati Hospital, for patient care.

Conflict of interest

The author declares no conflict of interest.

Author details

Hemant J. Mehta[1,2]

1 Lilavati Hospital and Research Center, Mumbai, India

2 AVATAR Foundation (Association of Vascular and Interventional Renal Physicians), India

*Address all correspondence to: drhmehta@hotmail.com

References

[1] Agrawal A. Endovascular interventions for central vein stenosis. Kidney Research and Clinical Practice. 2015;**34**(4):228-232

[2] USRDS. Ch. 4: Vascular access. In: United States Renal Data System. Vol. 2. 2015. pp. 359-376. DOI: 10.1053/j.ajkd.2017.01.023

[3] Lopez-Vargas PA, Craig JC, Gallagher MP, Walker RG, Snelling PL, Padagogos E, et al. Barriers to timely arteriovenous fistula creation: A study of providers and patients. American Journal of Kidney Diseases. 2011;**57**(6):873-882

[4] Forauer AR, Theoharis C. Histologic changes in the human vein wall adjacent to indwelling central venous catheters. Journal of Vascular and Interventional Radiology. 2013;**14**(9mPt 1):1163-1168

[5] Roy-Chaudhury P, Lee TC. Vascular stenosis: Biology and interventions. Current Opinion in Nephrology and Hypertension. 2007;**16**:516-522

[6] Tedla FM, Clerger G, Distant D, Salifu M. Prevalence of central vein stenosis in patients referred for vein mapping. Clinical Journal of the American Society of Nephrology. 2018;**13**(7):1063-1068

[7] Beathard G. Percutaneous angioplasty for the treatment of venous stenosis: A nephrologist's view. Seminars in Dialysis. 1995;**8**:166-170

[8] Adwaney A, Lim C, Blakey S, Duncan N, Ashby DR. Central venous stenosis, access outcome and survival in patients undergoing maintenance hemodialysis. Clinical Journal of the American Society of Nephrology. 2019;**14**(3):378-384

[9] Mehta HJ. Central venous stenosis: What should a nephrologist know? Indian Journal of Nephrology. 2017;**27**(6):427-429

[10] Tordoir J, Canaud B, Haage P, Konner K, Basci A, Fouque D, et al. EBPG on vascular access. Nephrology, Dialysis, Transplantation. 2007;**22**(Suppl 2):ii88-ii117

[11] Levit RD, Cohen RM, Kwak A, Shlansky-Goldberg RD, Clark TWI, Patel AA, et al. Asymptomatic central venous stenosis in hemodialysis patients. Radiology. 2006;**238**:1051-1056

[12] Ehrie JM, Sammarco TE, Chittams JL, Trerotola SO. Unmasking of previously asymptomatic central venous stenosis following percutaneous transluminal angioplasty of hemodialysis access. Journal of Vascular and Interventional Radiology. 2017;**28**:1409-1414

[13] Yan Y, Sudheendra D, Dagli MS, Stavropoulos SW, Clark TW, Soulen MC, et al. Effect of central venous angioplasty on hemodialysis access circuit flow: Prospective study of 25 symptomatic patients. Journal of Vascular and Interventional Radiology. 2015;**26**:984-991

[14] Kovalik EC, Newman GE, Suhocki P, Knelson M, Schwab SJ. Correction of central venous stenoses: Use of angioplasty and vascular Wallstents. Kidney International. 1994;**45**(4):1177-1181

[15] Horita Y. Percutaneous transluminal angioplasty for central venous stenosis or occlusion in hemodialysis patients. The Journal of Vascular Access. 2019;**20**(Suppl 1):87-92

[16] Al Shakarchi J, Houston JG, Jones RG, Inston N. A review on the hemodialysis reliable outflow (HeRO) graft for haemodialysis vascular access. European Journal of Vascular and Endovascular Surgery. 2015;**50**(1):108-113

[17] Dolmatch BL, Gurley JC, Baskin KM, Nikolic B, Lawson JH, Shenoy S, et al. Society of Interventional Radiology reporting standards for thoracic central vein obstruction: endorsed by the American Society of Diagnostic and Interventional Nephrology (ASDIN), British Society of Interventional Radiology (BSIR), Canadian Interventional Radiology Association (CIRA), Heart Rhythm Society (HRS), Indian Society of Vascular and Interventional Radiology (ISVIR), Vascular Access Society of the Americas (VASA), and Vascular Access Society of Britain and Ireland (VASBI). Journal of Vascular and Interventional Radiology. 2018;**29**:454.e3-460.e3

[18] Hentschel DM, Minarsch L, Vega F, Ebner A. The Surfacer® Inside-Out® Access System for right-sided catheter placement in dialysis patients with thoracic venous obstruction [published online ahead of print, 2019 Sep 20]. Journal of Vascular Access. 2019:1129729819867547. DOI: 10.1177/1129729819867547

[19] Reindl-Schwaighofer R, Matoussevitch V, Winnicki W, Kalmykov E, Gilbert J, Matzek W, et al. A novel inside-out access approach for hemodialysis catheter placement in patients with thoracic central venous occlusion. American Journal of Kidney Diseases. 2020;**75**(4):480-487

[20] deGraaf R, van Laanen J, Peppelenbosch N, van Loon M, Tordoir J. The value of intravascular ultrasound in the treatment of central venous obstructions in hemodialysis patients. The Journal of Vascular Access. 2016;**17**(Suppl 1):S12-S15

[21] Haskal ZJ, Trerotola S, Dolmatch B, Schuman E, Altman S, Mietling S, et al. Stent graft versus balloon angioplasty for failing dialysis-access grafts. The New England Journal of Medicine. 2010;**362**:494-503

[22] Salman L, Asif A. Stent graft for nephrologists: Concerns and consensus. Clinical Journal of the American Society of Nephrology. 2010;**5**:1347-1352

[23] Donaldson CW, Baker JN, Narayan RL, Provias TS, Rassi AN, Giri JS, et al. Thrombectomy using suction filtration and veno-venous bypass: Single center experience with a novel device. Catheterization and Cardiovascular Interventions. 2015;**86**:E81-E87

[24] Alkhouli M, Paul Sandhu P, Boobes K, Hatahet K, Raza F, Boobes Y. Cardiac complications of arteriovenous fistulas in patients with end-stage renal disease. Nefrología. 2015;**35**(3):234-245

Chapter 11

Early Detection and Endovascular Intervention to Correct Dialysis Vascular Access Malfunction

Pedro Ponce and Ana Mateus

Abstract

Endovascular intervention in hemodialysis vascular access is among the most frequent interventions performed in an angiography suite. Vascular stenosis is the most prevalent lesion causing vascular access malfunction. Vascular access pathology and the outcomes in response to endovascular treatment are quite different from the arterial territory. Treatment strategy must be integrated, multidisciplinary, and with a long-term perspective, as recurrence rates of malfunction are quite common. We will detail our experience managing an extremely busy vascular access center serving a population of 4000 dialysis patients, performing all endovascular techniques in close coordination with the surgical team.

Keywords: hemodialysis, vascular access, angioplasty

1. Introduction

Endovascular interventions have substituted surgical repair as the primary treatment of failing or thrombosed vascular access (VA). Endovascular and surgical techniques, however, are complementary. Optimizing endovascular interventions of VA malfunction is a crucial component for a successful vascular access program. The identification and early treatment of stenosis are essential to prevent access thrombosis and ultimate failure.

Despite recent advances in endovascular techniques and devices, angioplasty continues to be the primary method for the treatment of access-related stenosis. Not all stenosis needs to be treated. When timely applied, angioplasty is a fast, easy, and safe procedure that can extend the patency of a hemodialysis graft or fistula.

The *early detection and endovascular intervention to correct dialysis vascular access malfunction* are reviewed in this chapter, describing the authors' experience in a highly active Vascular Access Center in Lisbon, integrated in a large outpatient dialysis network. We will cover the following topics: (1) vascular access options and its selection, (2) vascular access morbidity and complications, (3) vascular access malfunction detection, (4) endovascular interventions to correct dialysis vascular access malfunction, and (5) endovascular intervention outcomes.

2. Vascular access options and its selection

The VA constitutes the interface between chronic kidney disease (CKD) patient and machine (the dialysis monitor); its function is a key factor that affects most

IntechOpen

dialysis treatment quality indicators, such as dialysis dose and adequacy (Kt/V), substitution volume during hemodiafiltration, operating costs, and vital prognosis of the dialysis patient.

In this chapter, we deal only with long-term arteriovenous accesses:

A. The native AV fistula (nAVF), usually result from an end-to-side anastomosis of a vein to an artery, either at the wrist (distal fistula), most commonly a radio-cephalic fistula, or at the elbow/upper arm level (proximal fistula), in this position most commonly a brachiocephalic fistula, or a brachio-basilic fistula, this last one requiring a second procedure the transposition to the surface of the arterialized vein.

B. The arteriovenous graft (AVG), usually a second choice in patients not suitable for a nAVF fistula, has better mechanical strength, can be used earlier, and has lower primary failure rates when compared with nAVF, but has a much higher infection risk, a poorer primary long-term patency, and needs many more interventions to remain functional.

The VA dysfunction and its complications, such as low access flow (Qa), infection, loss of dialysis adequacy, or thrombosis, are the major single cause of hospitalization and morbidity requiring endovascular intervention, as well as one of the most important drivers of the total cost of an end-stage renal failure program.

Whenever a native arteriovenous fistula (AVF) can be built and is able to mature in no more than 8 weeks, it is considered the first and best choice as a vascular access. It results in higher long-term longevity and less thrombotic or infectious morbidity, needs fewer procedures for maintenance, and is overall a big life and money saver.

The nAVF, however, comes with its own set of disadvantages. There is a higher risk of primary failure (nonmaturation) up to 60% prior to cannulation, requiring frequent angiographic procedures to assist maturation [1–3]. Studies have shown that the primary failure rate is two times greater for fistulas (40%) than grafts (19%), with similar cumulative patency; in addition, the number of catheter days before AV access use was more than double in those using a fistula (81 days) than those with AV grafts (38 days); however, grafts require more angioplasties (1.4 vs. 3.2 events) and thrombolysis (0.05 vs. 0.98 events) interventions per 1000 patient-days [2, 4]. The risk of primary fistula failure is much higher for lower arm fistula (28%) than with upper arm fistula (20%), although these last ones produce more than 90% of all cephalic arch stenosis [1].

The secondary patency rates of AV grafts (total life span even if requiring several interventions to maintain its function) are on average around 3 years, all in all identical to AV fistulas, but those improved rates are achieved at the expense of three- to six-fold greater reintervention rates.

There has never been a randomized control trial (RCT) comparing different VA choices regarding mortality or other hard outcomes. All large observational trials compared accesses achieved as opposed to the accesses that were intended (as in intention to treat). As 25–60% of all AVFs created either fail or need several procedures to mature and the central venous catheter (CVC) group in most studies were people in whom AVF failed or CVC was chosen because of a predictable bad prognosis (age, congestive heart failure, short life expectancy, etc.), we really cannot answer the question on which VA is the best. If we exclude patients that begin hemodialysis urgently, mortality between nAVF and CVC patients becomes identical. Using a decision analysis model (fed with data extracted from DOPPS 2, the

REDUCE FTM study, the DAC study, and CMS data) for choosing the best option for patients initiating hemodialysis (HD) with a CVC, a nAVF attempt strategy is associated with better survival and lower annual cost, but that advantage is progressively lost in patients above 60 years or diabetics [5, 6].

Access malfunction is a source of tremendous emotional and physical suffering, dialysis treatments loss, low treatment adequacy, urgent need for a central catheter as a substitution access, and referral for new angiography or surgical procedures at huge costs.

In this chapter, we basically describe our experience on VA management in our dialysis network treating approximately 5000 patients in our Vascular Access Center (VAC) that performs more than 1000 VA surgeries and more than 1600 endovascular interventions per year.

3. Vascular access morbidity and complications

The most common VA complications are failure to mature, persistently low Qa, suboptimal dialysis adequacy, pain, aneurysms, rupture/hemorrhage, infection, and thrombosis. Endovascular stenosis is the underlying lesion and the direct culprit behind most of these complications.

Neointimal hyperplasia is the common pathogenic mechanism inducing stenosis, and stenosis is the underlying promoter of thrombosis. Stenotic plaques are composed of myofibroblasts (smooth muscle cells) surrounded by extracellular matrix and macrophages. This cell proliferation begins in the adventitia and migrates toward the lumen of anastomotic areas or endothelial segments exposed to several stresses, such as surgical trauma, shear stress, wall stress, diameter and compliance mismatch, uremic endothelial dysfunction, and wall lesion secondary to repeated needle punctures.

Stenosis is necessary for thrombosis, but it is not enough. Only 30% of stenosis above 50% of lumen compromise will cause thrombosis in the next 6 months; we just do not know which ones. On the other hand, angioplasty induces accelerated NH with recurrent stenosis [7]. In 20% of the cases, recurrent stenosis occurs in 1 week and in 40% in 1 month [8], and although stenosis stenting may delay stenosis recurrence, it did not reduce the incidence of thrombosis [9].

As in other vascular territories, we do not know and have no biomarkers to decide which stenosis will progress to cause thrombosis, which stenosis if dilated will prevent thrombosis, which stenosis once dilated will suffer early recurrence, which is the best option to prevent recurrence, and how to define the successful angioplasty.

4. Vascular access malfunction detection

In hemodialysis vascular access management, just as in general medicine, an early diagnosis of malfunction and prevention of definite failure is considered the best approach to diminish morbidity and costs. This axiom was strongly suggested in several seminal studies [10, 11] and is expressed in most guidelines of scientific societies in this field.

It is recommended that regular monitoring of access function should be performed, preferably by measuring vascular access flow (Qa), and when access stenosis is present, preemptive intervention should be performed percutaneously without further delay. In support of these level 2 recommendations, we can quote: "All types of pressure measurement should be abandoned in favor of access flow measurement," and "Monitoring plus intervention reduces thrombotic rates, morbidity and costs" [11, 12].

Consensual recommendations for preemptive intervention in malfunctioning grafts are (a) Qa measurement <600 ml/min for grafts or <400 ml/min for native fistulas and (b) a Qa drop higher than 25% over two consecutive measurements [13].

However, recent and quite relevant information has questioned those recommendations, and scanning through recent prospective randomized controlled trials in this field reveals some discordant opinions.

No matter if we are looking at native fistulas or PTFE grafts, using only Qa measurements, or its association with Doppler studies or dynamic venous pressure as surveillance techniques, it is believed that VA stenosis is now very effectively detected and responsible for a large increase in percutaneous vascular access procedures. Surprisingly, however, it has been found that all these diagnostic and therapeutic procedures fail to reduce the thrombosis rate or prolong access longevity, fueling an ongoing controversy regarding its beneficial effects, both in terms of overall access survival and associated costs [6, 8, 14–20].

All presently approved clinical guidelines recommend performing surveillance of vascular access quality and performance, aiming at early detection of access stenosis, which induced a global trend toward implementation of Qa-based monitoring programs in many dialysis units.

The recommended Qa thresholds for angiography referral are based on its putative predictive power of access malfunction and/or failure.

However, even before the final decision on the clinical relevance of periodic Qa determination, the quality and accuracy of the Qa measurements methods must be questioned, as most techniques have a good correlation among them, but high variation in absolute terms (±200 ml/min) [21–30].

We are now in a position where we feel that we must do some form of VA surveillance, but do not know exactly which. Qa, although not perfect, with results that are hard to interpret and need specific calibration to fine tune appropriate alarm thresholds for each measurement technique, is probably the best hemodynamic parameter to follow.

In our unit, we evaluate monthly Qa, together with a trend analysis of other equally not perfect parameters, like physical examination [31], Kt/V in all dialysis treatments, recirculation, and maximum obtainable Qb with circuit arterial pressure above −250 mmHg, and then decide empirically, as physicians always do, when to refer to angiography.

A successful program of surveillance should reduce thrombosis rate by an amount identical to the angioplasty rate it induces. The key to measure surveillance effectiveness is avoidance of thrombosis; no other surrogate is acceptable.

As a matter of fact, absolute flow (Qa) and drop in flow, measured using several different flow indicators (ultrasound, thermal dilution, ionic dilution), are inaccurate predictors of thrombosis. Most thromboses are unpredictable, and interventions based on surveillance likely yield many unnecessary procedures at high cost.

We do not know if a vascular access defined by us as well functioning actually looks normal in angiography. Without that, it is difficult to really appreciate the specificity of our monitoring indicators and, most of all, the meaning of stenosis in the natural history of the VA.

Our data suggest that the presence of what we call a significant stenosis is not correlated with measured Qa and it might not be associated with early thrombosis deserving immediate intervention [20]. Further studies are needed to clarify the best surveillance protocol and the role of preemptive intervention in significant stenosis.

A proposal for surveillance could well include the following:

A. Each unit should perform sequential measurement and trend analysis of the parameters of their choice.

B. Physical examination done and recorded before each dialysis by the R.N., in an access without dressings and needles. Signs to be looked for include a pounding pulse, an intermittent thrill, arm swelling, increment in collateral veins, difficult hemostasis, a new or an enlarging aneurysm, and pain during treatment, reaching an agreement rate with angiogram to detect stenosis of 80% [31].

C. Access flow measurement (Qa) in:

i. High-risk grafts—Every 2 weeks.

ii. Other grafts—Quarterly.

iii. Native fistulas with a Qa < 1000 ml/min—Quarterly.

iv. Native fistulas with a previous Qa ≥ 1000 ml/min—Once a year or whenever clinically indicated.

We consider high-risk grafts:

a. "Last" available vascular access site of that patient.

b. Frequent clotter.

c. Frequent recurrence of significant stenosis (less than 3 months apart).

Patients are referred from the dialysis unit to our VAC by their nephrologists, the indication for intervention is confirmed upon arrival, and an ultrasound/Doppler study will be performed if needed, to decide if it should be referred to the surgical or endovascular arm of the VAC and to help planning the endovascular approach localizing eventual stenotic lesions, their location, and preferred puncture site.

Our referral criteria to surgery: (a) Native AVF thrombosis; (b) VA rupture; (c) infection with visible abscesses or purulent discharge at puncture sites; (d) need for a new VA; (e) steal syndrome, VA limb distal ischemia; (f) primary malfunction of a VA created or submitted to open surgery less than 1 month ago; (g) growing aneurysm; and (h) hemorrhage.

Referral criteria to endovascular intervention: (a) Growing edema of the VA limb, (b) VA pain during dialysis treatment, (c) recent increment of VA venous pressure associated with a drop in dialysis adequacy, (d) unexplained drop in dialysis adequacy, (e) a drop of VA flow (Qa) in 2 measurements <600 ml/min in a AVG or <400 ml/min a nAVF, (f) need for assisted maturation of a nAVF, (g) superior vena cava syndrome, and (h) AVG thrombosis.

The techniques we perform in the angiography suite are (a) diagnostic angiography in no more than 7% of all cases, (b) percutaneous angioplasty (PTA) of stenotic lesions, (c) thrombolysis for thrombosed AVGs, and (d) stenting of elastic or frequently relapsed stenosis.

In our unit, prospective results of 1-year follow-up in 71 new AV grafts with monthly surveillance revealed the following:

a. A Qa < 600 ml/min had the same predictive value with that ΔQa of 25%, and dynamic venous pressure was useless.

b. After 1 year only 35% of PTFEs did not need any kind of intervention. We demonstrated then a sensitivity of 82% and a specificity of 90% to detect stenosis.

c. "Successful" PTA in 91% and Qa↑ on average 142%.

d. A sensitivity of 39% and a specificity of 21% to detect thrombosis.

e. A thrombosis rate—0.46 thru/pt. year.

f. In 60% of cases, previous monitoring was normal.

5. Endovascular intervention to correct dialysis vascular access malfunction

The initial treatment recommended for stenotic lesions in both nAVF and AVG is endovascular intervention, primarily angioplasty. Endovascular intervention is employed to maintain or even rescue AV access [32].

The recommendation within the K/DOQI guidelines is to treat hemodialysis access stenosis of more than 50% of the vessel lumen, if those are related with reduced flow rate and high venous pressure. PTA is considered a standard of care in failing hemodialysis access due to its high rates of success and satisfactory patency rate [33].

5.1 Stenosis location

The stenotic lesions in an AV fistula can occur in any location of the access system, with a higher incidence in specific spots for each type of VA. This is the case of stenosis at the proximal "swing segment" (the vein segment immediately after the arteriovenous anastomosis of a nAVF, which was dissected and brought close to the artery to create the anastomosis) either in the upper arm in transposed brachio-basilic fistulas, or in the lower forearm, in radio-cephalic fistulas, which are relatively more frequent than lesions at any other site [34]. Another example is the cephalic arch region, in patients with brachiocephalic fistulas [32].

Below we describe some types of stenosis of the vascular circuit, selected for their particularities, namely, their frequency, risk of restenosis, and predictable danger of VA failure.

5.2 Cephalic arch stenosis

The proximal cephalic vein is characterized by a curved shape, which occurs as the cephalic arch passes though the coracoclavicular ligament, just before joining the subclavian vein.

Several reasons have been put forward to justify the development of cephalic arch stenosis, such as increased blood flow rates, hemodynamic factors associated with the vessel shape, external compression by the outer structures surrounding the vein, and hypertrophy of valves that are often present in the cephalic arch.

Although angioplasty is the accepted initial treatment of cephalic arch stenosis, it can be problematic because lesions in that location are more resistant to dilatation. When dealing with resistant stenotic lesions, it is shown that employing cutting balloons (see below) may improve outcomes. On the other hand, complications are more likely (vein rupture), and patency is reduced compared with other vein location. Stent placement in the arch is a delicate task because the stent should invade the subclavian vein lumen, which can result in its partial or total occlusion, impeding the future creation of an AVF or AVG using the basilic or axillary vein, thereby consuming vascular patrimony. In view of the recurrent problems with angioplasty of the cephalic arch, the stent placement can be an alternative to rescue the vascular access (**Figure 1**).

For several reasons, it is not possible to make any evidence-based recommendations on best practices for management of CAS (endovascular or surgical). There is profound heterogeneity in the studies retrieved, from their initial design to their presentation of data. Few studies were prospective, few studies involved more than one or two centers, and the lack of uniformity of outcomes is another weakness of current published studies. CAS is often managed alternatively by interventionists and surgeons, in our experience with identical success.

5.3 Central vein stenosis

The prior placement of a central venous catheter is by far the most common cause of central vein stenosis (CVS) in dialysis patients. Transvenous wires of cardiac rhythm devices are more and more related with central veins stenosis in this population of high cardiovascular morbidity. Hemodialysis patients are, therefore, primary candidates for new wireless pacemakers or epicardial pacemaker leads.

The surgical approach to central vein stenosis is difficult because they can hide behind the bone structure. Therefore, endovascular intervention with angioplasty and/or stent placement becomes a logistically more receptive proposal for treatment of CVS. Still, anatomically and functionally, central veins have several specific characteristics including the diameter, angle, and elasticity that make treatment and maintenance of their patency after intervention difficult.

Some central vein stenoses are not symptomatic. Asymptomatic central veins stenosis, involving less than 50% of the vessel lumen, does not require treatment and is best managed by simple supervision [35].

Angioplasty with or without stent placement has been the recommended preferred approach to CVS. The guideline 20 NKF-K/DOQI suggests that the percutaneous intervention with transluminal angioplasty is the preferred treatment for CVS [36]. PTA has very high initial technical success rates, ranging from 70 to 90% [37, 38]. Primary and cumulative patency rates are widely variable and can

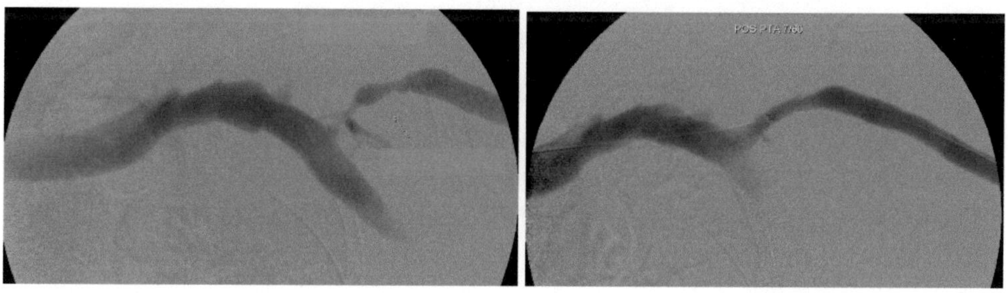

(a) (b)

Figure 1.
(a) and (b). Stenosis affecting cephalic arch; this lesion responded well to balloon angioplasty.

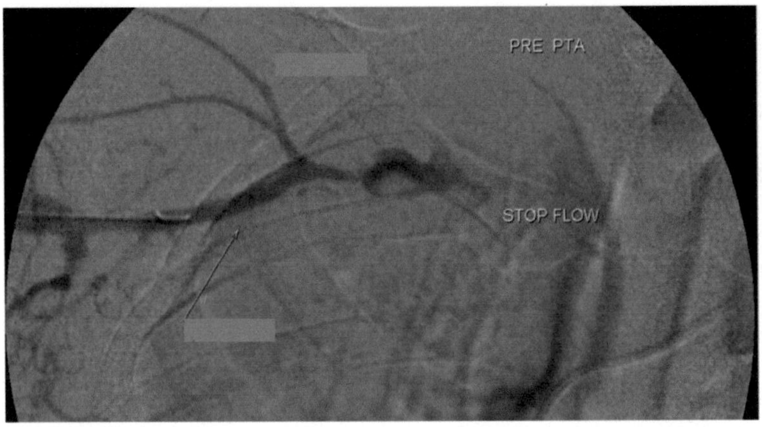

(a)

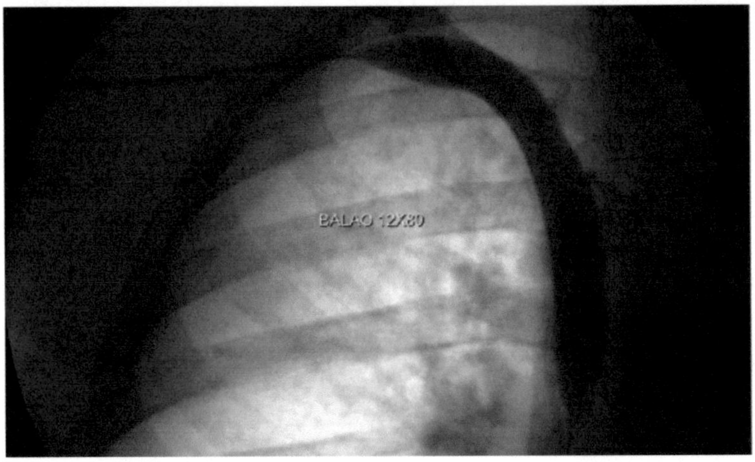

(b)

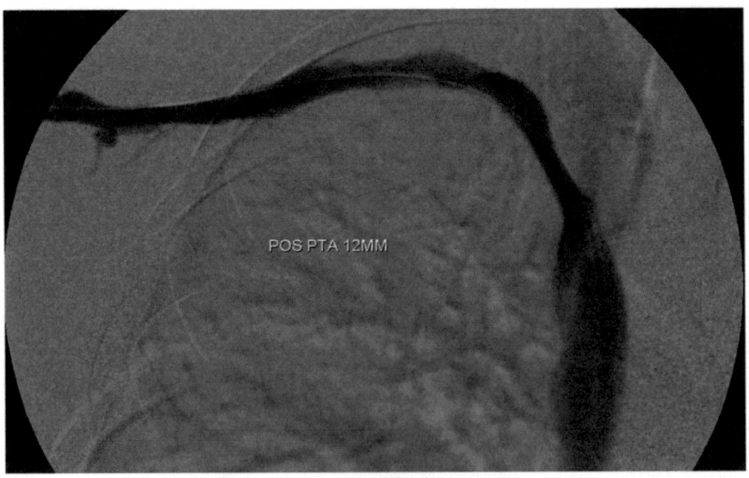

(c)

Figure 2.
(a) Right brachiocephalic trunk stop flow. (b) PTA of stenosis with 12 mm balloon. (c) Final angiogram result.

range between 23 and 63% at 6 months and 12 and 50% at 12 months in the case of primary patency rate, as well as 29 and 100% at 6 months and 13 and 100% at 12 months in the case of cumulative patency rate (**Figure 2**) [36, 39–42].

Our cumulative experience shows that angioplasty and stent placement is undermined by frequent and rapid recurrence. It can also happen that an asymptomatic lesion can become symptomatic upon intervention. Indeed, one study showed that stenosis can progress faster after intervention [37]. The venous response may be worsening, and the stenosis process can be accelerated due to angioplasty.

Correction of CVS with endovascular approaches remains therefore limited and suboptimal and may even be harmful in certain cases. After angioplasty, more aggressive neointimal hyperplasia and proliferative lesions were found in restenosis areas than in the original stenotic lesions [38].

A major problem with lesions in the central veins is that many are quite elastic. For this reason, endovascular stents are used more frequently for central veins stenosis than for other types of dialysis access lesions. Cost considerations are highly relevant and also the fact that we are left without any option to treat effectively a restenosis inside a stent. Even if we extend 100% the half-life of a recurrent stenotic access (from a procedure every 3 months to every 6 months), it may look as an impressive achievement, but with little clinical relevance.

5.4 Juxta-anastomotic location

The vein immediately adjacent to the arteriovenous anastomosis (commonly referred to as juxta-anastomosis) is a common location of stenosis. This is in part due to injury, which occurred while "swinging" the vein to form the AV anastomosis. Some studies demonstrate that the frequency of juxta-anastomotic stenosis may be up to 55% [43].

Angioplasty and surgery are two treatment options. Percutaneous angioplasty has 1-year patency rates of 44–79% [44–46]. For surgery, 1-year patency rates are between 64 and 88% [45–47]. In this location, we usually need very high-pressure balloons to deal with very hard lesions. If we elect a surgical solution, we get better results at the expense of a few more centimeters of vascular territory. Regrettably, randomized studies comparing endovascular treatment and surgery for this lesion are not available (**Figure 3**).

5.5 Type of angioplasty balloons

There are several types of balloons that we can use in angioplasty: (i) "high-pressure," (ii) "ultrahigh-pressure (UHP)," (iii) "cutting," and (iv) "drug-eluting."

5.5.1 High-pressure balloons

High-pressure, noncompliant balloons (e.g., Conquest from Bard Peripheral Vascular Inc., Tempe, Arizona) have rated burst pressures of 20 to 24 atm and are used to treat dialysis vascular access stenosis.

5.5.2 Ultrahigh-pressure balloons

Venous stenosis is characterized by extensive fibrosis and the need for ultrahigh-pressure balloon inflations [48] or cutting balloon atherotomy for optimal treatment [49, 50].

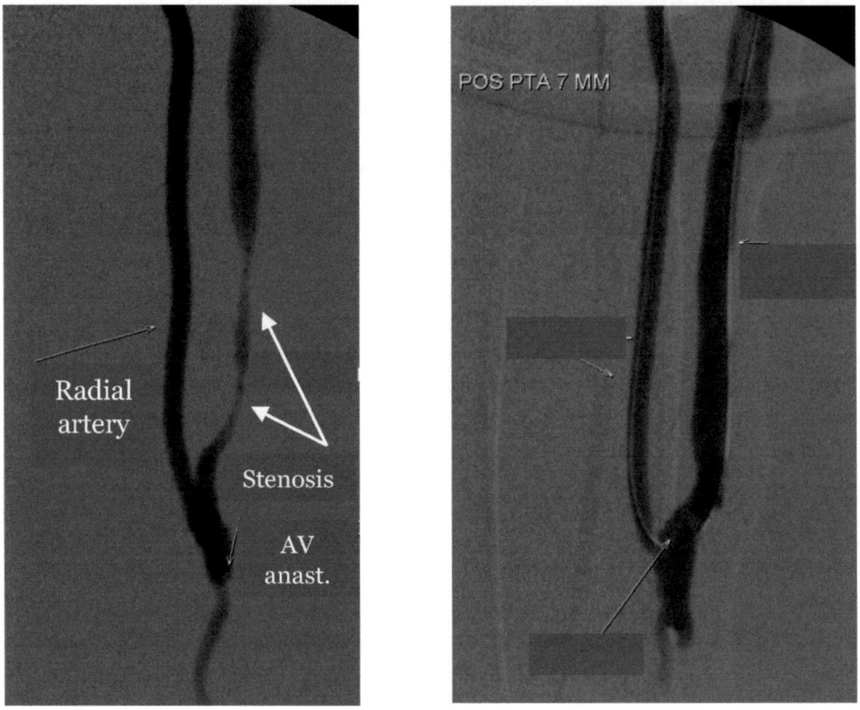

(a) (b)

Figure 3.
(a) Severe stenosis in juxta-anastomotic radio-cephalic fistula. (b) Angiogram result after angioplasty with 7 mm PTA balloon.

An UHP balloon is certified for a burst pressure of 27 atm, but higher inflation pressures are possible. Although those balloons do not provide better results in terms of permeability, when compared to conventional ones, it has been suggested that such devices may achieve better patency rates than traditional HP angioplasty balloons [51]. Its use is indicated in the treatment of symptomatic stenosis not responding to conventional high-pressure balloon. The high price of UHP balloon, the need for use thicker inserts, the difficulty of emptying, and its lower compliance and flexibility make it advisable that UHP balloons should not be a first choice in stenosis treatment.

Despite that, ultrahigh-pressure balloons have significantly reduced the incidence of "resistant" lesions [52].

5.5.3 Cutting balloons

The cutting balloons are special angioplasty balloons with three or four cutting edges (atherotomes) fixed longitudinally to its surface. The atherotomes expand radially with balloon inflation and provide longitudinal incisions into the lesion cutting into tenacious neointima. Using cutting balloons has the advantage that disruption of the lesion occurs in a more controlled manner and at lower balloon inflation pressure than with conventional angioplasty.

The use of a cutting angioplasty balloon (CAB) to treat resistant lesions can be found in several reports [49, 51]. Most of these reports are constrained because they are retrospective, lack control, or the size is too small to allow meaningful conclusions. Taking into account the data reported in the literature and also considering the authors experience, it can be stated that angioplasty with a cutting balloon is safe and can be considered as an alternative treatment for stenosis of hemodialysis AVFs that do not respond to conventional balloons.

There are serious methodologic limitations in the published reports describing the use of cutting balloon angioplasty to treat hemodialysis vascular access stenosis [53–56]. Studies include the concurrent use of cutting and conventional balloon angioplasty, the use of a high-pressure balloon, or a combination with placement of a stent after cutting balloon angioplasty. In other studies, cutting PTA was used only after the failure of high-pressure balloon angioplasty. In these reports, the long-term patency rate does not reflect the results obtainable with cutting balloon angioplasty as a primary, stand-alone treatment. The cutting balloon was designed primarily to reduce vascular trauma, thereby diminishing neointimal hyperplasia, thereby improving hemodialysis access long-term patency. It should be noted that studies comparing cutting balloon and conventional balloon angioplasty in the treatment of vascular access stenosis are fraught with conflicting results.

5.6 Drug-coated balloons

Good results have been obtained with drug-coated balloon (DCB) angioplasty used to prevent restenosis in the treatment of arterial stenosis. This approach (using paclitaxel-coated balloons) was extended to the treatment of stenosis associated with hemodialysis AV access, with mixed results [57].

Drug-coated balloon endovascular technology merges the dilating properties of angioplasty with local drug delivery. Balloon surface excipients enable drug-eluting within the vessel wall, inhibiting cell proliferation, and reducing neointimal hyperplasia, while avoiding the use of permanent metal stents.

DCB angioplasty of vascular access stenosis seem to be safe and effective, providing superior reintervention-free intervals compared to conventional plain balloon angioplasty [58–60]. Recently, Yan and others published a meta-analysis that reveals that DCB is an effective and safe method that can significantly prolong 6-month and 1-year target lesion primary patency for failing hemodialysis access, as compared to conventional plain balloon angioplasty. However, their study was limited by the small number of patients enrolled in each trial, the diversity characteristics of the lesions, the vintage of the dialysis access, and the formulations of paclitaxel (different dose or excipients used). A very heterogeneous group of studies lumped together [61].

The reported number of dialysis patients treated with DCBs is low, and several concerns remain unanswered. First of all, it is uncertain which lesions will benefit from the use of this balloon device. Lesion preparation is another issue that deserves further investigation. Manufacturing companies suggest pre-dilation with a shorter balloon, with the same diameter, to promote drug diffusion within the deeper layers of the vessel wall and to improve the restenosis rate. However, in some RCTs published, pre-dilation was not even performed. Last but not least, although the long-term safety of PCBs in dialysis access treatment has been proven, preclinical and experimental studies in animal models are lacking; consequently, we have no available information on the posttreatment lesion pathology, degree of drug diffusion, and the extent of paclitaxel fixation within the venous wall.

It should be noted that the use of drug-eluting balloons is a novel medical device that aims to decrease the trauma in the endothelium of the vascular wall of a fistula. Although more expensive than the conventional balloon, it is much cheaper than a bare metal stent, and repeated procedures can be performed in case of recurrences. More trials are needed to find out if this more expensive material can really increase the patency of venous lesions.

5.7 Stent placement

Several challenges must be faced by resistant or recurrent stenosis throughout the access circuit in terms of providing optimal hemodialysis treatment. Those stenoses can be successfully treated by endovascular stent placement, although it usually requires multiple procedures to maintain patency.

Indeed, bare metal stents and covered stents have emerged as a potential additional therapeutic intervention in vascular access dysfunction. However, results are not encouraging. For example, bare stents are seldom used due to a high incidence of in-stent stenosis, and covered stents also have problems.

There are three mostly accepted indications for stent deployment: (i) a stenotic lesion that recurs within a 3-month period after initially successful balloon angioplasty in a patient with *exhausted VA sites*, (ii) a stenotic lesion with high elastic recoil (usually in central veins), and (iii) rupture of an outflow vein after balloon angioplasty that cannot be handled using more conventional actions (balloon tamponade). Other special conditions where a stent implantation should be considered include (i) venous outflow stenosis, (ii) pseudo-aneurysms, and (iii) cephalic arch stenosis.

We must take special care not to occlude important collateral veins with implanted stent, namely, the homolateral internal jugular vein, always required for future central vein catheters.

There are several reported complications associated with stent placement, such as stent migration, or stent fracture, which is usually seen on control angiograms. Infection is also a significant complication with potentially tragic outcomes. It should be noted that the combination of the immune-compromised status of patients with ESRD and repetitive cannulations for dialysis treatments is likely factors leading to infection. One unique complication is stent struts protrusion, which results from placing stents in cannulation sites [62]. Damage of the metal part of the stents (struts) can result from repetitive cannulation.

The high cost of stents has to be taken into account, raising the question whether the benefits obtained by placing stents at stenotic lesions outweigh the costs associated with such treatment [9]. One should reflect if the option of creating a secondary AVF should be considered as an alternative treatment for placing a stent (**Figure 4**).

5.8 AVG thrombolysis

Graft thrombosis occurs in one-third of all AVG per year, and of those that thrombose, 60% have more than two episodes per year. Ninety percent of all AVG thrombosis are associated with a stenotic lesion, most commonly in the venous anastomosis, but can occur in any location, in 36% of the cases in more than one site.

In our VAC, AVG thrombosis is primarily referred to interventional nephrology for endovascular thrombectomy, combining pharmaco-mechanical thrombolysis with a multiperforated catheter occluded at its tip, allowing high-pressure lateral injection of heparinized saline to dislodge wall adherent clots, followed by angioplasty with a 8 mm balloon of all stenotic lesions and finally embolectomy of the arterial anastomosis with a 4 French Fogarty catheter, to remove a more adherent, residual, fibrin "white" clot. Alternatively, some of us may use a mechanical device, the Arrow-Trerotola©, that combines clot fragmentation and aspiration, adding quite a substantial extra cost, without improving outcomes.

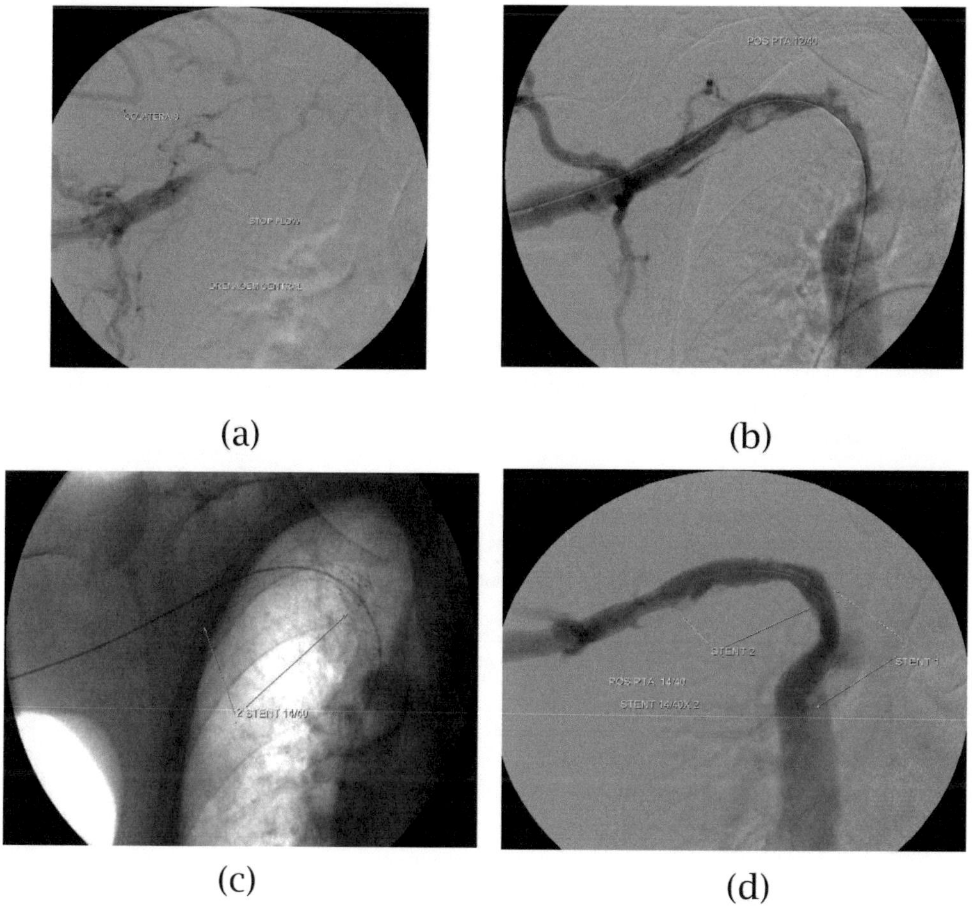

Figure 4.
(a) Stop flow at right BCT. (b) Placement of a stent. (c) Angiogram after 12 mm PTA balloon. (d) Final angiogram result.

The procedure should not be performed if the AVG is suspected to be infected or a graft rupture is detected. At the end of the procedure, we must check AVG flow, the presence of residual clot inside the VA, and the most dreadful complication, symptomatic hand ischemia due to distal arterial embolization, which must be resolved with embolectomy in the angiographic suite or urgently referred to surgery.

6. Endovascular intervention outcomes

The quality indicators achieved in our VAC include: (a) creation of a nAVF as first access in 80% of all patients and in 60% of subsequent accesses, (b) less than 40% primary failure of nAVF at 3 months, (c) less than 55% secondary failure of nAVF at 12 months, (d) less than 30% primary failure of AVGs at 3 months, (e) percent of functioning AVG post-thrombolysis >75% at 7 days and >50% at 3 months, and (f) no VA infections 15 days post-intervention. Regarding VA, the dialysis unit quality indicators are (a) percent of prevalent patients with nAVF >65%, (b) percent of patients with long-term tunneled catheters <20%, and (c) referral's rate to the VAC <0.8/patient years.

Procedures	At 30 days (%)	At 90 days (%)	At 180 days (%)
Diagnostic angiography	83	55	45
Angioplasty	92	60	45
Thrombolysis + angioplasty (AVG)	86	51	40

Table 1.
Primary patency in our VAC at 30, 90, and 180 days, in line with most literature in the field.

In intervening in a nAVF, use when available ultrasound localization of stenosis to plan the best place and direction to puncture the access
In intervening in a AVG, always puncture close to the arterial anastomosis in the direction of the flow toward the venous anastomosis
Use a 7F sheath and a hydrophilic guide wire. It allows balloons up to 14 mm to be inserted more than once
Do not miss any step even when it seems unnecessary. Always check AV anastomosis in nAVFs and arterial and venous anastomosis in AVGs, as well as central venous drainage
Do not accept incomplete balloon dilation. If necessary, use high-pressure balloons or cutting balloons
Avoid stents, only as a last resort
In AVG thrombolysis, after dealing with the venous anastomosis, even if the graft is already working, do approach with a Fogarty the arterial anastomosis
Always test flow at the end of a procedure. An eyeball test as the TIMI for cardiologists. If flow does not look great, it is because there is something else to fix

Table 2.
Clinical pearls to take home.

The technical details of all procedures we perform in our VAC are thoroughly described in a recent textbook [63, 64].

The National Kidney Foundation (KDOQI) guidelines [65] define a successful angioplasty a residual stenosis <30%, with return to acceptable levels of the parameters used to place the indication for angioplasty. Initial success rates using anatomical criteria ranged from 80 to 98%, but in some reports, 20–30% of these patients with anatomical success fail to increase blood flow (residual stenosis, a missed lesion, or elasticity). Primary patency rates are 41–76% at 6 months and 31–45% at 1 year.

Long-term primary patency rates for thrombectomy are not as good as for angioplasty; therefore every effort should be made to prevent thrombosis by the prospective diagnosis and treatment of venous stenosis.

In a thrombosed access, the treatment must be timely to avoid catheters, done as an outpatient, venous stenosis must be detected and corrected, hemodynamic parameters should return to baseline, and patient should be evaluated for a secondary arteriovenous native fistula, created using upper arm veins that have become dilated because of the functioning graft.

In 2019, 139 surgical thrombectomies were performed in 127 patients (69 in nAVF and 70 in AVG). In 49.6%, no new intervention was required, and the average time until a new intervention was 46.7 days. Primary patency at 1 month was 66%, at 3 months 54.4%, and at 6 months 17.5%. In that same period, the angiography suite received 134 patients for 179 procedures (171 in AVGs, 8 with a nAVF), there was immediate success in 159 patients, the average time until a new intervention was 58.1-day, and primary patency at 1 month was 71.6% and at 6 months 42.5%. In our case, Qa average improvement is >50%, and we expect a Kt/V above 1.4.

The immediate success rate of thrombolysis should be 85% or greater according to the NKF/KDOQI guidelines and the primary (unassisted) patency goals at 3 months at least 40% (**Tables 1** and **2**).

7. Conclusion

In conclusion, we are still dealing with quite a number of known unknowns. There has been no RCT to elucidate which percentage of lumen compromise should dictate the indication for angioplasty, and most operators choose 50%. Not all stenotic plaques were created equal, and some will never progress, but we cannot guess which ones. We also have no proof that a successful PTA in a graft improves long-term patency rate [14], angiographic criteria to assess the success of angioplasty are not predictive of changes in blood flow, and there is no correlation between changes in blood flow and changes in the percent of stenosis post-PTA [66]. In an era characterized by less is more, under the imperative of being useful for our patients, creating long-term solutions at sustainable costs, we feel a desperate need for robust scientific evidence to support our decision process and the procedures we perform. Just because it can be done, does not mean it should be done, our intervention is no more a question of know-how, but of know-when.

Author details

Pedro Ponce[1,2]* and Ana Mateus[2]

1 Nephrologist, General ICU of Hospital Cuf, Lisbon, Portugal

2 Vascular Access Centers, NephroCare, Portugal

*Address all correspondence to: pedro.ponce@fmc-ag.com

References

[1] Al-Jaishi A, Oliver M, Thomas S, Lok C, Zhang J, Garg A, et al. Patency rates of the arteriovenous fistula for hemodialysis: A systematic review and meta-analysis. American Journal of Kidney Diseases. 2014;**63**(3):464-478

[2] Lok C, Sontrop J, Tomlinson G, et al. Cumulative patency of contemporary fistulas versus grafts. Clinical Journal of the American Society of Nephrology. 2013;**8**:1-9

[3] Lok C. Fistula first initiative: Advantages and pitfalls. Clinical Journal of the American Society of Nephrology. 2007;**2**:1043-1053

[4] Al-Jaishi A, Moist L. Fistula eligibility: A work in progress. Seminars in Dialysis. 2014;**27**:173-178

[5] Drew D, Lok C, Cohen J, et al. Vascular access choice in incident hemodialysis patients: A decision analysis. Journal of the American Society of Nephrology. 2015;**26**:183-191

[6] Lumsden A, MacDonald M, Kikeri D, et al. Prophylactic balloon angioplasty fails to prolong the patency of expanded PTFE arteriovenous grafts. Journal of Vascular Surgery. 1997;**26**:382-390

[7] Chang C, Ko P, Hsu L, et al. Highly increased cell proliferation activity in the restenotic hemodialysis vascular access after percutaneous transluminal angioplasty. American Journal of Kidney Diseases. 2004;**43**:74-84

[8] Moist L, Churchill D, House A, et al. Regular monitoring of access flow compared with monitoring of venous pressure fails to improve graft survival. Journal of the American Society of Nephrology. 2003;**14**:2645-2653

[9] Salman L, Asif A. Stent graft for nephrologists: Concerns and consensus. Clinical Journal of the American Society of Nephrology. 2010;**5**:1347-1352

[10] Tessitore N, Bedogna V, Gammaro L, et al. Diagnostic accuracy of ultrasound dilution access blood flow measurement in detecting stenosis and predicting thrombosis in native forearm arteriovenous fistulae for hemodialysis. American Journal of Kidney Diseases. 2003;**42**:331-341

[11] McCarley P, Wingard R, Shyr Y, et al. Vascular access blood flow monitoring reduces access morbidity and costs. Kidney International. 2001;**60**:1164-1172

[12] Tonelli M, Jindal K, Hirsch D, et al. Screening for subclinical stenosis in native vessel arteriovenous fistulae. Journal of the American Society of Nephrology. 2001;**12**:1729-1733

[13] Tessitore N, Mansueto G, Bedogna V, et al. A prospective controlled trial on effect of percutaneous transluminal angioplasty on functioning arteriovenous fistulae survival. Journal of the American Society of Nephrology. 2003;**14**:1623-1627

[14] Dember L, Holmberg E, Kaufman J. Randomized controlled trial of prophylactic repair of hemodialysis arteriovenous graft stenosis. Kidney International. 2004;**66**:390-398

[15] Ikizler T, Himmelfarb J. Trials and trade-offs in hemodialysis vascular access monitoring. Nephrology, Dialysis, Transplantation. 2006;**21**:3362-3363

[16] Shahin H, Reddy G, Sharafuddin M, et al. Monthly access flow monitoring with increased prophylactic angioplasty did not improve fistula patency. Kidney International. 2005;**68**:2352-2361

[17] Robbin ML, Oser RF, Lee JY, et al. Randomized comparison of ultrasound

surveillance and clinical monitoring on arteriovenous graft outcomes. Kidney International. 2006;**69**:730-735

[18] Lok CE, Bhola C, Croxford R, et al. Reducing vascular access morbidity: A comparative trial of two vascular access monitoring strategies. Nephrology, Dialysis, Transplantation. 2003;**18**:1174-1180

[19] Ram SJ, Work J, Caldito GC, et al. A randomized controlled trial of blood flow and stenosis surveillance of haemodialysis grafts. Kidney International. 2003;**64**:272-280

[20] Ponce P, Mateus A, Santos L. Anatomical correlation of a well-functioning access graft for haemodialysis. Nephrology, Dialysis, Transplantation. 2009;**24**:535-538

[21] Ponce P, Pinto B. Measuring vascular access flow: The accuracy of different methods. Portuguese Journal of Nephrology & Hypertension. 2011;**25**:151-155

[22] Krivitski N. Theory and validation of access flow measurement by dilution technique during hemodialysis. Kidney International. 1995;**48**:244-250

[23] Mercadal L, Hamani A, Bene B, Petclerc T. Determination of access flow from ionic dialysance: Theory and validation. Kidney International. 1999;**56**:1560-1565

[24] Lindsay R, Huang S, Sternby J, Hertz T. The measurement of hemodialysis access blood flow by a conductivity step method. Clinical Journal of the American Society of Nephrology. 2010;**5**:1602-1606

[25] Schneditz D, Wang E, Levin N. Validation of haemodialysis recirculation and access blood flow measured by thermodilution. Nephrology, Dialysis, Transplantation. 1999;**14**:376-383

[26] Lacson E, Lazarus J, Panlilio R, Gotch F. Comparisons of hemodialysis blood access flow rates using online measurement of conductivity dialysance and ultrasound dilution. American Journal of Kidney Diseases. 2008;**51**:99-106

[27] Lopot F, Nejedly B, Sulkova S, Blaha J. Comparison of different techniques of haemodialysis vascular access flow evaluation. The Journal of Vascular Access. 2004;**5**:25-32

[28] Fontseré N, Blasco M, Maduell F, et al. Practical utility of online clearance and blood temperature monitors as non-invasive techniques to measure hemodialysis blood access flow. Blood Purification. 2011;**31**:1-8

[29] Bosman P, Boereboom F, Bakker C, et al. Access flow measurement in hemodialysis patients. Journal of the American Society of Nephrology. 1996;**7**:966-969

[30] Tonelli M, Klarenbach S, Jindal K, et al. Access flow in arteriovenous accesses by optodilutional and ultrasound dilution methods. American Journal of Kidney Diseases. 2005;**46**:933-937

[31] Asif A, Leon C, Vargas L, et al. Accuracy of physical examination in the detection of arteriovenous fistula stenosis. Clinical Journal of the American Society of Nephrology. 2007;**2**:1191-1194

[32] Turmel-Rodrigues L, Pengloan J, Baudin S, Testou D, Abaza M, Dahdah G, et al. Treatment of stenosis and thrombosis in hemodialysis fistulas and grafts by interventional radiology. Nephrology, Dialysis, Transplantation. 2000;**15**:2029-2036

[33] Tordoir J, Mickley V. NKF-K/DOQI clinical practice guidelines for vascular access: Update 2000. American Journal of Kidney Diseases. 2001;**37**:S137-S181

[34] Cui J, Xu D, Ma J, Liu B, Kawai T, Yeh H, et al. Stenoses in the surgically manipulated segment have better angioplasty response compared to the surgically naive segment in fistulas. The Journal of Vascular Access. 2017;**18**:192-199

[35] Vascular Access 2006 Work Group. Clinical practice guidelines for vascular access. American Journal of Kidney Diseases. 2006;**48**(Suppl 1):S176

[36] Bakken AM, Protack CD, Saad WE, Lee DE, Waldman DL, Davies MG. Long-term outcomes of primary angioplasty and primary stenting of central venous stenosis in hemodialysis patients. Journal of Vascular Surgery. 2007;**45**:776-783

[37] Levit RD, Cohen RM, Kwak A, Shlansky-Goldberg RD, Clark TW, Patel AA, et al. Asymptomatic central venous stenosis in hemodialysis patients. Radiology. 2006;**238**:1051-1056

[38] Chang CJ, Ko PJ, Hsu LA, Ko YS, Ko YL, Chen CF, et al. Highly increased cell proliferation activity in the restenotic hemodialysis vascular access after percutaneous transluminal angioplasty: Implication in prevention of restenosis. American Journal of Kidney Diseases. 2004;**43**:74-84

[39] Tordoir J, Mickley V. National Kidney Foundation Guideline 20. K/DOQI Clinical Practice Guidelines for Vascular Access, 2000. American Journal of Kidney Diseases. 2001;**37**(Suppl 1):S137-S181

[40] Dammers R, de Haan MW, Planken NR, van der Sande FM, Tordoir JH. Central vein obstruction in hemodialysis patients: Results of radiological and surgical intervention. European Journal of Vascular and Endovascular Surgery. 2003;**26**:317-321

[41] Beathard GA. Percutaneous transvenous angioplasty in the treatment of vascular access stenosis. Kidney International. 1992;**42**:1390

[42] Quinn SF, Schuman ES, Demlow TA, et al. Percutaneous transluminal angioplasty versus endovascular stent placement in the treatment of venous stenoses in patients undergoing hemodialysis: Intermediate results. Journal of Vascular and Interventional Radiology. 1995;**6**:851

[43] Turmel-Rodrigues L, Mouton A, Birmelé B, et al. Salvage of immature forearm fistulas for hemodialysis by interventional radiology. Nephrology, Dialysis, Transplantation. 2001;**16**:2365

[44] Mortamais J, Papillard M, Girouin N, et al. Endovascular treatment of juxta-anastomotic venous stenoses of forearm radiocephalic fistulas: Long-term results and prognostic factors. Journal of Vascular and Interventional Radiology. 2013;**24**:558

[45] Manninen HI, Kaukanen ET, Ikaheimo R, et al. Brachial arterial access: Endovascular treatment of failling Brescia-Cimino hemodialysis fistulas - Initial success and long-term results. Radiology. 2001;**218**:711

[46] Clark TWI, Hirsch DA, Jindal KJ, Veugelers PJ, LeBlanc J. Outcome and prognostic factors of restenosis after percutaneous treatment of native hemodialysis fistulas. Journal of Vascular and Interventional Radiology. 2002;**13**(1):51-59

[47] Tessitore N, Mansueto G, Lipari G, et al. Endovascular versus surgical preemptive repair of forearm arteriovenous fistula juxta-anastomotic stenosis: Analysis of data collected prospectively from 1999 to 2004. Clinical Journal of the American Society of Nephrology. 2006;**1**:448-454

[48] Trerotola SO, Kwak A, Clark TW, et al. Prospective study of balloon inflation pressures and other technical aspects of hemodialysis angioplasty. Journal of Vascular and Interventional Radiology. 2005;**16**:1613-1618

[49] Vesely TM, Siegel JB. Use of the peripheral cutting balloon to treat hemodialysis-related stenoses. Journal of Vascular and Interventional Radiology. 2005;**16**:1593-1603

[50] Kariya S, Tanigawa N, Kojima H, Komemushi A, Shomura Y, Shiraishi T, et al. Primary patency with cutting and conventional balloon angioplasty for different types of hemodialysis access stenosis. Radiology. 2007;**243**:578-587

[51] Rajan D, Platzker T, Lok C, Beecroft JR, Tan KT, Sniderman KW, et al. Ultrahigh pressure versus high-pressure angioplasty for treatment of venous anastomotic stenosis in hemodialysis grafts: Is there a difference in patency? Journal of Vascular and Interventional Radiology. 2007;**18**:709-714

[52] Trerotola SO, Stavropoulos SW, Shlansky-Goldberg R, Tuite CM, Kobrin S, Rudnick MR. Hemodialysis-related venous stenosis: Treatment with ultrahigh-pressure angioplasty balloons. Radiology. 2004;**231**:259-262

[53] Bittl JA. Venous rupture during percutaneous treatment of hemodialysis fistulas and grafts. Catheterization and Cardiovascular Interventions. 2009;**74**:1097-1101

[54] Ryan JM, Dumbleton SA, Smith TP. Using a cutting balloon to treat resistant high-grade dialysis graft stenosis. AJR. American Journal of Roentgenology. 2003;**180**:1072-1074

[55] Singer-Jordan J, Papura S. Cutting balloon angioplasty for primary treatment of hemodialysis fistula venous stenoses: Preliminary results. Journal of Vascular and Interventional Radiology. 2005;**16**:25-29

[56] Song HH, Kim KT, Chung SK, Kim YO, Yoon SA. Cutting balloon angioplasty for resistant venous stenoses of Brescia-Cimino fistulas. Journal of Vascular and Interventional Radiology. 2004;**15**:1463-1467

[57] Khawaja AZ, Cassidy DB, Al Shakarchi J, et al. Systemic review of drug eluting balloon angioplasty for arteriovenous haemodialysis access stenosis. The Journal of Vascular Access. 2016;**17**:103-110

[58] Katsanos K, Karnabatidis D, Kitrou P, et al. Paclitaxel-coated balloon angioplasty vs. plain balloon dilation for the treatment of failing dialysis access: 6-month interim results from a prospective randomized controlled trial. Journal of Endovascular Therapy. 2012;**19**:263-272

[59] Lai CC, Fang HC, Tseng CJ, et al. Percutaneous angioplasty using a paclitaxel-coated balloon improves target lesion restenosis on inflow lesions of autogenous radiocephalic fistulas: A pilot study. Journal of Vascular and Interventional Radiology. 2014;**25**:535-541

[60] Massmann A, Fries P, Obst-Gleditsch K, et al. Paclitaxel-coated balloon angioplasty for symptomatic central vein restenosis in patients with hemodialysis fistulas. Journal of Endovascular Therapy. 2015;**22**:74-79

[61] Yuan Y, Cheng W, Lu H. Drug-eluting balloon versus plain balloon angioplasty for the treatment of failing hemodialysis access: A systematic review and meta-analysis. Annals of Vascular Surgery. 2019;**64**:389-396

[62] Asif A, Gadalean F, Eid N, Merrill D, Salman L. Stent graft infection and protrusion through

the skin: Clinical considerations and potential medico-legal ramifications. Seminars in Dialysis. 2010;**23**(5):540-542

[63] Beathard G. "Arteriovenous grafts stenosis and thrombosis" in Interventional Nephrology. China: The McGraw-Hill Companies Inc.; 2012. p. 179

[64] Beathard G. Venous angioplasty. In: Interventional Nephrology. China: The McGraw-Hill Companies Inc.; 2012. p. 199

[65] NKF. KDOQI clinical practice guidelines for vascular access. American Journal of Kidney Diseases. 2006;**48**(Suppl 1):S248-S272

[66] Ahya S, Windus D, Vesely T, et al. Flow in hemodialysis grafts after angioplasty. Kidney International. 2001;**59**:1974

Section 3

Cardiovascular Interventions

Chapter 12

Coronary Artery Intervention Techniques

Imran Khalil

Abstract

The topic of coronary artery intervention techniques is very complex. This chapter's goal is to discuss basic to complex techniques summarized to help coronary operators at all levels to understand the practical aspects of daily coronary interventions using a noncomplex approach. With the revolution of percutaneous cardiovascular and valvular interventions, more patients with complex coronary lesions are treated with percutaneous coronary intervention (PCI) over coronary artery bypass graft (CABG) surgery. Thus, mastering all approaches, techniques of PCI, being comfortable with performing high risk PCIs, and using hemodynamic support devices have become very important. While the basics of coronary interventions have not changed, equipment innovation has a very rapid pace with almost daily additions to the arsenal of coronary interventions, in particular, stent development. Stent therapy for coronary interventions especially in acute coronary syndrome is a proven concept. This created a race to develop a perfect stent that allows for physiological healing of the coronaries and avoid their use in long-term issues. With each addition to the equipment collection comes a learning curve on both technical and clinical evidence aspects, all which make coronary intervention a more specialized and rapidly progressive field.

Keywords: percutaneous coronary interventions, techniques, complex, high risk, equipment, radial approach, bifurcations stenting, coronary guidewires, coronary guide catheters, left main, venous graft interventions, instent restenosis

1. Introduction

For daily planned procedures, there are several approaches for coronary interventions. In reality and especially an emergency situation, any kind of arterial approach that can reach the coronary tree can be used as long as emergency percutaneous coronary interventions could be successfully and safely performed.

These common approaches include radial right and left, ulnar right and left, distal radial right and left, femoral, and brachial. Carotid, axillary approaches might be necessary in the right clinical presentation. For each approach, operators need to be familiar with the limitations, advantages, disadvantages, access and closure techniques, potential complications, and their management. Knowledge of arterial and venous anatomy and its possible anomalies are basic requirements of any vascular operator.

This chapter is focusing on PCI technical aspects and high-risk interventions. Reader is redirected to other resources that focus on performing diagnostic left heart catheterization (LHC) as it is crucial to understand everything about diagnostic catheters, procedure, and equipment before proceeding with PCI.

Table 1 includes a required checklist of equipment needed in any catheterization lab performing PCI, especially high-risk PCI.

2. Percutaneous coronary interventions

Performing successful PCI requires good planning. Access site, anticoagulation, antiplatelet therapy, good assessment of target lesions, intravascular imaging, adjunct therapies (i.e. atherectomy or other plaque modification procedures), and instruments necessary to perform the procedure and handle complications should be available.

The main simple steps for any PCI are engaging the target system with the guide catheter, wiring the lesion, preparing the lesion for stenting and finally deploying the stent. Every step can be a challenge by itself.

2.1 Radial approach

Over the last two decades, radial approach for coronary interventions has developed significantly. It has become the standard of care in any catheterization lab.

In addition to growing evidence that supports this approach of safety and better outcome in coronary interventions [1–4], it is also significantly evolving as a great approach for peripheral arterial interventions, including abdominal vessel interventions and even lower extremity interventions.

With obesity pandemic, operators need to perform LHC/PCI using a radial approach and avoid femoral at all prices, and we will discuss the femoral approach in obese patients. Obese patients can be very challenging patients for radial approach, but it is definitely worth it to avoid using femoral approach and dealing with access and potential complications that rise especially in obese diabetic patients [5].

For our topic of coronary interventions, radial approach especially right radial approach is the main approach for any patient; first time coronary angiogram and PCI patients or returning patients, chronic total obstruction interventions and even patients with prior CABG [6].

In case of suspected acute stent thrombosis after completing PCI, radial access at the same site can be safely performed. While in femoral approach, it depends on the closure device that has been used.

It has proven that it is safer than any other approach with less bleeding, access complications, and outcome at least in STEMI patients [3].

Even in post-CABG patients, right radial approach can be used effectively. All aortic grafts can be imaged easily. Even the left internal mammillary artery LIMA can be reached but requires manipulating across the aortic arch to reach left subclavian and wiring it. Meaning crossing all the head vessel which in diseased aortic arch might not be a smart idea as it could increase risk of emboli ischemic stroke significantly. That is where left radial approach comes handy.

In elderly small size females, radial approach for LHC/PCI is a priority as this category of patients carries the highest risk of vascular complications and bleeding using femoral approach. 5Fr radial sheath is considered in general safer to perform LHC and even simple PCI that does not require 6F guide catheters.

Sheaths	6–8 French standard (short and supportive long 23, 45, 65 cm for support of a tortuous, iliac and aorta for femoral approach). Multiple sheaths available: pinnacle, bright tip, braided and destinations Radial sheaths 6–7 French; several available sheaths: slender sheath most commonly used Sheathless 7Fr system like RailWay system
Injection system	Manifold 4 valve system or Acist device. At least Manifold should be available
Y-connector with hemostatic valve	Regular Tuohy, Co-pilot, or Guardian
Guide catheters	Multiple available guide catheters available from different companies and for right and left system; differences are minimal. Starting from less support to maximum support. More support is provided with contralateral support guide catheters against the contralateral aortic wall or aortic valve For the right: Judkins right 4, IMA, Amplatz right, Multipurpose, KR4, IKARI left, Voda right, Amplatz left For the left system: Judkins left, IKAR left, Kimny, Voda left, EBU, XB, CLS, SAL, Amplatz left etc.
Guide catheter extensions	Guideliner, Guidezilla, Guidion, Trapliner
Guide wires	Vascular wires and catheters: 0.035 or 0.038 J tip wire, wholey wire, glide wire, glide wire advantage wire, super stiff or extra stiff wire (help advance sheath through scar tissue and straighten tortuous large vessels), glide straight and angled tip catheters For coronary wires: see **Table 2** for list of available wires
Intravascular diagnostic imaging	IVUS, OCT
Micro-catheters/support catheters	See **Table 3** for list of available micro catheters
Lesion crossing/ preparation for stenting	Small balloons, over the wire or rapid exchange Tornus or Turnpike Gold Threader LASER Atherectomy systems (rotational, orbital)
Dissection/reentry equipment	CrossBoss Catheter/Stingray LP balloon and wire
Balloons and stents	Compliant and noncompliant balloons of all different sizes and lengths, cutting balloons, Ostial Flash Bare metal stents, drug eluting stents and Covered stents
Complications management	Covered stents (Graftmaster or PK Papyrus) Vascular coils: better if detachable and 0.014 compatible such as Axium coils. Other 0.018 pushable coils could be used if there are the only available ones but they require higher profile micro catheters like Progreat or Renegade Pericardiocentesis tray, echo contrast Echocardiogram probe and vascular probe Thrombin Snares: Esnare or Atrieve 18–30 mm or 27–45 mm Vascular balloons and stents for vascular access complications
Hemodynamics support	Impella 2,5, CP, Impella RP, IABP and VA ECMO
Radiation protection	

Table 1.
Necessary equipment for successful PCI program.

In chronic total occlusion (CTO) interventions, radial approach can be used as a single access in antegrade approach or in retrograde approach with another access that could be femoral or even left radial depending on the clinical scenario.

Radial approach is very convenient for patients, allowing them to move as soon as possible and avoid prolonged bed rest and recurrent need for applying pressure in case of recurrent bleeding.

Initially, radial approach had increased radiation exposure and time compared to femoral approach. As it has a learning curve, this is not true anymore due to increase in operators' experience. Still, left radial approach has more operator radiation compared to femoral and right radial but less complications compared to femoral approach [7–9]. Using appropriate radiation protection could decrease operator's radiation exposure [10].

As in any artery, radial artery can dilate, but the dilation ratio depends on the baseline size, presence of atherosclerosis disease, and calcifications. Complications can occur when inappropriate dilation is performed. Specific medication mix is used to avoid spasm of radial or ulnar artery after getting access and sheath inserted. Still, some patients have significant spasm which can make radial approach very hard and even impossible to complete the requiring switching to femoral approach.

When facing any resistance advancing the wire, operator should perform an angiogram especially if 7F system is planned.

Sheath-less technique is encouraged when using larger than 6 F. 7Fr and can be performed in most patients. 8F requires large radial artery. Female patients with small size and short status are more likely to not have a radial vessel that accommodates larger than 6Fr system.

Ulnar artery can be dominant or the same size and can be used for PCI easily and safely. There is no significant data to compare radial and ulnar approaches.

2.2 Understanding coronary artery lesions

Atherosclerosis is the most common etiology for coronary artery disease. However, operator should understand the difference in physiology and invasive management of other etiologies such in inflammatory post-transplant vasculopathy (Cardiac Allograft Vasculopathy CAV) (**Tables 2** and **3**), vasculitis, aneurysms, and spontaneous coronary artery dissections (**Table 4**). Although the main principles of interventions are similar, these special etiologies require special considerations.

National American College of Cardiology/American Heart Association/Society for Cardiovascular Angiography and Interventions ACC/AHA/SCAI and international societies of cardiovascular diseases European Society of Cardiology ESC have their classifications of lesions risk of interventions for each coronary lesion based on

Type A	Discrete, tubular, or multiple stenosis	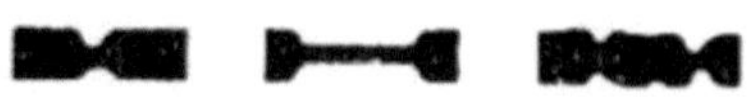
Type B1	Abrupt onset with distal diffuse concentric narrowing and obliterated vessels	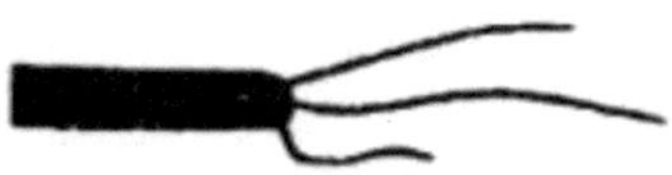
Type B2	Gradual, concentric tapering with distal portion having some residual lumen	
Type C	Narrowed irregular distal branches with terminations that are often none-tapered and squared off, ending abruptly	

Table 2.
Types of cardiac allograft vasculopathy lesions.

	Class I	Class II	Class III	Class IV
Severity	Minimal	Mild	Moderate	Severe
Intimal thickness	<0.3 mm	<0.3 mm	0.3–0.5 mm	>1 mm
Or			Or	Or
Extent of plaque	<180	>180	>0.5 mm, <180	>0.5 mm, >180

Table 3.
Duke classification of cardiac allograft vasculopathy on IVUS.

Type 1	Multiple radiolucent lumen
Type 2	Long diffuse and smooth narrowing of the body or distal end of the vessel
Type 3	Focal or tubular stenosis

Table 4.
Classification of spontaneous coronary artery dissection.

specific characteristics and success rate of intervention (**Tables 5** and **6**), Systemic evaluation of coronary lesion and understanding of the anatomical and physiological characteristics for each lesion are essential for successful intervention.

Syntax score is an additional tool that was developed to stratify patients based on the complexity of their coronary artery disease (CAD) and identify patients who benefit from different revascularizations options (CABG and PCI) based on their score. Similar to ACC/AHA classification of lesions, Syntax score is calculated based on each lesion characteristics with more details (**Figure 1** and **Table 7**). It is another available tool to evaluate the risk of lesions and subsequently the outcome of procedure.

Type A lesions: high success rate > 85%; low risk	
Discrete <10 mm length	Little or no calcification
Concentric	Less than total occlusion
Readily accessible	Not ostial location
None-angulated segment <45°	No major branch involvement
Smooth contour	Absence of thrombus
Type B lesions: moderate success 60–85%: moderate risk	
Tubular 10–20 mm length	Ostial in location
Eccentric	Bifurcation lesions requiring double guidewires
Moderate tortuosity of proximal segment	Some thrombus
Moderately angulated 45–90°	Total occlusion <3 months old
Irregular contour	Moderate to heavy calcifications
Type C lesions: low success <60%; high risk	
Diffuse lesion >20 mm length	Degenerated venous graft with friable lesions
Excessive tortuosity of proximal segment	Total occlusion >3 months old
Extremely angulated segment >90°	Inability to protect side branch

Table 5.
ACC/AHA classification of coronary lesions and outcome predictors.

SCAI Type I: highest success rate and lowest risk
Does not meet the criteria for ACC/AHA type C lesion
Patent
SCAI Type II lesion
Diffuse lesion >20 mm length
Excessive tortuosity of proximal segment
Extremely angulated segment >90°
Inability to protect major side branch
Degenerated venous graft with friable lesions
Patent
SCAI Type III lesion
Does not meet the criteria for ACC/AHA type C lesion
Occluded
SCAI Type IV lesion
Diffuse lesion >20 mm length
Excessive tortuosity of proximal segment
Extremely angulated segment >90°
Inability to protect major side branch
Degenerated venous graft with friable lesions
And occluded OR occluded more than 3 months alone

Table 6.
SCAI classification of coronary lesions.

Bifurcation lesions are one of the most challenging lesions for intervention. Multiple classifications have been developed with Medina being the most used one (**Figure 2**).

All classifications are meant to help operator to address the risk of intervention, success rate, potential complications and outcome. Operator should always keep in mind that coronary angiograms are only two dimensional images of three dimensional lesions. Baseline orthogonal and multiple projections angiogram should be used as possible to help achieve best angiographic results.

Deciding the need for hemodynamic support is not only related to the lesion characteristics. It is also based on the whole picture of the patient presentation, coronary and peripheral anatomy, comorbidities and evidence-based outcome. In some cases, the decision is clear whether to use hemodynamic mechanical support or not but in most of the cases, the answer is not clear.

Available mechanical hemodynamic support devices (left ventricular assist device LVAD) are intra-aortic balloon pump IABP, Impella (which comes in different sizes depending on the cardiac output they provide Impella 2.5, Impella CP, Impella 5), RP Impella (right ventricular Impella), venous arterial Extracorporeal membrane oxygenation (ECMO) (which also can provide different cardiac output depending on cannula size but also provide oxygenation which Impella does not) and Tandem heart. The discussion of each device indications, advantage and disadvantages is beyond this chapter.

The timing of hemodynamic support in acute setting (not planned PCI) before or after restoration of coronary flow is controversial and depends on several

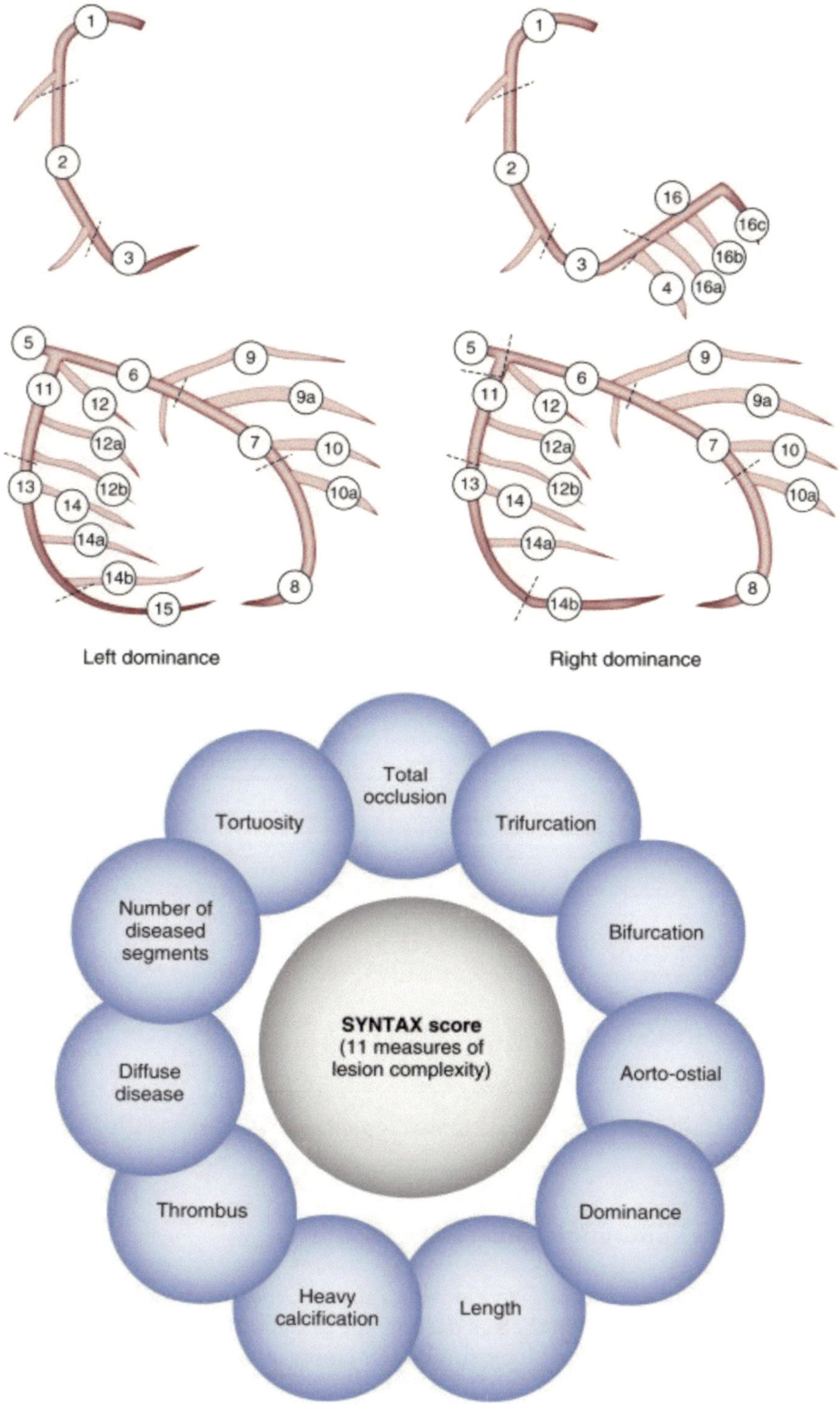

Figure 1.
Syntax score: top shows the dominance and numbering of coronaries segments, bottom: characteristics of each segment.

cofounders such as the presence of cardiogenic shock and the expected time to restore coronary flow in challenging lesions. Ongoing clinical trial are trying to address these questions. So far, there is no strong data to support placement

Lesion characteristics	Impact on syntax score
Diameter reduction	
Total occlusion	X5
Significant lesion (50–99%)	X2
Total occlusion	
Age > 3 months	+1
Blunt stump	+1
Bridging	+1
First segment visible beyond total occlusion	+1 per nonvisible segment
Side branch present	+1
Trifurcations	
1 diseased segment	+3
2 diseased segments	+4
3 diseased segments	+5
4 diseased segments	+6
Bifurcations	
Type A, B, C	+1
Type D, E, F, G	+2
Angulated <70°	+1
Aorto-ostial lesions	+1
Severe tortuosity	+2
Length > 2 cm	+1
Heavy calcifications	+2
Thrombus	+1
Diffuse disease/small vessels	+1 per segment number

Table 7.
Factors affecting lesion scoring in the syntax score.

of any hemodynamic support device in cardiogenic shock in the setting of acute coronary syndrome.

2.3 Choosing the appropriate guide catheter

Several medical companies provide wide range of options for guide catheters designs. Each has their own catheters designs for radial or femoral approach. They share the general principle and look similar. Operator should be knowledgeable of advantages and disadvantages of each and be comfortable to deal with challenges and complications as they appear.

Choosing the appropriate guide catheter is a very important step. It can make the intervention significantly easier and smother than using inappropriate guide catheter.

Goals of guide catheter:

Engage target coronary coaxially to avoid damage of the engagement and deep intubation.

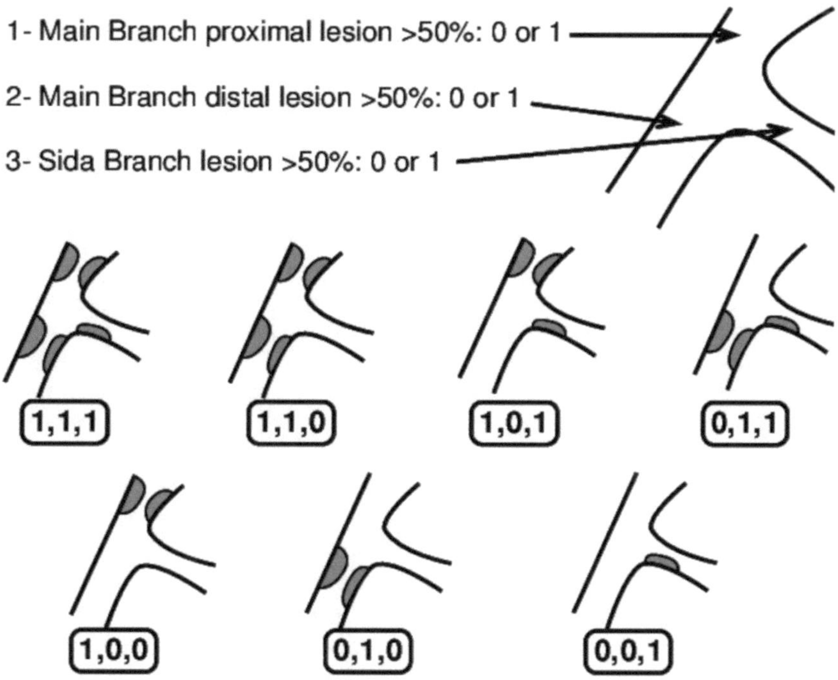

Figure 2.
Medina classification.

Provide support for intervention and stability with multiple exchanges of balloons, stent, guide extensions, and adjunct therapies.

Allow coronary flow during intervention.

2.3.1 Basic information to help operator handling guide catheters

Guide catheters although have three layers (diagnostic have two layers); they have thinner walls than diagnostic catheters to allow larger lumen. This makes them prone to kinking and weakening, and the middle layer is usually braided wire to minimize this risk. The tip of guide catheter is not tapered (diagnostic catheters have tapered tip).

Moving/rotating the guide catheter similar to diagnostic catheters with slower speed and patience to transmit torque (1 to 1 torque transmission) when withdrawing or advancing.

Advancing guide catheter slowly to avoid deep coronary intubation and damage.

Live monitoring of pressure wave to notice any change (ventricularization, damping or disappearance).

Guide catheters are used with hemostasis valve to allow instrumentation and imaging at the same time.

A lot of operators and some companies recommend keeping the 0.035″ guide wire inside while trying to engage the target coronary and adjust the location of the wire based on the operator assessment of the guide segment that need more support to stay straight. This only possible with a hemostasis valve (Tuohy) in place. Operator should make sure to de-air the system well while using this technique and assure good seal that prevents air from entering the system. Most operators keep the main 0.035″ guide wire in till they wire the coronary with 0.014 guide wire and secure guide engagement. This technique is mostly used for radial approach especially in patients with extensive tortuous vessels.

Consider longer sheath to provide good support through tortuous vessels. This is mainly a femoral approach option.

Bleed back from the hemostasis valve after performing exchanges to avoid introducing air or building clots in the system. This is very important while performing complex interventions with multiple wires and balloons and after aspiration thrombectomy.

If more support is needed and guide catheter needed to be advanced inside the coronary, operator should perform that over a wire or a balloon.

Advancing any instrument can push the guide out (especially if not a good support guide) causing disengagement and vice versa; pulling instruments can create a suction mechanism and advance the guide catheter deep inside the coronary and cause complications (dissection, perforation, and ischemia). Operators can use this mechanism to their benefit to provide more support or disengage the guide when needed (i.e. stenting ostial left main).

Guide catheters are available with or without side holes. Side holes purpose to prevent coronary obstruction by allowing some blood flow especially when using severe ostial lesions. Some operators argue that although using side holes can help avoid dampening of pressure, it does not support much coronary support and only give operators a false sense of comfort. Interventional guide wires can come out of these side holes and make it to coronary and unless operators are aware of that potential issue, complications can occur. Lastly, side holes can increase contrast volume used and weaken the tip of the guide catheter and make it prone to kink.

In addition to tip shape and length, shaft length is another important characteristic. Shorter guide catheters are used in CTO, bypass grafts and internal mammillary artery IMA interventions to allow for more wire to reach lesions in retrograde CTO approach and distal lesion in the grafts, anastomosis or target bypassed vessel. Longer shafts are used in tall patients or patients with significant tortuous aorto-femoral vessels. Standard shaft length is 100 cm, short is 80 or 90 cm, and long is 110–115 cm. Operators can shorten the guide by cutting a segment of the guide and connect them using sheath segment.

2.3.2 Sizing of guide catheter

There are four available sizes for coronary interventions (**Table 8**). Amount of contrast used in PCI increases with increasing guide catheter size.5Fr guide catheters: rarely used. Allows for simple single vessel PCI.

Outer lumen size (French)	5	6	7	8
Manufacturer/guide design		**Inner lumen size (inch)**		
Boston Scientific/Wiseguide	NA	0.066	0.076	0.086
Abbott/Viking	NA	0.068	0.078	0.091
Boston Scientific/Mach1	NA	0.070	0.081	0.091
Cordis/Vista Brite Tip	0.056	0.070	0.078	0.088
Medtronic/Launcher	NA	0.071	0.081	0.090

Table 8.
Different guide catheter designs per company and sizes.

6Fr guide catheters:

The workhorse size for most of PCI cases.
Allow for performing kissing rapid exchange balloons of almost any coronary size.
Does not allow simultaneous double stenting techniques.
Allow for simultaneous balloon and stent deployments but with limitation of size related to stent size.
Allow for rotational atherectomy max size Rotablator 1.5.
Limited on the size of covered stent that can be used. For Graftmaster covered stent (Max size 3.5 mm stent). Newer PK papyrus covered stent can fit in 5Fr for sizes up t0 4.0 mm and requires 6Fr guide for >4.0 mm stents.

7Fr guide catheters:

The most commonly used size in high risk interventions for technical support or in preparation to deal with complications:
Allow for simultaneous double stenting techniques.
Allow for rotational atherectomy max size Rotablator 1.75.
Allows for two over the wire balloons.

8Fr guide catheter:

Limited in availability.
Used for high risk interventions and CTO.
Allow for rotational atherectomy max size Rotablator 2.0.
Required for complex CTO intervention where intravascular ultrasound (IVUS) directed true lumen reentry and balloon are required.

2.3.3 Choice for guide catheter tip curve, shape and length for PCI depends on several factors

The access approach: radial right, left or femoral. Technically, most of femoral guide catheters could be used in radial approach and vice versa. However, some guide catheters are originally designed for radial approach (i.e. XB) and would be more effective if it is used for the same purpose especially nonexperience operators and in challenging interventions. A big advantage of radial approach is the availability of multiple guide catheter that can be used as a single catheter to perform diagnostic and intervention using same catheter for left and right with very good support and without the need to exchange. Some of these guide catheters are: EBU, Kimny, Q-Curve, Multi-Aortic Curve MAC and even Amplatz left. Manipulating and adjusting the guide bend with 0.035″ wire might be required to achieve that (Wire assisted guide engagement technique). Using the guide wire can make any left contralateral support catheter (EBU, XB, Kimny, Voda, Q-Curve, FCL, MAC, CLS, Kiesz left, Amplatz left) a single catheter for both left and right but this requires caution and experience to avoid advancing the 0.035″ wire inside the coronary (**Figure 3**). Left radial approach is similar to femoral approach in regard to guide catheter choice.

Anatomical factors:

The diagnostic catheter used to perform diagnostic angiogram is one of the most important factors. The diagnostic angiogram procedure is very important in general in deciding the choice for interventional guide catheter as it provides information about the difficulty of vessel engagement, vessel take off, position of the heart in the chest, ascending aortic length, width and orientation in chest, length and degree

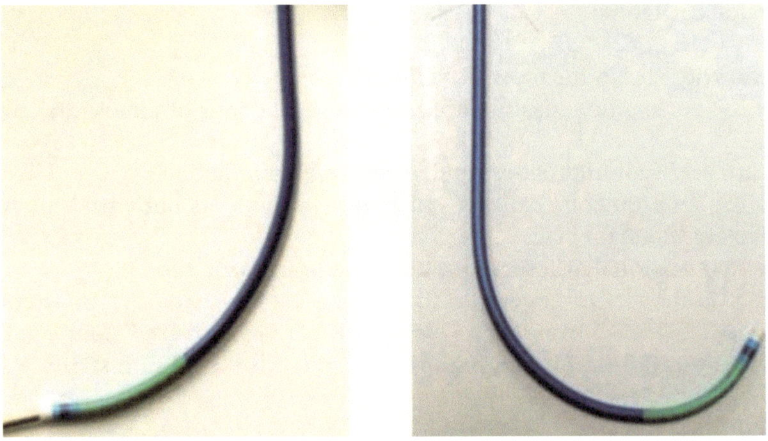

Figure 3.
Changing catheter tip shape with wire assist.

of required support of the guide catheter. In femoral and radial approaches using pre-shaped diagnostic catheters, guide catheter length is usually 0.5 shorter than the diagnostic catheter used. This rule does not apply for radial approach when a single diagnostic catheter is used. In this case, operator makes the choice based on the diagnostic catheter used and the other factors.

The vessel involved; left anterior descending (LAD) or left circumflex (LCX), or right coronary artery (RCA), the location of takeoff of the vessel, presence of anomalous coronary and the shape of coronary or graft takeoff.

Lesion specific factors: the location of the lesion (ostial or not), the difficulty of the lesion and the need for support (tortuous, calcified coronary) (**Tables 9** and **10**), setting of intervention CTO vs. acute vs. elective case.

For left system: shorter guides will selectively engage LAD and longer guides will electively engage and support LCX like Voda left (VL) and Amplatz left (AL).

2.3.4 Special cases for choosing appropriate guide catheters

Left coronary system: there are large range of guide catheters GC especially for left system catheters and all of them can be used in all different left system variable anatomies. XB, EBU, CLS, VL, SAL, MAC, Q-wave and AL catheters can provide good contralateral aortic or leaflet support especially during radial approach. JL/FL guide catheter are the old typical GC used in femoral approach. It provides minimal support from femoral approach. However, during radial approach, support of this GC can varies depending on the brachiocephalic and aortic anatomy. There are variable take offs and length of the left main. Superior take off would require longer GC to engage and at the same time achieve good support from aortic leaflet with or without contralateral aortic support. Horizontal take off could be engaged from the top by JL/FL GCs or by contralateral support GC. Short left main and separate ostia of LAD/LCX poses more challenge. Longer GC could engage either LAD or LCX selectively which could be a significant advantage when the target lesion is beyond the ostium. This provides much strong support for intervention but might occludes the other vessel and induces ischemia. This challenge is sometime unavoidable and thus could be managed by careful intermittent engagement and disengagement as needed during intervention. On the other hand, shorter GCs are needed for ostial target lesions.

For ostial left main interventions, a guide with side holes and easy way to disengage is preferred. JL/FL are good guide catheters for that. Still, contralateral

Judkins Left (least support)		Catheter with two bends the sort bend does not provide much support. Can have some advantage for ostial and proximal left main lesions where deep engagement is contraindicated
Ikari Left	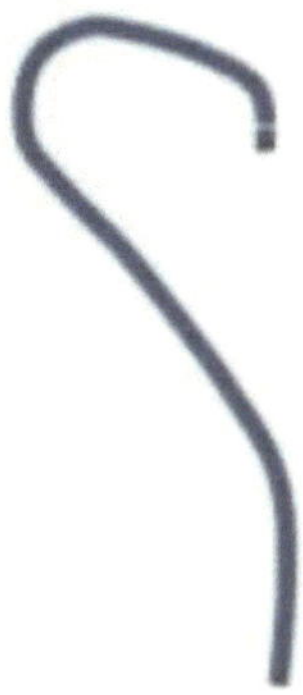	Radial guide: can be used for both left and right interventions as a single catheter technique (Useful in STEMI). Better support that JL but for the same double curve reason
Kimny	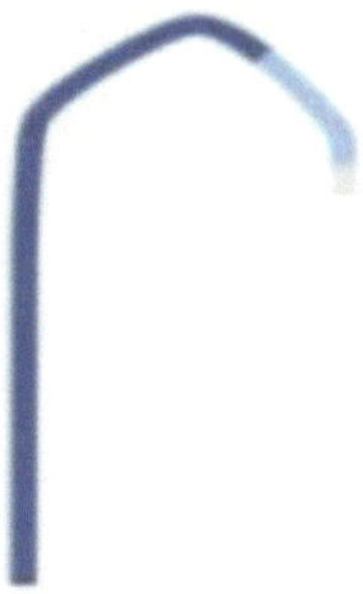	Similar to Ikari but more support
Contralateral Support Catheters (EBU, XB, Voda left, CLS, Q Curve, Kiesz left)	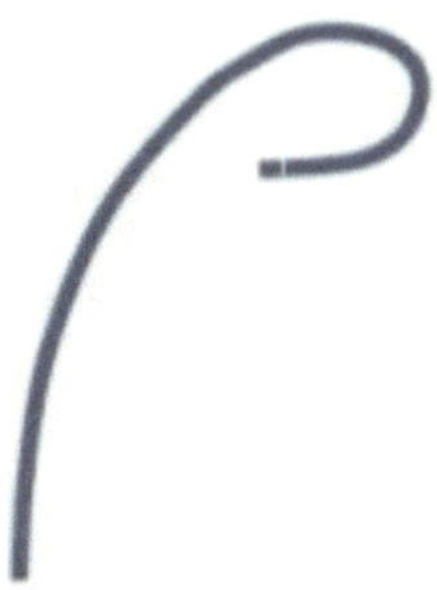	Very good support from contralateral aortic wall or sinus of Valsalva. EBU and Q curve can be used as a single catheter for left and right (STEMI cases). A workhorse guide catheter Voda left is a good support catheter for LCX interventions
Amplatz Left, SAL (Best support)	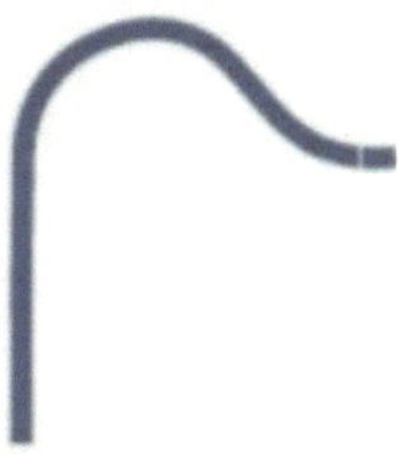	Best support guide catheter. Deep engagement. Very useful for complex PCI and CTO interventions

Table 9.
Classification of left coronary system guide catheters by level of support.

Judkins Right (least support)	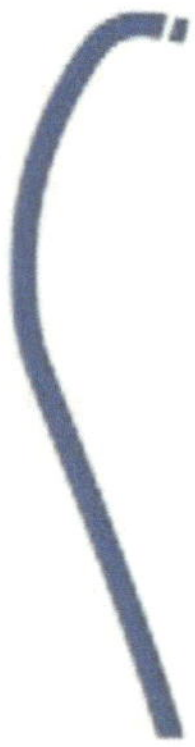	A workhorse guide catheter. Very useful for all types of take offs Very useful for engaging all venous grafts and head vessels IMA guide catheter is similar with more acute distal bend
Amplatz Right, KR (Kiesz Right), Hockey stick	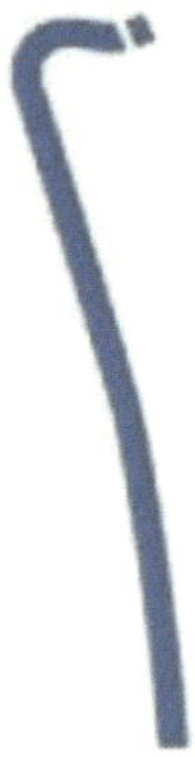	A little better support than JR but still passive support with no contralateral support Also can be used for engaging venous grafts
Multipurpose	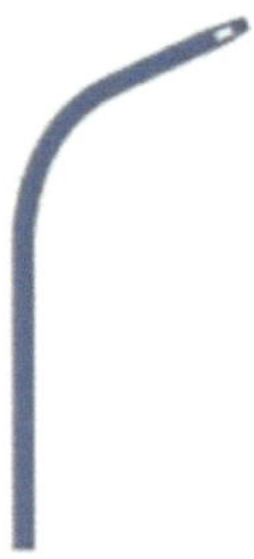	Requires significant manipulation and use f wire to support it. Very helpful in most downward pointing vessels like RCA and right venous grafts and anomalous LCX
Ikari Left, Ikari Right	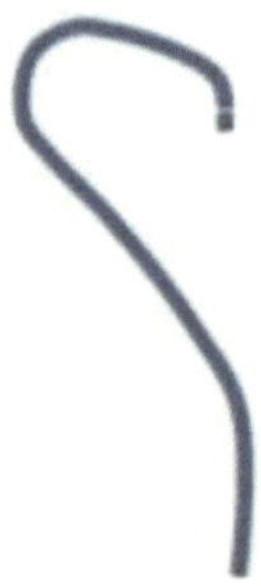	Radial guide: can be used for both left and right interventions as a single catheter technique (Useful in STEMI). Provide contralateral and better support for right interventions than left
Contralateral Support Catheters (EBU, XB, Voda, CLS, Q-Curve MAC)	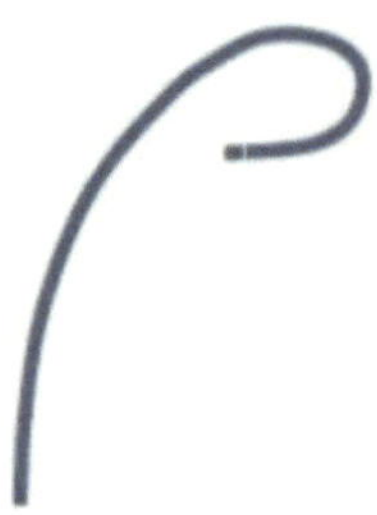	Very good support from contralateral aortic wall or sinus of Valsalva EBU, Q curve and MAC (Multi-Aortic Curve) guide catheter can be used as a single catheter for left and right using radial approach (STEMI cases). Another advantage of radial approach to make these guides workhorse guide catheters Voda right is a specific for RCA

Amplatz Left, (Best support)	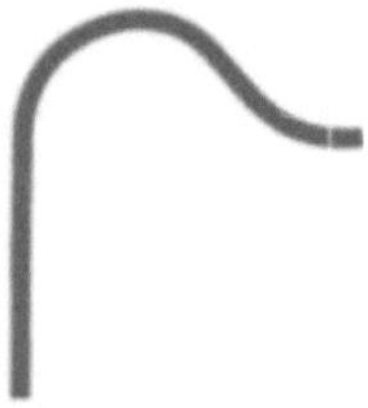	Best support guide catheter. Deep engagement. Very useful for complex PCI and CTO interventions A very good support guide catheter for all venous graft interventions and for the same reason, it is good for abnormal take off of the RCA (anterior, superior, and posterior)

Table 10.
Classification of right coronary system guide catheters by level of support.

aortic support GC can be used especially when additional interventions with support is required.

RCA system: because of the variable origin and takeoff of the RCA (posterior, anterior, superior anterior origins, inferior, horizontal, superior, Shepherd's Crook take offs), contralateral support guides for RCA interventions are less available, but some of the left guides can be used for the right interventions with aortic contralateral wall support like EBU, Voda, SAL, Q-Curve, MAC, and AL. Some companies have more specific right guide catheter with contralateral aortic wall support (Voda with right curve).

Contralateral support is very important for RCA interventions that needs significant support. However, workhorse guide catheters (JR/FR/IMA/3RDC/AR) are still mostly used due to their availability and operators' comfort level using them especially in challenging RCA take offs. Coaxial engagement and good support are two qualities for good interventions that are difficult to obtain at the same time in abnormal RCA take off using especially using workhorse GCs. For example: inferior take off engagement with multipurpose GC would provide good engagement but minimal support. Superior and Shepherd's Crook take off are one of the most challenging cases for any operator. Special radial designed GCs (KR superior, Voda right, RCA Shepher's Crook RC4SC, Ikari right) also can be very helpful. Posterior origin of the RCA can be reached with WRP, multipurpose AR and AL GCs. Anterior origin of the RCA would require long GC such as AL. Using RAO projections can be very helpful to engage posterior and anterior origin.

For the most common coronary anomaly (LCX origin from RCA): multipurpose GC and JR short tip are good options. However, due to poor support, aforementioned contralateral aortic GCs can provide significant support with deep engagement that can cause pressure dampening and decrease coronary flow.

Grafts: internal thoracic artery or internal mammillary artery IMA has special diagnostic catheters with similar guide catheters like regular IMA tip and LIMA VB-1 that can be used. JR, 3RDC, Cobra and LCB guides can be used too and all depends on the LIMA take off left subclavian.

Venous grafts can be engaged and intervene on using multiple catheters depending on their take off: JR, AL, IMA, special RCB, LCB right and left coronary bypass catheters, MPA, Hockey stick or even JL. Some operators use catheters used to engage abdominal aorta branches like Cobra, Renal catheters RC, Contralateral, MIK, HK1.0 or SHK. Amplatz left is a workhorse GC that can be used in all venous grafts and almost any types of origins or take offs while providing best support.

RIMA: free RIMA is imaged and intervene on similar to venous grafts depending on its origin from the aorta. Pedicle RIMA can be reached by right radial approach or femoral approach. JR, Barbeau or special RIMA guide catheter can be helpful in femoral approach.

Thrombotic lesions are common findings in ACS especially STEMIs and venous grafts lesions. There are multiple available catheters approved for cardiac vessels interventions (**Table 11**). They share the same principle of mechanical aspiration embolectomy that depends on manual or machine assisted aspiration of the clot. Multiple passes might be required for some cases. No blood return while aspirating is a sign of either poor flow triggered by clot occluding the catheter or suctioning against the vessel wall. When no blood return is seen, the catheter should be withdrawn till blood return is seen. If blood return still not seen, the catheter should be removed out of the body and examined for clot at the tip. It is very important to keep negative pressure while withdrawing the catheter out of the GC followed by bleed back of the GC to remove any potential clot left within the GC.

Aspiration thrombectomy can aspirate the clots from the coronaries and displace it to systemic circulation. The data of using aspiration embolectomy is controversial. Most recent guidelines recommend against their routine use due to increased risk of embolic strokes and no clinical outcome benefit. However, some cases with significant thrombosis cannot be resolved without their use.

Coronary micro-catheters are small catheters compatible with 0.014″ coronary wires. There is a wide spectrum of micro-catheters with different designs (**Table 12**). They provide operators with significant ability to provide wire exchanges, crossing difficult lesions, assist wiring difficult angulated lesions (**Table 13**) and many other technical advantages especially in CTO interventions.

Upsizing or exchanging GC to provide more support during procedure is challenging after crossing a difficult lesion or any case where guide wire position is critical. The risk of losing guide wire position while loading the new GC is high. Long guide wire or adding extension wire is first step. More support with additional buddy wire and/or using micro catheter inside the new GC could be helpful.

Manufacturer	Catheter name	Compatibility	Length	Note
Pneumbra	Indigo CAT RX	5.3 Fr	140 cm	Aspiration catheter of CAT RX SEPC4 catheter can be used to break the clots (200 cm)
Medtronic	Export Advance	6.0 Fr	140 cm	
	Export AP	6.0 Fr	140 cm	
Vascular solutions/ Teleflex	Pronto	5.0 to 10 Fr	Pronto V4 (138 cm) Pronto V3 (140 cm) Pronto LP (138 cm)	Pronto V4 and V3 are available with 5.5, 6, and 8Fr Pronto LP available with 5, 6 Fr Pronto 0.03 is peripheral catheter 10 Fr, 120° angled 4 cm tip
Terumo	Priority one	6 and 7FR	140 cm	
Spectranetics	Quick Cat	6Fr	145 cm	
Atrium	Xpress-Way	6 and 7 Fr	140 cm	
Boston Scientific	Fetch 2	6Fr	135 cm	
Stron Medical	Vmax	5, 6 and 7Fr	135–141 cm	
Tsuna Med	Emax	5, 6 and 7Fr	136.5–141 cm	

Table 11.
Coronary Embolectomy Catheters.

Manufacturer	Catheter name	Length	Distal shaft outer diameter (French)	Notes
CSI cardiovascular systems	Teleport Teleport Control	135 cm, 150 cm	2.0 Proximal shaft 2.6 2.1 Proximal shaft 2.7	Advanced both by clock and counterclockwise rotation
Terumo	Progreat	110 cm, 130 cm	2.4 and 2.7	Used for coiling with large coils and 0.018 wires
	Finecross MG	130 cm, 150 cm	1.8	Very small, not much support to cross any lesion
Spectranetics	Quick Cross	135 cm, 150 cm	2.0	
Boston Scientific	Renegade 18	105 cm, 114 cm, 135 cm	2.5	Used for coiling with large coils and 0.018 wires
	Mamba	135 cm	2.3	
	Mamba Flex	135 cm, 150 cm	2.1	
Cordis	Transit	135 cm	2.5	
	Prowler	150 cm	1.9	
Raxwood	MicroCross 14 MicroCross 14 es	155 cm	1.6	
Vascular solutions	Minnie	90 cm, 135 cm, 150 cm	2.2	
	Turnpike	135 cm, 150 cm	2.6	
	Turnpike LP	135 cm, 150 cm	2.2	
	Turnpike Spiral	135 cm, 150 cm	3.1	
	Turnpike Gold	135 cm	3.2	
Asahi	Tornus	135 cm	2.1 and 2.6	To advance it, counterclockwise rotation
	Corsair Corsair Pro	135 cm, 150 cm	2.6	
	Caravel	135 cm, 150 cm	1.9	
Volcano	Valet	135 cm, 150 cm	1.8	Shapeable distal tip

Table 12.
Coronary micro catheters.

2.4 Choosing the appropriate guide wire

There are large number of guide wires from different companies with different characteristics. Operator should be comfortable and familiar with design, characteristics, advantages, and disadvantages of at least workhorse wires and special wires especially high risk and CTO operators.

Manufacturer	Catheter name	Length	Distal shaft outer diameter (French)	Notes
Vascular solutions	SuperCross	130 cm, 150 cm	2.1	Preformed angled catheter; straight, 45, 90, 120°
	Venture	145 cm (rapid exchange) 140 cm (over the wire)	2.2	Steerable micro catheter to help change the angle
	Twin Pass Twin Pass Torque	140 cm	1.9 distal tip and 3Fr crossing profile	
	NinjaSwift			Steerable micro catheter to help change the angle

Table 13.
Steerable, angled, dual lumen micro-catheters.

Every wire has unique characteristics: the easiest way to remember the details of each wire is dividing them into groups with shared characteristics (**Table 14**).

There are three basic components of guide wires: central core (Stainless steel or Nitinol) and form the first 145 cm (or 140 cm) of guide wires, the distal 40 cm (or 35 cm) which has thinner extension part of the central core covered by polymer sleeve or coil-spring (platinum, tungsten, and stainless steel) and finally the tip which is usually covered by lubricious coating that define the wire as hydrophobic or hydrophilic. The tip is usually radiopaque and varies in length (20 mm–25 cm).

Last few decades have introduced nitinol to wires' design instead of stainless steel. This advancement has shown significant improvement in wires' design. Nitinol is a unique element that allows wires' tip to be more flexible, kink resistance, durable (retain the shape), and reshapable, all of which allow wires to be used several times to cross/wire different lesions and vessels. A very practical and time-saving tool especially in complex, bifurcation, and multivessel interventions.

Guide wire comes in two lengths. Long wires of 300 cm are used to perform exchanges, using micro-catheters, using over the wire balloons, CTO retrograde approaches (and externalization), or while using adjunct therapy like atherectomy. Regular length guide wires of 180 cm are of the workhorse wire length and used with rapid exchange balloons and stents. Few extension wires (Doc wire, Add Wire, Cynch) are available and can be attached to all guide wires when needed.

The goals of guide wires are to cross the target lesion safely without causing any damage to the vessel or alternating of the plaque in addition to providing good support to deliver other equipment (balloons and stents).

The operator's choice of guide wire is dependent mainly on two factors: lesions/vessel related factors and wire characteristics.

Wire characteristics: shaft characteristics are mainly related to the support and stiffness they provide. Most important characteristics are related to guide wires' tip:

Wire tip's strength, shape, and coating: tip can be straight or tapered, have polymer coating or not, have coil support or not, hydrophilic, or hydrophobic. Tapered, polymer coating, coiled, and hydrophilic tips can cross difficult lesion while increasing the risk of vessel injury.

Strength of the tip: it is how many grams of power is required to bend the tip when applied against the surface of the vessel wire. Multiple wires have a

Manufacturer	Tip style	Commercial name	Tip stiffness (gf)	Clinical tips
Boston Scientific	Hydrophilic polymer, straight (nontapered)	Samurai	0.5	Workhorse wire. Longer radiopaque segment 4 cm, longer coil 20 cm, which provides more support for tortuous vessels and makes it a good buddy wire
Boston Scientific		Marvel	0.9	Workhorse wire. Longer radiopaque segment (3 cm), more slippery than other work hose wires
Abbott		BALANCE MIDDLEWEIGHT UNIVERSAL II	0.7	Hi Torque workhorse wire
Asahi	Hydrophobic tip (But the coil is coated with hydrophilic coating), straight (nontapered)	ProWater	0.8	Good Workhorse wire with good torque control and support. Has transition point to the stiff part 10 cm to distal tip that operator would feel challenge advancing the wire distally and can cause Wire artifact if it was at a bend. Longer coil (20 cm)
Asahi	Hydrophilic polymer, tapered	Fielder XT Fielder XT-A Fielder XT-R	0.8 1.0 0.6 1.2	More used in CTO PCI for antegrade crossing and Knuckle technique, retrograde crossing. Fielder XT-R is used for wiring retrograde collaterals
Boston Scientific		Fighters	1.2	Same as above
Asahi	Hydrophilic coated, straight nontapered,	Fielder FC	0.8	Can be used as a workhorse wire, used more for retrograde approaches in CTO
Asahi		Sion Black	0.8	Mostly used for retrograde approaches in CTO
Abbott		Whisper LS Whisper MS Whisper ES	0.8 1.0 1.2	Slippery and can wire very small vessels and cause perforation if operator has limited experience
Abbott		Pilot 50	1.5	Stronger tip stiffness with hydrophilic coating that can be used to cross difficult branches but carries higher risk of dissection and that's why it can be used for CTO dissection and reentry techniques
Boston Scientific		Choice PT Floppy	2.1	Same as above
Abbott		Pilot 150/200	2.7/4.1	Same as above with stiffer tip
Asahi		Gladius	3	
Terumo		Crosswire NT	7.7	
Boston Scientific		PT Graphic Intermediate	1.7	
Boston Scientific		PT2 Moderate support	2.9	

Manufacturer	Tip style	Commercial name	Tip stiffness (gf)	Clinical tips
Cordis		Shinobi	7.0	
Cordis		Shinobi Plus	6.8	
Asahi	No polymer, Hydrophilic, Straight	Suoh 03	0.3	Very low profile wire so best to wire EPICARDIAL collaterals and minimize risk of perforation
Asahi		SION	0.7	Most common wire used for wiring collaterals
Asahi		SION blue (less hydrophilic)	0.5	Good Workhorse wire
Boston Scientific		Samurai RC	1.2	More support than Samurai with longer coil 24 cm and much higher tip stiffness
Terumo	Tapered, M-coating hydrophilic/ hydrophobic coating	Runthrough NS Extra Floppy (Tip 0.008) RUNTHROUGH NS HYPERCOAT	1.o 0.7	"M-coat" technology hydrophilic coating over the distal 24.8 cm of the distal tip enables smooth tractability in the tortuous anatomy while the silicone tip on the distal 2 mm Recently became one of the workhorse wires given its favorable crossing profile for complex PCI and ability to use same wire for different lesions and reshaping the tip
Abbott	Tapered	Cross it 100XT (0.010″)	1.7	
Asahi	Tapered, no polymer, hydrophilic	Gaia 1st (0.010″) Gaia 2nd (0.011″) Gaia 3rd (0.012″)	1.7 3.5 4.5	High stiffness tip so used for crossing CTO in a vessel with known course or retrograde known course without significant tortuosity
Asahi		Confianza Pro 9, 12 (0.009″)	9.3 12	
Asahi		Astato 20 (0.008″)	20	
Abbot		Progress 140 T (0.0105″) Progress 200 T (0.009″)	12. 13.3	
Medtronic		Persuader 9 (0.011″)	9.1	
Medtronic		ProVia 9, 12 (0.009″)	11.8, 13.5	
Boston Scientific		Hornet 10, 14 (0.00″)	10, 14	
Asahi	Straight tip, no polymer	MiracleBros, 3, 4.5, 6	3.9, 4.4, 8.8	High tip stiffness, Antegrade crossing for CTO when vessel course is known
		MiracleBros 12	13	
Abbott		Ultimate 3	3	
Abbott		Progress 40, 80, 120	5.5, 9.7, 13.9	

Manufacturer	Tip style	Commercial name	Tip stiffness (gf)	Clinical tips
Medtronic		Persuader 3, 6 (philic and phobic)	5.1, 8.0	
Medtronic		ProVia 3, 6 (philic and phobic)	8.3, 9.1	
Asahi	Tapered, no polymer, hydrophobic	Confianza Pro 9, 12 (0.009″) Hydrophobic	8.6, 12	
Medtronic		Persuader 9 Hydrophobic	9.1	
Medtronic		ProVia 9, 12 Hydrophobic	11.8, 13.	
Abbott	Soft, nontapered	Iron Man	1	Extra support wire, good buddy wires
Asahi		Grand Slam	0.7	
Boston Scientific		Mailman		
Asahi	Externalization wires (most common used ones)	RG3		Only for CTO retrograde interventions
Vascular solutions		R350		

Table 14.
Coronaries guide wires 0.014.

number that determine the strength of the tip. The highest the number the stronger the tip.

Steer-ability, tip control, tracking, support (push-ability), lubricity: optimal wire has best steer-ability, tip control, tracking and support to cross a lesion or branch vessel jailed by stent without vessel damage. Ability to provide accurate transmit of torque to the tip of the wire and direct it to where operator needed to be is one of the most important characteristics for any wire.

Tips for guide wire handling:

Always start with a workhorse wire and escalate the strength as needed (Prowater, BMW, Runthrough, etc.).

Avoid using polymer coated wire at the beginning. Polymer coated wires become stiffer in a warm environment, and pre-shaped ones have no secondary curve.

Advance wire slowly and freely. Assure tip of the wire is free by performing continuous spinning and advancing slowly.

Find the best safest lumen or micro-channel to cross the lesion using multiple orthogonal views and direct the tip to it while rotating and advancing to cross the lesion. This becomes very important while crossing an occluded vessel (STEMIs) or CTOs to avoid disturbing plaque or wiring sub-intimal space and cause thrombosis or dissection/perforation.

Never cross a lesion after the tip bends (Knuckled wire). Pull to straighten the tip and rotate to find the micro-channel. Advancing the wire after bending can cross to sub-intimal space and causes dissection (it is a technique for CTO interventions using specific wires and the goal is to cross to sub-intimal space and re-cross to true lumen). One exception is presence of large burden of thrombus and unclear trajectory of the vessel. In such case, operator might use the knuckle technique to minimize the risk of vessel injury as knuckled workhorse wire can pass easily through thrombus and allow safely the true lumen and trajectory of the vessel. Still, this technique is better performed by experienced operator.

Pull the branch wire before performing optimization of stent apposition when a stent is jailing a branch wire.

Develop a tactile feed-back for wires to avoid wiring small branch vessel or wiring under stent (between stent and vessel's wall).

To avoid perforation: keep a wire in a main large vessel (not small branch) and be aware of the distal tip of the wire at all times especially while performing multiple over the wire exchanges where the wire can travel distally and cause perforations. These kinds of distal perforation can be missed easily unless operator pays a good attention to angiograms. Also, the distal perforation causes slow bleeding that can take hours to manifest as tamponade. Thus, early detection and prevention are very important.

Any wire can cause perforation especially distal end perforation.

Wire effect or pseudo stenosis (Accordion's effect): occurs more in tortuous vessels and wires with strong shaft that can straighten the vessel at the tortuous segments and cause pseudo-stenosis (lesions) and even dissections. Examining baseline images can help distinguish this effect in addition to repeat angiogram after pulling the stiff segment of the wire out of the tortuous segment of the vessel. This way, operator can be assured that it is a wire effect and at the same time in safe position to re-advance the wire if the repeat angiogram revealed true damage (dissection or plaque shifting) that requires further intervention.

In cases that require more guide wires support, operators can use buddy wire technique by using additional wire with good support or (if the support wire can be advanced) exchanging the workhorse wire for a strong support wire using over the wire balloon or micro-catheter.

For cases where wiring a jailed vessel through stent struts, operator would choose a wire with good tip control, tracking and lubricity to direct the wire toward the vessel lumen jailed by stent. Strength here is not necessary and wires with high strength should be avoided as it carries higher risk of perforation or crossing under stent struts and dissect the branch vessel that supposed to be wired. However, some strength might be required in case of significant lesion in the branch vessel. That is why the operator should always plan the techniques for bifurcation stenting that requires rewiring based on the easiest vessel to rewire in addition to other factors will discuss later. To avoid under stent wiring, operator can use the main vessel wire and use it to wire the branch vessel. As long as operator does not withdraw the wire beyond the stent proximal edge level, operator can be comfortable that the wire is not under stent.

Strength is important in CTO or heavy calcified/organized thrombus lesions. Wires with higher strength tip should be used when the vessel track/trajectory is easy to see. Having a balloon or micro catheter close to the tip to increase support can increase the strength of the tip by 10 times and even more depending on the wire.

Shaping the tip of the wire: also an important step to get to the lesion especially in tortuous vessels and to cross the target lesion. Operators have different ways to approach the best shape for a specific lesion. Primary curve is the bend closer to the tip. A secondary curve is the bend distal to the tip. Basic rule for shaping is making primary curve mates most angulated vessel bend and secondary curve matches the vessel size. A simple primary curve is enough in most cases. A primary 120 angle curve is usually referred to as a CTO curve because it provides a good strength to cross the lesion and mainly used in CTO lesions. When operator is working on a distal lesion with tortuous vessel a secondary curve is required most of the time to reach the distal lesion. In left system interventions, a lot of the times the LAD and/or LCX comes out with very acute angle. Such case would require mainly a secondary curve to cross the first angle of takeoff unless further tortuosity distally is present then another curve is required. The more acute the curve and especially secondary curve, the more likely that the wire would be entering the branch vessels. That is because a secondary curve is more likely to be larger than the width of the vessel which makes the wire easier to reach branches. For the same reason, if the vessel is straight, a simple short primary curve is sufficient to reach a distal lesion without difficulty wiring all branches across the vessel.

Extension wires are very helpful when a long wire is needed in cases that require the use of over the wire balloon, micro catheter, or atherectomy. To perform catheter exchanges (micro catheter or OTW balloon) over a regular length wire while assuring minimal or no movement of the wire, there are few techniques:

To avoid withdrawing the wire and losing wire position:

A trapper catheter which is special catheter with a balloon designed to trap the wire. Sometimes this catheter can be too short to trap the wire.

Advancing an extra balloon inside the GC close to the tip without getting out of the guide catheter then inflating the balloon to trap the wire while performing the exchange then it is deflated and pulled out.

A 3 cc syringe filled of heparinized saline is attached to the catheter hub and continuous slow injection is performed after assuring no air in the system. That generates enough energy to prevent the wire from being withdrawn while pulling the catheter are pulled out of guide. This technique is least successful and requires a lot of experience and luck. It is not a trusted technique, so it is not encouraged to be used in critical scenarios where losing wire position is critical.

To avoid wire migration distally while advancing the catheter, a 10 cc syringe is attached to the catheter hub then a slow negative pressure is applied while the it is advanced till the wire is seen coming out of the hub inside the syringe. At this point the syringe is disconnected, the wire is railed, and the catheter is advanced in a usual manner.

2.5 Balloons and angioplasty

Multiple balloons with different designs from multiple companies are available. Main important characteristics for balloons are: balloon diameter, length, compliance, rupture pressure, tip designs, crossing profile, shaft diameter and length. Standard diameter for coronary interventions starts from 1.2 mm and goes up. However, there are commercially available smaller balloons: nano-balloon 0.85 and 1 mm balloons (Sapphire Pro, Ikazuchi Zero, Ryurel). If necessary, even large diameter peripheral balloons can be used.

Selection of Balloons: after wiring the target vessel and lesion, balloon can be advanced and inflated to perform angioplasty. The goal of pre-dilatation of lesion is to prepare lesion for stenting and assess whether the lesion/plaque would response to balloon and stenting afterwards would have a good results or further plaque modification is needed. Balloons are also used for post stenting optimization of stents size and assuring stent well apposition. Inflation should always be started at the target lesion and monitored under fluoroscopy.

There are two general balloons designs: one over the wire and would require long wire and one referred to as rapid exchange which allows loading over the wire without long wire. Rapid exchange balloon is the first choice usually and considered the workhorse balloon design. Regular balloons have two radio-opaque markers at both ends. Smaller balloons ≤1.2 mm diameter and ≤ 8 mm have a single marker in the middle.

Balloon compliance: compliance is one of the most important factors to select the appropriate balloon. More compliance allows for more adoption to vessel morphology without damaging normal vessel. Compliant balloons can extend as much as it is inflated till they reach rupture pressure so they are limited by pressure range that can be used safely without rupture, whereas less compliant balloons can take high pressure and technically they are not supposed to expand beyond the size they are designed for (limited by diameter). Still, even noncompliant balloons can rupture if inflated beyond their rupture pressure. Operators develop experience and remember rupture pressure so they anticipate rupture based on the balloons and avoid it. Each balloon comes with instructions about inflation pressures and diameters and rupture pressure. Rupture should be avoided unless it is intentional (in some CTO techniques) as the rapid release in pressure can cause dissections, perforations, and air embolism. Risk of rupture increases with calcified tortuous severe lesions and using high inflation pressures. Operator can recognize rupture easily by feeling sudden drop in balloon pressure and can be seen on fluoroscopy. If balloon rupture occurs, negative pressure should be applied rapidly, and balloon should be withdrawn. Follow up angiogram and assessing for complication should be performed. Semi-compliant balloons are mostly used for pre-dilatation and preparation of the lesion.

Balloon length is determined mainly by the lesion length (should match). It is usually shorter than the final stent which covers the proximal and distal edge of the lesion. Shorter balloons can be considered for resistant lesions. For post stenting dilation, balloon length matches the stent length.

Balloon diameter: for pre-dilatation, balloon diameters are based on the target vessel. The role is 0.9–1.1 balloon to vessel ratio. However, there are multiple exceptions to the role. Resistance lesion does not allow using this role. Starting with small balloon and escalating diameter is necessary. This approach is also helpful to avoid complications in cases of total occlusion of the vessel and especially if vessel trajectory is not clear and suspicion of being in small branch.

Best balloons for pre-dilatation are balloons with the lowest crossing profiles: crossing profile has direct effect on a balloon's ability to cross the lesion. It is related to specific balloon design, balloon tip diameter in addition to diameter (balloon and shaft), and length. Shorter, smaller balloons have lower crossing profiles.

Plain Old Balloon Angioplasty POBA is still performed even with rapid development of stents. The indication for POBA is limited to recurrent instent restenosis in small vessel and especially in diabetic patient where the risk of restenosis is very high in case of adding additional layer of stent. In rare indication, pre op POBA is performed for severe stenosis to avoid stenting and the need for dual anti-platelets therapy.

Cutting or scoring balloons are noncompliant balloons surrounded by metal wires or microtomes that can help in preparation resistance calcified lesions. Several designs are available. In general, cutting balloons are available in limited sizes and lengths. They have high crossing profile which make their use challenging especially where they are needed the most. This makes their use not common and mainly indicated in ostial lesions. Some operators use it for resistant lesions not amendable to other adjunct lesion modifications and instent restenosis due to new atherosclerosis where the stent struts are not close to the lumen. Other instent restenosis mechanisms where the stent struts are close to the lumen, it is not recommended to use cutting balloons.

Withdrawing balloons should be performed after full deflation and confirmed re-wrapping of the balloon using fluoroscopy.

2.6 Stents

There are several stents from several medical companies with variable designs and engineering. Operator should be familiar with the basics of stent design, engineering, and generations. Stent design's topic is extensive, and reader is referred to dedicated stent chapter.

Similar to balloons: crossing profiles, stents design/generation, struts characteristics, stent drug, presence of polymer, sizes (diameter and length), clinical safety data and outcome all factors that affect operator choice of stent. Smallest stent diameter is 2 mm. Stenting vessel <2 mm size is not recommended as the value and long-term outcome is significantly questionable. However, balloon angioplasty of small vessels is recommended especially when these vessels supply a significant territory of the myocardium and when their occlusion cause significant symptoms or hemodynamic effect such as in cases of some septal perforators and right ventricular branch which could cause right ventricular infarction, shock and even death. These branches could shut down when jailed by stents and so it is recommended to avoid multiple layers of stents or stents overlap when jailing a branch vessel. In cases where multiple stents are needed in the main vessel, operator should plan to avoid multiple layers of stents jailing the branch vessel.

In coronary world, all available stents are rapid exchange balloon expanded design. In rare cases, it is necessary to use a peripheral size or self-expandable stent such in very large coronaries >6 mm or in cases of complications like perforations in a large coronary. Balloon expandable stents are semi-compliant balloons that can expand by increasing inflation pressure but there a max stent size for each design. As in balloons, each stent has a table for inflation pressure and correlating diameter as part of their design.

The old and still active role is to use stent length that covers the lesion with both proximal and distal stent edges at normal segment of the coronary. This is the role that current evidence support. However, with rapid progress in coronary stents design, wide spread of stent use, and expansion of stent indications such in diabetic patients with diffuse coronary disease, this role might not be applicable anymore.

Stent size topic is more complicated than balloon. The technical goal of stenting is to achieve a good coverage of the plaque, restore the vessel lumen, allow covering of struts with endothelium and prevent restenosis by using stent with strong radial force to prevent recoil and assuring well apposed struts. Operator should be knowledgeable of available stent sizes and design that allow them to expand beyond their original size by inflating the balloon beyond the design pressure or by post dilatation using larger balloon. For example: if an operator used a 3.0 mm stent that is designed to expand only to 3.5 mm and tried to expanded the stent to match the vessel size of 4 mm, that might be unsuccessful, cause struts fracture, significant recoil and restenosis. At the same time, using inappropriately large stent size, can cause edge dissection, perforation, rapid atherosclerosis at the edges due to inflammation and under expansion of the stent and restenosis. Stent size should be based on the size of reference vessel diameter RVD proximal and distal to the lesion to match the vessel size as close as possible. Operator can use several techniques to choose the appropriate stent size: using the balloon size used to prepare the lesion, compare vessel size to the guide catheter diameter, performing angiogram after lesion preparation and intra-coronary Nitroglycerin, fluoroscopy based quantitative measurement and using intravascular imaging (IVUS or OCT).

To assure good results, operator can use stent imaging enhancement technology (Available on Phillips Fluoroscopy system) and intravascular imaging. Most operators use post dilatation with balloon to achieve good angiographic results. This step has been shown to improve angiographic results. Clinically, the benefit and long-term outcome of this step is a complex question to answer as it has multiple variables and cofounders. It is related to the clinical presentation acute myocardial infarction vs. stable angina, type of lesion and stent generation. Best data support this step for bare metal stents and first-generation drug eluting stents. For second and third generation DES, the data are controversial [11–13]. Significant evidence supports this step [14]. However, some question it as it might lead to microvascular injury or distal embolization in the setting of acute myocardial infarction. It is best to make individual decision to perform post dilatation in acute myocardial infarction cases.

Operator should minimize the number of stents used by using single stent and avoid stents overlap. This can be challenging in long lesions with significant discrepancy between proximal and distal vessel size or in challenging distal lesion in tortuous vessel. Using shorter and multiple stents might be required if other techniques for increasing support for delivery are not successful.

Stent restenosis is related to target vessel size (smaller have higher risk), stent length (longer higher risk), small diameter stents, undersized stent, stent drug type and body response (inflammation), ostial lesions, venous grafts lesions especially distal anastomosis to target vessel, presence of diabetes mellitus and calcifications. Appropriate oversizing might have beneficial results and reduce target lesion revascularization.

Stents thrombosis risk increases with premature stopping of anti-platelets therapy, stents overlap, bifurcation lesions, stent edge dissection, stent's struts malapposition, time from implantation, poor distal flow post intervention, presence of diabetes mellitus and chronic kidney disease, reduced left ventricular systolic function. There are some data to subject larger vessel and especially RCA has more risk of thrombosis.

3. Helpful tips to address difficulties performing basic steps of PCI

3.1 Difficulty wiring

Wiring the true lumen during PCI is the initial and most important step. Operators can face several difficulties and some solutions are listed:

1. Severe stenotic lesions:

   Find the microchannel using multiple views and use escalating wire technique to provide more support to the wire tip.

   Use a micro catheter or balloon to support wire's tip.

2. Tortuous vessels and lesions: use wires with strong shaft support and torque transmission.

3. Angulated target vessels:

   Adjust the wire tip to the most angulated vessel.

   Use angulated micro-catheter like super cross 45-90-120° or steerable micro-catheter.

   Use dual lumen micro-catheter.

   Use knuckled wire retro wiring technique: advancing knuckled wire in the main vessel beyond the takeoff of the branch angulated vessel then withdrawing slowly toward till the tip of the wire engage the target vessel. This technique is helpful to wire a jailed branch vessel and assuring the wire is not between stent and vessel wall (under stent).

3.2 Difficulty delivering balloons and stents

First step to recognize if the difficulty is related to the lesion itself or difficulty due to the target vessel (severe tortuosity or calcifications)

Use a buddy wire technique.

Use a wire with strong shaft (Grandslam, ironman, mailman) that provide more support. If not able to deliver such wire, use special wire that can navigate tortuous vessels (Suoh, Sion blue or Black, Samurai) and exchange for stiffer wire using over the wire balloon or micro-catheter.

Use a guide extension: guide extensions should be advanced carefully over a balloon or stent using balloon-assisted tracking technique to avoid vessel injury especially at vessel bends. Guide extension shaft is to one side (not centered like balloons or stents) and their lumen is on the other side which make them biased to one side and that's the reason the tip can damage the intima and cause dissection while advancing them. Guide extensions will cause pressure dampening and can increase ischemia as they get advanced within the coronary. Operator should avoid advancing them to a target vessel smaller than the size of guide extension to avoid vessel injury. Contrast injection with high pressure through a guide extension can cause dissection.

Deep guide intubation.

Using anchor balloon. A small compliant balloon in a proximal branch is usually used to provide support.

If the difficulty *is more related to the lesion itself:*

Use simultaneous two small balloons inflations.

Use glide balloon.

Grenadoplasty: intentionally inflating small balloon to rupture which could affect the lesion integrity.

Wire cutting technique: using two wires across the lesion, passing small balloon over one wire, and performing tugging and pushing on the balloon or the other wire that can act as a saw cutting the lesion.

Use lesion modification techniques such as atherectomy, LASER, Intra vascular lithotripsy, brachytherapy.

More aggressive techniques involve sub-intimal access to perform external crush or distal anchoring.

Combination of above techniques is needed in difficult cases.

3.3 Difficulty with stent delivery

In addition to techniques above:

Use shorter stent with smaller struts.

Administration of Rota glide/Viper glide while advancing the stent toward the lesion.

4. Special challenging cases of PCIs

4.1 Aorto-ostial lesions

Aorto-ostial lesions (RCA, left main, and bypass grafts) can be challenging for several reasons:

Engaging challenges: after selecting appropriate guide shape, engaging severe lesions most likely would cause dampening, possibly ischemia, dangerous arrhythmias, and subsequent hemodynamic effect. To avoid these issues or in cases with challenging coronary take offs, operators can use one or more of the following techniques:

Using a GC with side holes. Again, side holes can cause a false sense of assurance.

Quick engagement and wiring followed by disengagement to minimize ischemia.

Phishing technique: it involves having the tip of the guide few millimeters close to the ostium without engagement then attempting to wire the coronary. If the ostium lumen can accommodate a micro catheter, then micro catheter can be used to approach the ostium with long wire to facilitate wiring the coronary. Steerable micro catheters are the most helpful when using this technique.

Using a small 4 or 5Fr diagnostic catheter to engage and wire the coronary with a long wire then exchange with the appropriate guide catheter over the long wire.

Calcified ostial lesions that requires adjunct plaque modification such as atherectomy carries risk of causing aortic dissections. This can occur with simple angioplasty. The inflations time while performing angioplasty or stenting should be short as these vessels might be the only perfusion source of the heart.

Missing the target: as operators try to match the proximal end of the stent to the ostium, it is not uncommon to miss the target ostial lesions. Locating the ostium is challenging and appropriate imaging views are critical here. To assure best view of ostial lesion, orthogonal views should be used. For ostial left main, superficial LAO/cranial and for RCA steep RAO and even lateral views are required depending on its origin. It is essential to know where the stent ends in regard to its radiopaque markers in order not to miss the ostium as some stents ends at the distant end of the radiopaque marker and others at the proximal end of the marker. In order to achieve good lesion coverage, stents are deployed to protrude couple of millimeters out of the coronary and inside the ascending aorta. A lot of operators recommend flaring the protruding part with large balloon and high pressure to make the stent take the shape of the internal aorta. This step is important especially when future interventions are anticipated. Without this step, future engagement of the stent and PCI becomes a very difficult mission and almost impossible. There are special designed balloons that can help with achieving this step. A catheter with two balloons, two inflating ports, and three markers that identify the edges of the two balloons. Operators should use caution while using these double balloons as inflating proximal balloon inside the vessel can cause vessel injury. Sbazo technique is a unique technique where another wire is passed through the proximal stent cell and while advancing the stent the wire stops the advancement while assuring covering the ostium. The same technique can be used at a bifurcation ostium lesion while avoiding jailing the branch vessel.

4.2 Bifurcation lesion techniques

Bifurcation of lesions in general is one of the most technically complex coronary interventions. Multiple classifications for bifurcation coronary lesions are available. The most common one is Medina classification which has three digits depending on true lesion involvement of vessels around bifurcation.

In order to make bifurcation stenting simpler, the first decision is to decide whether the single-stent (provisional stenting) or the two-stent approach is the appropriate technique. There are significant data comparing provisional stenting to other two stent techniques. Both are acceptable techniques with good outcome and the decision to choose one is related to several factors.

Several techniques are used for bifurcation lesions. Deciding the best technique to use depends on multiple factors: medina classification, the angle between main and branch vessels, size difference of main and branch vessels, difficulty to rewire the sent struts, expected plaques shifting/angle changes post stenting and need for branch stenting distal to the bifurcation lesion, size and territory size of branch vessel and presence of trifurcation or proximal lesion.

Proximal optimization technique POT is an important step while performing any PCI and especially in the setting of bifurcation stenting. It refers to performing angioplasty inside the proximal segment of the stent/stents (making sure the distal end of the balloon at the level of side branch) to make sure proximal stent are well apposed and dilated to match the proximal vessel size. Injecting contrast while the balloon is inflated can help assuring well stent apposition when no contrast leak to distal vessel. POT allows safe rewiring and further intervention of the SB when required. It is important to perform POT at the right level, repeat it or perform kissing balloons if the SB was ballooned to optimize any possible distortion of the stent and to remove the SB wire before repeating POT or performing kissing balloons to avoid wire trapping complications.

Final kissing balloon is recommended in all two stents techniques. Kissing balloons goal is to optimize the bifurcation carina and lumens of both vessel at this level without compromise one of the bifurcation lumens.

IVUS-assisted bifurcation stenting has better outcome especially in distal left main bifurcation lesion. Because fluoroscopy angiogram provides only two-dimensional images, intravascular imaging with IVUS and/or OCT can be very helpful to understand the morphology of bifurcation stenosis if performed before and after to evaluate the results and need for further intervention.

For any bifurcation lesion, protecting both vessels, branch vessel (side branch SB) and main vessel (MV) by wiring them is recommended especially when branch vessel is 2 mm and larger in diameter. Even in Medina 0.1.0 lesions, wiring both vessel for protection is recommended. Acute vessel closure of large branch could occur when least expected especially in the setting of small bifurcation angle.

It is very important to pre-determine the best views that allow the operator to evaluate the bifurcations accurately and assess the changes in both branches and main vessel at the same time with each step. Orthogonal views are important during all steps.

There is no available guide catheter that allows simultaneous three balloon inflations or stent deployments. There are techniques that use two guide catheters one 7Fr and the other 6 or Fr to treat trifurcation lesion with the risk of inducing ischemia by completely obstructing the coronary ostium.

Bifurcation lesions that carry the highest risk are true bifurcation lesions Medina 1.1.1 of distal left main involving ostial LAD and LCX. Unprotected left main is referred to any left main with no bypass to the LAD or LCX. It is important to recognize that intervention on unprotected left main carries a higher risk especially in the setting of left dominant system. Although recent emerging data suggest a similar outcome comparing PCI to CABG in such lesions even in diabetic patients, CABG still has the best data [11–13]. Discussion of the data is beyond this chapter. However, a simple decision-making approach is that the more complex anatomy, the more benefit CABG can provide especially in diabetic patients with low left ventricular ejection fractions [14]. It is important to recognize that diabetic patients have higher risk of restenosis and tend to have smaller vessels' lumen due to diffuse disease which in turn increases the need for vessel revascularization due to more hemodynamically significant restenosis. The same percentage of stenosis could be tolerated better with less hemodynamic effect in larger non-diabetic vessels. If a patient is not a candidate for CABG, a hemodynamic support device should be considered depending on the severity of stenosis, calcification, the need for atherectomy or other lesion modification techniques, presence of aortic valve stenosis, and LV function. Even with normal LV function, operator should consider mechanical support with severe calcified lesions with high risk of acute vessel closure, low LVEF, prolonged ischemia or complication. Simultaneous kissing stents to minimize ischemia time is a good option especially in Medina 0.1.1 lesions. **Figure 4** shows a simple decision-making approach for bifurcation stenting.

4.2.1 Provisional stenting

Stenting from main vessel to main vessel or branch depends on size differences, angulation of the SB, and the easier vessel to rewire after jailing it in case further intervention is needed.

When the size difference is less between the SB and proximal MV compared to difference between distal lesion of MV and proximal vessel, then stenting from main vessel to the SB is a good option, otherwise, stenting from proximal to distal MV is most common especially in LAD bifurcation lesions. Stenting to SB like from proximal LCX to branch obtuse marginal is more common than stenting from proximal to distal LCX. Evaluating the SB flow is very important to make a decision whether it requires angioplasty or stenting. Before judging the branch flow, it is recommended to administer intracoronary nitroglycerin.

As long as SB has normal flow and is not at risk of closure, no further intervention is required. If SB flow is impaired, performing angioplasty of stent struts the next step. If the results of angioplasty weren't successful to improve the flow, or caused SB injury, stenting becomes required. For the same reason SB with normal flow or small lumen <2 mm should not be rewired unless poor flow is present as rewiring with or without angioplasty might cause more complications than benefits. When attempting to rewire the jailed SB through stent struts, there is always a concern of wiring under the stent or not able to wire the SB especially when POT is not performed. To avoid that, the MV wire can be used to rewire the SB as long as the operator does not withdraw the wire beyond the proximal edge of the stent. In this way, the operator can be assured that the wire is inside the stent. Another approach is to reverse wire the SB by wiring the MV stent with J tip wire and then the wire is withdrawn to the origin of SB. Lastly, a special twin pass micro-catheter loaded on the MV wire and passed till

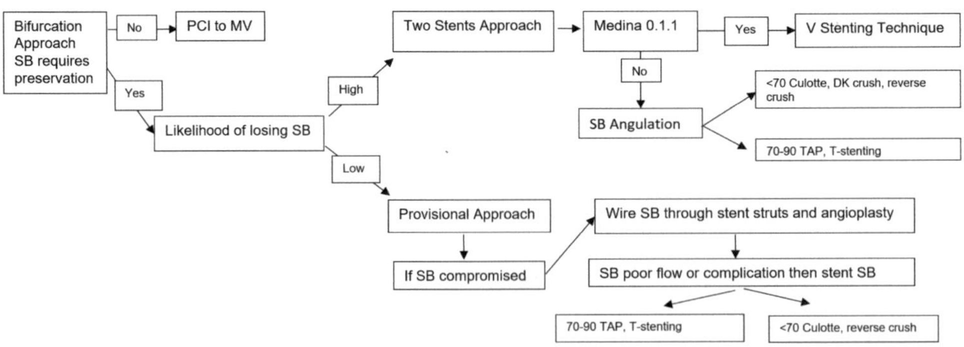

Figure 4.
A simple decision-making approach for bifurcation stenting.

the bifurcation. The second lumen can be used to wire the branch safely within the stent and provide support in challenging SB rewiring cases. However, this technique requires long wire (or extension wires) to make exchanges.

When SB stenting is required, reverse crush, T-stenting, TAP or Culottes techniques could be used.

4.2.2 Mini crush technique

After wiring both the main vessel and its branch. A stent sized to the SB is placed into the branch vessel. To assure complete coverage of the lesion, part of the stent protrudes insides the MV. As the goal is to cover the whole bifurcation, the length of the protruding segment of stent correlates with the angulation angle. The smaller the angle the longer this protruding segment inside the MV. If the SB is taking off at 80° then theoretically, no part of stent should be protruding inside the MV. After SB stenting, a balloon loaded on the wire of the MV is used to crush the protruding segment of stent followed by stenting of the MV. The goal of mini crush that protruding segment of the stent would not jail the SB completely so if post stenting intra vascular imaging is performed, the distal part of the SB takeoff lumen will have two layers of stent, the protruding crushed segment of the SB stent and the MV stent while the proximal part will have only the MV stent. Rewiring the branch through the main stent struts and performing kissing balloon creating new carina is recommended. The lesion under the carina will have two layers of stents. If the segment of stent protruding inside the MV is long enough that when it is crushed by angioplasty/stenting the MV, the technique turns to crush stenting technique.

4.2.3 Crush stenting technique

After wiring both vessels, loading a balloon on the MV wire, stenting the SB with significant part of stent protruding inside the MV is performed. The MV balloon then used to crush the protruding segment of the SB stent jailing the lumen of the branch completely with two layers of stents. Stenting of MV is then performed jailing the SB with additional layer of stent struts. Before that the SB wire is withdrawn to avoid wire trapping complications. Now, the SB is covered with three layers of stent struts which most likely will affect the flow of the SB. Thus, rewiring across these layers of stents is required and used to perform angioplasty to dilate the stent struts followed by performing kissing balloons.

4.2.4 Reverse crush technique

It is similar to the crush technique but in reverse sequences. After wiring both vessels, the MV is stented then the SB is rewired across the MV stent struts which maybe challenging especially in the setting of true SB severe stenosis, and rewiring becomes more difficult with plaque shifting/angulation angle changes after stenting the MV. A balloon angioplasty followed by stent that protrude partially or completely inside the MV is deployed. At this point, depending on the angiographic results and the covering of diseased, the operator might crush the SB stent performing angioplasty inside the MV stent (followed by the rest of crush technique) or perform kissing balloon leaving segment of the protruding stent hanging in the lumen of the MV.

4.2.5 Culottes' bifurcation stenting

It is the most complicated technique but has a good supportive data. After wiring both vessels. The vessel with the hardest to rewire is stented first. Then alternating wires positions to wire the SB through stent struts followed by performing angioplasty to dilate struts to the nonstented vessel. This step might require several balloons' angioplasty with escalating sizes. Then, stenting the SB jailing the first stented vessel. Again, here alternating wire positions are performed followed by final kissing balloon. The advantage of this technique is complete coverage of the lesions with stents. However, double coverage of proximal MV with two layers of stents and new carina have been controversial and suspected to increase risk of thrombosis. Most recent evidence suggests no difference between this technique and other two stents techniques in terms of stent thrombosis. Culottes' technique is best used when the branched vessels are close in diameter to the MV to avoid stent size mismatch and the angulation angle is acute below 70°.

4.2.6 V stenting

This technique is best used in bifurcation lesion Medina class 0.1.1 where the proximal MV is not involved or when the lesion is barely involving the proximal MV. After wiring both vessels, angioplasty of both vessels might be required regardless to pass stents followed by simultaneous kissing stenting. Stenting is step wise fashion with deploying one stent at time is feasible using 6F GC as long as it is followed by kissing balloons. Otherwise, performing kissing stent requires 7F GC.

4.2.7 Double barrel kissing stents technique

As in the case of V stenting, this technique requires 7F GC. It can be quick minimizing ischemia time and thus useful for large left main vessel with bifurcation disease involving LAD and LCX. After wiring both vessels, simultaneous stenting is performed creating double barrel in the proximal MV. Clearly, the stents in the proximal MV are not fully deployed and they are crushed against each other and the relationship between these barrels are not as simple it might appear. They are mostly twisted around each other and the size difference might affect the morphology of each stent within that part, i.e., one stent could be circle, the other is D shaped where in perfect scenario they both should have D shaped appearance with full apposition against the vessel. Clearly, re-accessing can be very challenging, which makes this technique less suitable for small vessel bifurcation lesions and for patients with expected need for further revascularization.

4.2.8 T-stenting technique

Bifurcation lesions that are appropriate for T stenting are lesions where the angulation angle is between 70 and 90°. The steps include wiring both vessels, performing necessary pre ballooning if needed, and then stenting the SB followed by stenting MV jailing the SB stent. A helpful technique to assure full coverage of bifurcation lesion is to leave inflated balloon inside the MV first then pulling he stent of the SB till it faces the resistance from the inflated MV balloon and then deflating that balloon followed by deploying the SB stent and finally stenting the MV. Depending on the results, rewiring through the MV stent struts might be necessary, followed by performing kissing balloons. When the angulation angle is less than 70, this approach is called TAP.

4.2.9 T-stenting and small protrusion technique TAP

It is a modification of the T-stenting technique aimed at optimizing "bail-out" SB stent implantation after MV treated by the "provisional" approach. Thus, it is applied after the MV stent has been deployed and kissing balloon inflation has been performed. In particular, TAP stenting was developed to ensure full SB ostium coverage by DES struts. To achieve this, the SB stent is delivered with intentional minimal protrusion inside the MV with an uninflated balloon positioned in the MV across the SB take-off. After SB stent deployment, kissing balloons inflation is immediately performed with the stent's balloon and the MV balloon. Further kissing balloon inflations with noncompliant balloons may be advisable in the case of suboptimal stent expansion. During the practice of TAP stenting, the operator should pay attention to and try to limit as much as possible the protrusion inside the MV which influences the length of the neo-carina. Nevertheless, similar to crush techniques, two main determinants of neo-carina length should be recognized: the SB take-off angle and the "quality" of pre-TAP kissing inflation. The impact of the SB take-off angle is quite intuitive: when the SB has a "T" shape take-off, small or absent SB stent protrusion inside the MV is needed to cover the SB ostium successfully. On the other hand, acute SB angles (Y-shapes) are associated with longer, oval-shaped SB ostia. Such an anatomic configuration implies the need for wider protrusion of the SB stent inside the MV, resulting in a longer neo-carina.

4.3 Grafts interventions

Engaging, performing angiogram and interventions on RIMA/LIMA carries higher risk for multiple reasons. LIMA is a vessel with high risk for dissection during any instrumentation. Most patients that requires LIMA interventions have significant underlying native vessel a baseline with possible occlusion of other bypass grafts. In a lot of clinical scenarios, LIMA could be the only source of perfusion for the heart.

Grafts/LIMA interventions could be performed via any approach. Left radial or distal left radial has the advantage of avoiding complications of femoral approaches and avoid left subclavian issues. Most common LIMA interventions are related to anastomosis at the LAD, left subclavian pseud or true stenosis, and ostial lesions at the takeoff from left subclavian. Lesions in the body of LIMA are less common. When using femoral approach, a lot of operators prefer to use a short LIMA guide which allows for more wire to reach distally to distal LAD after the anastomosis. Short GC usually is not required when using left radial approaches and if needed, shortening the guide catheter is a technique that can be used.

Distal anastomosis interventions: in early post-operative days, grafts angiogram (especially arterial grafts LIMA, RIMA, radial) might appear concerning for a dissection or spasm and this could be related to the post-operative shock or vasoactive medication. Most of the times, graft has not yet matured, and later imaging would confirm that. Stenosis at the anastomosis is mostly related to operative technical issues during post-operative period vs. true progression of CAD during the months or years after. Intervention if truly indicated should be performed quickly but safely specially in fresh LIMA-LAD anastomosis. Operator should minimize occluding the target grafts with the guide catheter as much as safely possible. Direct stenting is a good option if a stent could be passed without ballooning. Fresh anastomosis and sutures might be frail and over inflation of the balloon or stent should be avoided. Stent is sized based on the size of the bypassed vessel. One of the challenges in SVG anastomosis interventions is sizing the stent. It is very common that SVG is much larger than the target bypassed vessel. Proximal optimization technique using balloon diameter sized to SVG to dilate the segment of stent inside SVG. Data suggests good outcome post PCI of LIMA-LAD if performed by experience operator. Proximal optimization technique to the size of the LIMA has a lower risk especially in early days post bypass.

SVG are prone to thrombosis. Microvascular thrombosis can lead to bad outcomes. Using distal embolic protection (**Table 15**) in cardiac vessels interventions has showed benefits in interventions on SVGs especially with thrombotic lesions. The goal of distal embolic protection is to minimize/stop any thrombi from traveling distally to microvasculature. These devices cannot be used for all SVGs interventions. Distally to the target lesion, vessel should have about 4 cm safe landing segment where the device can be deployed. Severe stenotic lesions (especially aorto-ostial lesions) make using distal embolic protection technically challenging or impossible. Some operators advocate in such cases with difficulty passing the embolic protection device is to perform direct stenting if it allows. Fibrotic lesions (instent restenosis) with no friable thrombotic material, might not benefit from embolic protection. Direct stenting is another approach to minimize distal embolization and microvascular obstruction when feasible. Aneurysmal changes in SVG are very common which makes stent sizes difficult. Sizing should be based on the nonaneurysmal segment and post dilation can be used when needed. Proximal embolic protection devices are still available but are not used as much as the distal one during PCI on SVGs. The idea of these devices to reduce the thrombi that can travel upwards and cause organ ischemia specifically a stroke.

No reflow phenomena is common during any coronary or graft intervention. It is more common with thrombotic lesions and thought to be related to microvascular thrombosis and/or dysfunction. In addition to minimize clot burden with embolectomy, angioplasty and stenting to trap clots, administrating of microvascular active medications nitroprusside, verapamil and/or adenosine is necessary.

4.4 Instent restenosis treatment

Simple focal restenosis is usually treated with DES. The era of DES changed the approach of instent restenosis treatment. A second and a third layer of stents can be used to treat the lesion especially focal lesions in the body of the stent or edge of stent whether the prior used stent was a BMS or DES. Treatment of instent restenosis can be very challenging due to the variable potential underlying pathophysiology of stent restenosis: undersized, under expanded stent, presence of calcification, neoatherosclerosis, fibrotic tissue or presence of diffuse instent restenosis. Understanding the mechanism of restenosis is the main step to choose the appropriate treatment strategy. Intravascular imaging with IVUS or OCT if possible can be very helpful. However, most of the time these imaging catheters cannot cross the restenosis. In these setting, ballooning might be the only option.

In case of diffuse instent neoatherosclerosis cutting balloons is not a good option especially if the prior stents are well sized and fully apposed. The decision of adding a

Device	Guide compatibility	Crossing profile	Vessel size	Length of filter/ landing zone	Notes
Spider RX (ev3)	6Fr	3.2 Fr	3–6 mm	10 mm/39 mm,	Only one with wire of choice
FilterWire (Boston Scientific)	6Fr	3.2 Fr	2.5–5.5 mm	15 mm/39 mm	
GaurdWire	6Fr	2.1 and 2.8 Fr	3–6 mm		
Interceptor	6Fr	2.7 Fr	2.5–5.5 mm		Capture Small Particles <50 µm

Table 15.
Distal embolization protection devices.

second layer of stent depends on the results of angioplasty, size of the vessel, and long-term outcome. If the mechanism of restenosis is under expanded stent, fibrotic tissue, calcifications underneath the stent or hyper intimal hyperplasia, the treatment is targeting the underlying tissue. Available treatment options are those used for adjunct plaque modifications (brachytherapy, LASER, and intravascular lithotripsy).

4.5 Post aortic valve replacement coronary intervention

Supra-annular valves like CoreValve bio prosthetic makes coronary access challenging. The goal is to a use a guide catheter to cross the cells of the bio prosthetic valve at the level of the coronary. Best approach is to use a 0.5 shorter guide catheter than usually used. Wire assisted technique to manipulate the GC to sit within the bio prosthetic and at the appropriate cell level to cross toward the coronary ostium. Manipulating the GC with a 0.035″ guide wire should be performed within the lumen of the aorta and away from the aortic wall to avoid aortic or coronary ostium injury. Guide wire makes the GC stiff and moving the GC quickly could cause the GC to jump quickly and damage the coronary ostium. Once the GC is in a good trajectory and directed toward the coronary ostium, GC should be advanced slowly toward the ostium.

5. Conclusion

Percutaneous coronary interventions have always been crucial in medical care. Now more than ever, with rapidly evolving percutaneous interventions and less surgical interventions, coronary percutaneous interventions are priority. Developing required technical skills and mastering basic and complicated intervention techniques have never been as important as they are now. Before proceeding with any intervention, all necessary equipment and medications should be available. Other essential requirements for any successful intervention include planning, having competency in required techniques, early recognition, and being prepared to manage complications.

Conflict of interest

The author declares no conflict of interest.

Author details

Imran Khalil
Medicine (Interventional Cardiology), VA Medical Center, Indiana University School of Medicine, Indianapolis, Indiana

*Address all correspondence to: elimrans@hotmail.com

References

[1] Romagnoli E, Biondi-Zoccai G, Sciahbasi A, et al. Radial versus femoral randomized investigation in ST-segment elevation acute coronary syndrome: The RIFLE-STEACS (radial versus femoral randomized investigation in ST-elevation acute coronary syndrome) study. Journal of the American College of Cardiology. 2012;**60**(24):2481-2489. DOI: 10.1016/j.jacc.2012.06.017

[2] Jolly SS, Yusuf S, Cairns J, et al. Radial versus femoral access for coronary angiography and intervention in patients with acute coronary syndromes (RIVAL): A randomised, parallel group, multicentre trial [published correction appears in Lancet. 2011 Apr 23;377(9775): 1408] [published correction appears in Lancet. 2011 Jul 2;378(9785):30]. Lancet. 2011;**377**(9775):1409-1420. DOI: 10.1016/S0140-6736(11)60404-2

[3] Jolly SS, Amlani S, Hamon M, Yusuf S, Mehta SR. Radial versus femoral access for coronary angiography or intervention and the impact on major bleeding and ischemic events: A systematic review and meta-analysis of randomized trials. American Heart Journal. 2009;**157**(1):132-140. DOI: 10.1016/j.ahj.2008.08.023

[4] Ferrante G, Rao SV, Jüni P, et al. Radial versus femoral access for coronary interventions across the entire spectrum of patients with coronary artery disease: A meta-analysis of randomized trials. JACC. Cardiovascular Interventions. 2016;**9**(14):1419-1434. DOI: 10.1016/j.jcin.2016.04.014Twenty

[5] Hibbert B, Simard T, Wilson KR, et al. Transradial versus transfemoral artery approach for coronary angiography and percutaneous coronary intervention in the extremely obese. JACC. Cardiovascular Interventions. 2012;**5**(8):819-826. DOI: 10.1016/j.jcin.2012.04.009

[6] Michael TT, Alomar M, Papayannis A, et al. A randomized comparison of the transradial and transfemoral approaches for coronary artery bypass graft angiography and intervention: The RADIAL-CABG trial (RADIAL versus femoral access for coronary artery bypass graft angiography and intervention). JACC. Cardiovascular Interventions. 2013;**6**(11):1138-1144. DOI: 10.1016/j.jcin.2013.08.004

[7] Pancholy SB, Joshi P, Shah S, Rao SV, Bertrand OF, Patel TM. Effect of vascular access site choice on radiation exposure during coronary angiography: The REVERE trial (randomized evaluation of vascular entry site and radiation exposure). JACC. Cardiovascular Interventions. 17 August 2015;**8**(9):1189-1196

[8] Shah RM, Patel D, Abbate A, Cowley MJ, Jovin IS. Comparison of transradial coronary procedures via right radial versus left radial artery approach: A meta-analysis. Catheterization and Cardiovascular Interventions. 2016;**88**(7):1027-1033. DOI: 10.1002/ccd.26519

[9] Plourde G, Pancholy SB, Nolan J, et al. Radiation exposure in relation to the arterial access site used for diagnostic coronary angiography and percutaneous coronary intervention: A systematic review and meta-analysis. Lancet. 2015;**386**(10009):2192-2203

[10] Anadol R, Brandt M, Merz N, Knorr M, Ahoopai M, Geyer M, et al. EffectivenesS of additional x-ray PRotection dEviceS in reducing scattered radiation in radial intervention: The ESPRESSO randomized trial. Open. 2019;**9**: e029509. DOI: 10.1136/bmjopen-2019-029509

[11] Thuijs DJFM, Kappetein AP, Serruys PW, et al. Percutaneous

coronary intervention versus coronary artery bypass grafting in patients with three-vessel or left main coronary artery disease: 10-year follow-up of the multicentre randomised controlled SYNTAX trial [published correction appears in Lancet. 14 March 2020;395 (10227):870]. Lancet. 2019;**394**(10206): 1325-1334. DOI: 10.1016/S0140-6736 (19)31997-X

[12] Yousif A, James PH, Ahran DA, et al. Mortality after drug-eluting stents vs. coronary artery bypass grafting for left main coronary artery disease: A meta-analysis of randomized controlled trials. European Heart Journal. 2020:1-8. DOI: 10.1093/eurheartj/ehaa135

[13] Duk-Woo P, Jung-Min A, Hanbit P, et al. On behalf of the PRECOMBAT investigators. Circulation. 2020;**141**: 1437-1446

[14] Niels RH, Timo M, Mitchell L, et al. Percutaneous coronary angioplasty versus coronary artery bypass grafting in the treatment of unprotected left main stenosis: Updated 5-year outcomes from the randomised, non-inferiority NOBLE trial. 2019. Lancet. 18-24 January 2020;**395**(10219):191-199. DOI: 10.1016/77S0140-6736(19)32972-1

Chapter 13

Primary Angioplasty: From the Artery to the Myocardium

Miguel Angel Farah, Franco Farah and Miguel Alejandro Farah

Abstract

The prognosis of patients suffering from acute myocardial infarction (AMI) is related to the amount of muscle loss and ventricular function deterioration caused by the event. Primary angioplasty is the most effective reperfusion strategy. Early reperfusion limits the size of the infarction and improves the prognosis. However, the incidence of death and post-AMI heart failure remains around 20% during the first year. Factors that contribute to myocardial damage are ischemia, mechanical forces, inflammation, and reperfusion injury. All those take a variable and sometimes unpredictable preponderance at different times during the evolution of acute myocardial infarction. The damage caused by the different mechanisms is irreversible; therefore, any therapeutic strategy must be preventive. Developed treatments for continuous myocardial protection could potentially preserve the myocardium during the delay of the system and during the early evolution of the event. Developed controlled reperfusion procedures where the interventional cardiologist assumes the treatment not only of the culprit vessel but also of the myocardium could potentially decrease myocardial damage, preserve ventricular function, and improve patients' prognosis.

Keywords: myocardial damage, acute myocardial infarction, ischemia, mechanical forces, inflammation, reperfusion injury, continuous myocardial protection, controlled reperfusion

1. Introduction

The prognosis of patients suffering from acute myocardial infarction (AMI) is directly related to the amount of muscle loss and the deterioration of ventricular function caused by the event [1–4]. Consequently, the goal of treatment in the initial phase, beyond preserving life, is to limit myocardial damage. Early reperfusion of the myocardium limits the size of the infarction and improves the prognosis of patients [3, 4]. Primary angioplasty is the most effective reperfusion strategy for the treatment of acute myocardial infarction [5–7]. From the first reports of mechanical reperfusion to the present, the primary angioplasty strategy continuously improved in different aspects such as greater accessibility to the method [8–10], safer vascular accesses [11, 12], and the use of drug-eluting stents that modulate the scarring of the coronary artery wall [13, 14] to prevent restenosis of the vessel or vessels treated. In addition, the development of antithrombotic and antiplatelet drugs also contributed to improving early and late artery permeability [15, 16]. The enormous effort focused on the treatment of the coronary artery has led to the fact that the success of primary angioplasty is now greater than 95% [7]. The angiographic success rate ceased to be a problem. However, the post-AMI incidence of death and heart failure remains around 20% during the first year [17], and as mentioned earlier this correlates directly with the amount of myocardium damaged and the deterioration of ventricular function.

2. The following case serves to illustrate the result of AMI usual treatment at present

52-year-old male, with grade II obesity, dyslipidemia, hypertension, and smoking history and with no previous cardiovascular events, arrives at the hospital 60 minutes after the onset of symptoms. The first electrocardiogram (ECG) shows rS in V1, V2, and V3 and ST-segment elevation from V1 to V6 (**Figure 1**).

At admission the arterial blood pressure was 145/80 mm of hg, the heart rate was 78 beats per minute, and the Killip Kimball grade was A. The patient received aspirin (250 mg), clopidogrel (600 mg), unfractionated heparin in intravenous bolus (5000 UI), and rosuvastatin (40 mg). At 80 minutes after admission, 140 minutes from the onset of symptoms, coronary angiography is performed showing single-vessel disease with thrombotic occlusion of the middle third of the anterior descending artery (ADA) and TIMI 0 flow. Primary angioplasty is performed to the middle third of the ADA with thromboaspiration and stent implantation achieving an adequate result with TIMI 3 flow, symptom relief, and absence of complications.

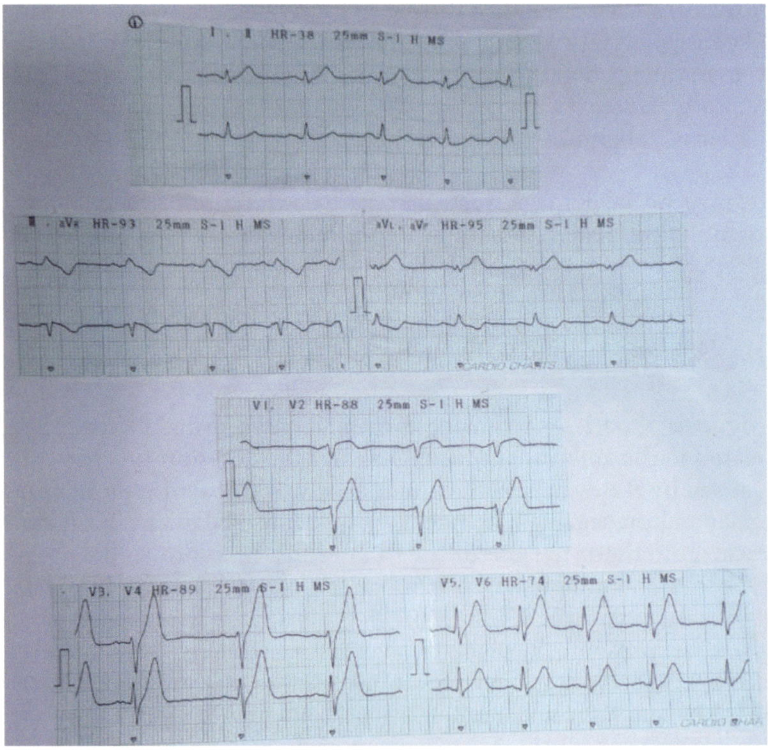

Figure 1.
ECG at admission.

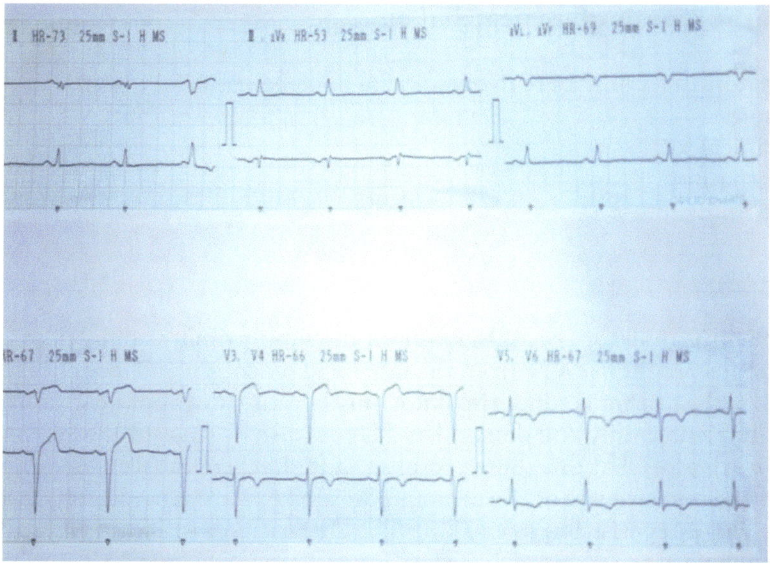

Figure 2.
ECG postprimary angioplasty.

The post-procedure ECG shows QS in V1, V2, and V3 and ST level and negative T from V1 to V6 (**Figure 2**).

IECA and B blockers are started. It evolves without recurrence of symptoms; however, at 48 hours, the ECG shows QS from V1 to V5 and low R in V6 (**Figure 3**).

Note that despite early assistance, it no longer has positive vectors in V1, V2, and V3, and after the usual successful treatment and aligned with the guidelines based on current evidence, it continues to lose precordial vectors after primary angioplasty. The echocardiogram shows antero-apical dyskinesia and impaired ventricular function, with an ejection fraction of 35% measured by the Simpson method. There are several mechanisms by which the myocardium is lost in the different phases of AMI.

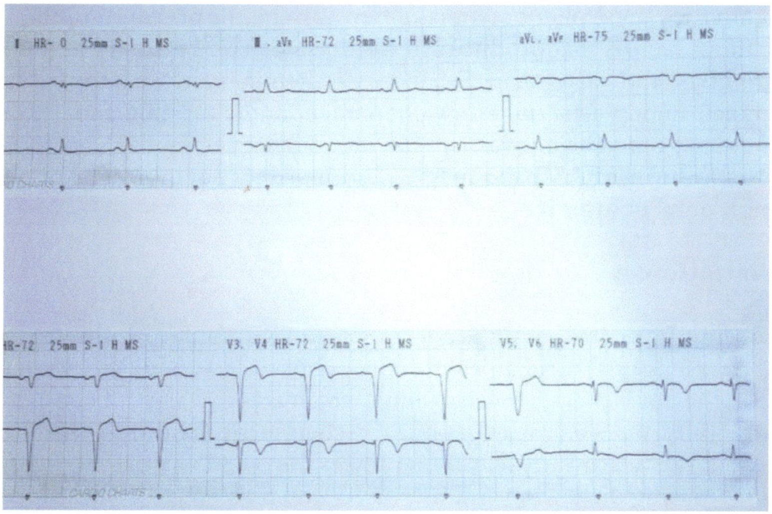

Figure 3.
ECG at 48 hours.

3. Etiopathogenesis of myocardial damage

The factors that contribute to myocardial damage are as follows:
Ischemia.
Mechanical forces.
Inflammation.
Reperfusion injury.

3.1 Ischemia

It implies the interruption of blood flow, the supply of O_2 and nutrients. The myocyte stops producing ATP from the fatty acid oxidation and switches to another metabolic pathway that is suboptimal not only because it cannot maintain a balance between nutrient supply and demand and O_2 but also because of the accumulation of metabolic wastes that this route produces, and that generates an environment harmful to the subsistence of the cells and the appropriate reperfusion, favoring the phenomenon of reperfusion injury [18]. The alternative route for ATP production during ischemia is anaerobic glycolysis; its potential to produce ATP is 20 times less than aerobic glucose metabolism and even less than the route commonly used by myocyte which is the aerobic metabolism of fatty acids. The glycogen reserve as a source of anaerobic ATP is depleted in 30–60 minutes and also generates lactic acidosis, high concentration of protons at tissue level, and excess of H_2O. The mechanisms of myocardial damage due to ischemia involve low production of ATP that is insufficient not only for myocyte function but also to preserve its structure and to maintain hydroelectrolytic balance by the Na-K ATPase pump, which implies an increase in Na and intracellular H_2O with tissue and cellular edema, vacuolization, and cell burst [19, 20]. Inactivation of the Na-K ATPase pump leads to the activation of the Na-Ca exchange, resulting in increased intracellular calcium with hypercontraction of myocytes (contraction band necrosis) [21, 22]. The entry of Ca into the cell is one of the mechanisms by which the permeability of the transition pores of the mitochondria increases and their destruction occurs [23]. Myocardial ischemia can be either primary before applying reperfusion therapy or secondary, that is, after recanalizing the occlusion. As for primary ischemia, it can occur in a sustained or episodic manner. In some cases, episodic primary ischemia can generate a protective myocyte phenomenon known as ischemic preconditioning [24]. The mechanical factors that produce arterial occlusion and primary ischemia are plaque thrombus, and vasospasm. Secondary ischemia is always harmful and may be due to failed angioplasty, no reflow phenomenon, distal embolism, thrombotic reocclusion, post-reperfusion, vasospasm, etc. Consequently, myocardial ischemia occurs from the onset of AMI and may end with primary angioplasty, or persist (not reflow), or recur after it.

3.2 Mechanical forces

The ischemic myocardium stops contracting and is distended; this situation subjects it to exceptional mechanical forces of tension, traction, and stretching. In each systole, the nonischemic myocardium, which acts in a state of compensatory hypercontractility, pulls on the edges of the ischemic myocardium. In addition, in each systole, the healthy myocardium presses the blood against the ischemic myocardium causing distension and increased wall tension [25]. These forces of stretching and traction produce direct tissue damage [26] but also by increasing the tumor necrosis factor trigger mechanisms of apoptosis [27] dependent on caspases that produce cell death in early and late stages of AMI. The strongest evidence of the damage that mechanical forces can produce is the rupture of the ventricular wall. As they are direct forces exerted on the ischemic myocardium, it is to be assumed that the damage is related to the magnitude and frequency of exposure; therefore, the higher the heart rate and inotropism, the greater the damage produced by this mechanism. This mechanism of myocardial damage begins immediately after the onset of ischemia and lasts beyond reperfusion.

3.3 Inflammation

The inflammatory response during the acute ischemic event plays a decisive role in the size of the infarction and the subsequent adverse left ventricle remodeling [28]. The onset of myocardial ischemia during AMI triggers a pro-inflammatory response whose initial objective is to eliminate damaged cells and tissue from the injured area. This initial pro-inflammatory phase contributes to myocyte death and tissue damage [29, 30]. This phase is followed by a repairing anti-inflammatory stage that leads to healing. Balance alterations and the transition between the pro-inflammatory phase and the anti-inflammatory phase can increase myocardial damage during the event and contribute to an adverse left ventricle remodeling after AMI [28]. In addition, the inflammatory response as an acute phase reactant is related to the location and size of AMI. Large and anterior infarct shoots a greater extent of acute phase reactants. The initial pro-inflammatory phase includes complement cascade activation and reactive oxygen species (ROS) production [28]. The damage-associated molecular patterns (DAMPs) production that binds to receptors in membranes cell and cytosolic proteins (inflammasomes), in either, circulating or myocardium resident cells. Inflammasomes cause caspase activation (which initiate the pyroptosis phenomenon, [apoptosis, and inflammatory necrosis]) and release pro-inflammatory cytokine as such as IL-1 and IL-8 and chemokines that recruit pro-inflammatory cells (polymorphonuclear, monocytes, macrophages, T and B lymphocytes) [28]. In addition, the inflammasomes activated during AMI induce ATP loss from the injured cells to the extracellular space, K outflow, lysosomal destabilization, and ROS generation by the mitochondria [28]. The anti-inflammatory phase begins with neutrophil and dendritic cell arrival; these cells secrete anti-inflammatory cytokines such as IL-10 and tissue growth factors that begin damaged tissue repair [28]. Monocytes and macrophages induced by interferon change their phenotype towards anti-inflammatory expressions [28]. Dendritic cells secrete chemotactic substances for regulatory T lymphocytes (CD4, CD25, and FOXP3) and T helper lymphocytes; these lymphocyte subtypes also secrete anti-inflammatory and reparative substances such as IL-10 and tissue growth factor and also induce the expression of anti-inflammatory macrophage phenotypes [28]. Although it is not proven, it is speculated that they could also activate pre- and post-conditioning mechanisms [28]. This myocardial damage mechanism is triggered in early stages after the onset of ischemia and continues beyond reperfusion.

3.4 Reperfusion injury

Myocardial reperfusion can itself produce more damage and cell death; this process defines the phenomenon of reperfusion injury [31–33] that could be prevented by applying additional therapies [34]. Reperfusion injury could be responsible for up to 50% of the final myocardial damage during acute myocardial infarction. The time elapsed since the onset of symptoms, diabetes, TIMI 0 flow in baseline angiography, DA involvement, and presentation with heart failure is associated with a greater chance of presenting reperfusion injury [35]. Elevation of white blood cells, greater activation (platelet size and reactivity), high levels of thromboxane

A2 and ET1, hyperglycemia associated or not with diabetes, and C-reactive protein before reperfusion are predictors of this phenomenon [36–38]. It is possible that there is always some degree of reperfusion damage, but the patients with little time of evolution of the symptoms and those who presented previous angina seem less susceptible [39, 40]. There is a useful premise to estimate its magnitude; the greater and more intense the ischemia, the greater the reperfusion injury [35, 41–43]. In daily practice, the lack of resolution of the ST segment after achieving epicardial coronary flow is used as a marker of reperfusion failure. In patients who do not correct the ST, the mortality of AMI triples beyond achieving adequate epicardial flow [44, 45]. The most important events that occur during reperfusion and trigger mechanisms of injury are the steep increase in oxygen content in a medium with a low PH (tissue acidosis caused by ischemia). In this scenario, O_2 binds to hydrogen protons generating reactive oxygen species that by themselves generate DNA, protein, and lipid damage to the membranes and consequently direct cell death [46, 47]. Besides, reactive oxygen species have pro-inflammatory effects mediated by cytokines that cause apoptosis and cellular necroptosis [48]. At the level of the mitochondria, ROS causes the opening of the transition pores of their membranes making them susceptible to irreversible damage [48]. At the endoplasmic reticulum level, the damage caused by ROS alters the dynamics of calcium, which in the context of reperfusion of an acidotic environment generates calcium entry into the sarcolemma, producing sustained hypercontraction that results in necrosis with contraction bands [47–49]. The calcium entry activates Ca-dependent proteases that degrade structural components of the cell [50]. The reperfusion injury affects not only the myocyte but also the microvasculature, where ROS not only produces direct damage to the endothelial cells causing increased permeability of the capillary wall resulting in edema but also is chemotactic for neutrophils, activates complement, and triggers pro-thrombotic phenomena [48–51]. In brief, microvascular occlusion occurs due to perivascular edema, cluster of neutrophils, and local thrombosis. Injury due to reperfusion occurs due to the arrival of saturated O_2 blood to myocardial tissue that is vulnerable to metabolic changes and the local internal environment, which occurred during ischemia. Reperfusion injury is a rapid and irreversible phenomenon [52].

The phenomena of ischemia, damage due to mechanical forces, inflammation, and reperfusion injury take a variable and sometimes unpredictable preponderance at different times during the evolution of AMI (**Figure 4**).

Also, the damage caused by the different mechanisms is irreversible; therefore, any therapeutic strategy must be preventive that implies pathophysiological

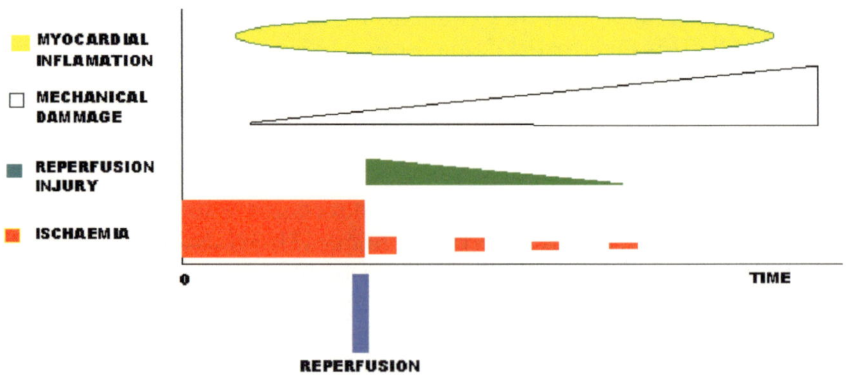

Figure 4.
Myocardial damage mechanism, importance, and development over time.

conditions that culminate in myocardial damage and act before the point of no return in the viability of the cell occurs.

4. Analysis of guidelines for AMI treatment

Both the AHA-ACC guidelines and the ESC guidelines for AMI treatment are strongly oriented to early and sustained reperfusion, which constitutes the most powerful resource for improving prognosis and saving lives during the event. The best way to show successful post-PCI or thrombolytic reperfusion is to verify the correction of the ST segment of the ECG performed after reperfusion therapy. Approximately 30% of patients receiving primary angioplasty in a timely manner do not correct ST elevation or initially correct it but continue to lose positive ECG vectors after apparently successful reperfusion. As we saw in the previous section, this happens because there is myocardial damage before, during, and after reperfusion [53]. However, the analysis of the guidelines shows that measures to reduce myocardial damage beyond reperfusion are poorly developed. The related items found in the current guides are reproduced below.

4.1 AHA-ACC guides 2013

4.1.1 Nitroglycerin

It improves the conditions of pre- and post-load of the ventricle and could also improve collateral flow and reduce BP which would improve the imbalance between supply and demand of O_2 in some patients. Based on the evidence provided by a meta-analysis that included 22 clinical trials and more than 80,000 patients, 3 or 4 deaths could be avoided per 1000 treated patients, which implies a net benefit. Nitroglycerin is a class I indication with a level of evidence C for patients with ischemic pain, hypertension, or pulmonary congestion [54].

4.1.2 B blockers

During the first hours of AMI, the B blockers can decrease the demand for O_2 by the myocardium by decreasing heart rate, blood pressure, and contractility and, additionally, by prolonging diastole, can improve ischemic myocardial perfusion, mainly of the subendocardium. As a consequence of this, B blockers can reduce the size of the AMI. Based on the clinical evidence provided by the ISIS I, MIAMI, TIMI II, and Taste I trials, the use of B blockers early, in the absence of contraindications, may offer benefits from the first day and in a sustained way avoiding around 6 deaths per 1000 patients treated. B oral blockers have class I indication level of evidence A, and in the form of intravenous administration, they have class IIa indication with level of evidence B [55–57].

4.1.3 Metabolic control

The metabolic modulation of the insulin glucose axis by infusion of glucose-insulin-potassium was evaluated in different trials with diverse and contradictory results that when taken together result in an intervention without net benefit compared to placebo. However, these guidelines suggest that it could be of benefit in patients with less than 12 hours of evolution, in Killip Kimball. Beyond that, the guidelines do not establish an indication with a level of evidence defined for this intervention [58].

4.1.4 Glycemia control

During AMI, the levels of catecholamines and cortisol increase, insulin decreases, and blood glucagon increase. This leads to a notable increase in blood glucose and decreased glucose utilization by cells. Free fatty acids and their metabolites are increased that increase myocardial damage by different mechanisms (direct inhibition of glucose oxidation, increased demand for O_2, direct toxicity). Insulin can reverse some of these mechanisms by inducing the production of ATP from aerobic glucose metabolism in the myocyte. Several studies mentioned in these guidelines demonstrated benefits in patients with hyperglycemia who received insulin infusion for strict glycemic control during the event. These guidelines establish that the normalization of insulin glycemia is a class I indication with a level of evidence B for patients with complicated AMI and class IIa with a level of evidence B for patients with uncomplicated AMI [59–61, 62].

4.2 ESC guides 2017

These guidelines mention, scarcely, that to reduce myocardial damage beyond reperfusion therapy, some strategies that include pharmacological and mechanical therapies have been demonstrating the potential to reduce the size of AMI by decreasing the impact of reperfusion injury in small clinical trials. But there is no large-scale clinical study that has demonstrated clinical benefit. Therefore, they make no recommendation regarding measures to limit reperfusion injury or any other therapy to reduce myocardial damage during the event, beyond reperfusion [63].

5. Current reperfusion adjuvant therapy status

The use of B blockers and nitrates is favorable to reduce myocardial damage caused by primary and secondary ischemia, reducing the imbalance between supply and demand of O_2 and nutrients until reperfusion. Beside, these drugs are useful to optimize the conditions of pre- and post-loading of LV, decrease heart rate and blood pressure, and thus limit the damage caused by mechanical stress. A wide variety of potent platelet antiplatelets such as clopidogrel, prasugrel, or ticagrelor added to the routine use of aspirin were shown to reduce the recurrence of ischemic events after reperfusion (secondary ischemia). Although it is not clearly established by evidence from clinical trials, thromboaspiration; potent vasodilators at the microvasculature level such as adenosine and calcium blockers, among others; and the use of IIb–IIIa glycoprotein inhibitors may be effective in prevention and treatment of no-reflow. The phenomenon of no-reflow can cause ischemia (secondary ischemia) to continue beyond the recanalization of the epicardial artery. However, reperfusion inflammation and injury are not prevented or treated in daily practice.

6. Perspectives

The development of reperfusion therapies for AMI was shown to reduce mortality strongly. There are possibilities to optimize its use. Health teams must continue fighting to shorten the system times and detect the best strategy according to the context in which they operate. There are working groups that carry out research in basic sciences, translational research, and clinical research and are making advances in myocardial protection. Cyclosporine and colchicine are currently evaluated for their ability to reduce the damage caused by inflammation. Developed treatments for *continuing myocardial protection* [52], which the clinical cardiologists administer from the moment of diagnosis until the convalescence of the patient in a critical unit, could potentially preserve myocardium during the delay of the system and the early evolution of the event. Developed *controlled reperfusion* [52] procedures where the interventional cardiologist assumes the treatment not only of the guilty vessel but also of the myocardium could potentially decrease myocardial damage, preserve ventricular function, and improve the prognosis of patients suffering from AMI. The concept of *controlled reperfusion* involves deciding how to reperfuse (e.g., post-conditioning) and with what to reperfuse (e.g., administering to the ischemic myocardium, through dedicated catheters, before the opening of the artery, blood modified or enriched with drugs), preparing the myocardium for a more complete and definitive recovery.

A wide field of research appears to improve the treatment outcome of patients suffering from AMI aiming not only at arterial recanalization but also at myocardial preservation.

Abbreviations

AMI	acute myocardial infarction
ECG	electrocardiogram
ROS	reactive oxygen species
ADA	anterior descending artery

Author details

Miguel Angel Farah*, Franco Farah and Miguel Alejandro Farah
MEDIS Institute, Salta, Argentina

*Address all correspondence to: farahale@yahoo.com

References

[1] Cohn JN, Ferrari R, Sharpe N, et al. Cardiac remodeling—Concepts and clinical implications: A consensus paper from an international forum on cardiac remodeling behalf of an International Forum on Cardiac Remodeling. Journal of the American College of Cardiology. 2000;**35**:569-582

[2] Sabbah HN, Goldstein S, et al. Ventricular remodelling: Consequences and therapy. European Heart Journal. 1993;**14**(suppl C):24-29

[3] Gibson CM et al. NRMI and current treatment patterns for ST-elevation myocardial infarction. American Heart Journal. 2004;**148**(5 Suppl):S29-S33

[4] Keeley EC, Hillis LD, et al. Primary PCI for myocardial infarction with ST-segment elevation. The New England Journal of Medicine. 2007;**356**(1):47-54

[5] Grines CL, Cox DA, Stone GW, et al. Coronary angioplasty with or without stent implantation for acute myocardial infarction. Stent primary angioplasty in myocardial infarction study group. The New England Journal of Medicine. 1999;**341**(26):1949-1956

[6] Stone GW, Brodie BR, Griffin JJ, et al. Prospective, multicenter study of the safety and feasibility of primary stenting in acute myocardial infarction: In-hospital and 30-day results of the PAMI stent pilot trial. Journal of the American College of Cardiology. 1998;**31**(1):23-30

[7] Keeley EC, Boura JA, Grines CL, et al. Primary angioplasty versus intravenous thrombolytic therapy for acute myocardial infarction: A quantitative review of 23 randomised trials. Lancet. 2003;**361**(9351):13-20

[8] Herrin J, Miller LE, Turkmani DF, et al. National performance on door-in to door-out time among patients transferred for primary percutaneous coronary intervention. Archives of Internal Medicine. 2011;**171**(21):1879-1886

[9] Sorensen JT, Terkelsen CJ, Norgaard BL, et al. Urban and rural implementation of pre-hospital diagnosis and direct referral for primary percutaneous coronary intervention in patients with acute ST-elevation myocardial infarction. European Heart Journal. 2011;**32**(4):430-436

[10] Wang TY, Nallamothu BK, Krumholz HM, et al. Association of door-in to door-out time with reperfusion delays and outcomes among patients transferred for primary percutaneous coronary intervention. Journal of the American Medical Association. 2011;**305**(24):2540-2547

[11] Karrowni W, Vyas A, Giacomino B, et al. Radial versus femoral access for primary percutaneous interventions in ST-segment elevation myocardial infarction patients: A meta-analysis of randomized controlled trials. JACC: Cardiovascular Interventions. 2013;**6**(8):814-823

[12] Vranckx P, Frigoli E, Valgimigli M, et al. Radial versus femoral access in patients with acute coronary syndromes with or without ST-segment elevation. European Heart Journal. 2017;**38**(14):1069-1080

[13] De Luca G, Stone GW, et al. Drug-eluting vs bare-metal stents in primary angioplasty: A pooled patient-level meta-analysis of randomized trials. Archives of Internal Medicine. 2012;**172**(8):611-621

[14] Wallace EL, Abdel-Latif A, et al. Meta-analysis of long-term outcomes for drug-eluting stents versus bare-metal stents in primary percutaneous coronary interventions for ST-segment

elevation myocardial infarction. The American Journal of Cardiology. 2012;**109**(7):932-940

[15] Braunwald E, McCabe CH, Montalescot G, Gibson CM, Antman EM, et al. Prasugrel versus clopidogrel in patients with acute coronary syndromes. The New England Journal of Medicine. 2007;**357**(20):2001-2015

[16] Wallentin L, Becker RC, Harrington RA, et al. Ticagrelor versus clopidogrel in patients with acute coronary syndromes. The New England Journal of Medicine. 2009;**361**(11):1045-1057

[17] Kochar A, Christopher B, et al. Post-myocardial infarction heart failure. Journal of the American College of Cardiology. 2018;**6**(3):179-186

[18] Piper HM, Garcia-Dorado D, Ovize M, et al. A fresh look at reperfusion injury. Cardiovascular Research. 1998;**38**:291-300

[19] Inserte J, Garcia-Dorado D, Ruiz-Meana M, Padilla F, Barrabés JA, Pina P, et al. Effect of inhibition of Na(+)/Ca(2+) exchanger at the time of myocardial reperfusion on hypercontracture and cell death. Cardiovascular Research. 2002;**55**:739-748

[20] Garcia-Dorado D, Theroux P, Munoz R, Alonso J, Elizaga J, Fernandez-Avilés F, et al. Favorable effects of hyperosmotic reperfusion on myocardial edema and infarct size. The American Journal of Physiology. 1992;**262**:H17-H22

[21] Siegmund B, Zude R, Piper HM, et al. Recovery of anoxic-reoxygenated cardiomyocytes from severe calcium overload. The American Journal of Physiology. 1992;**263**:H1262-H1269

[22] Barrabes JA, Garcia-Dorado D, Ruiz-Meana M, Piper HM, Solares J, Gonzalez MA, et al. Myocardial segment shrinkage during coronary reperfusion in situ. Relation to hypercontracture and myocardial necrosis. Pflügers Archiv. 1996;**431**:519-526

[23] Kingma JG et al. Acute myocardial injury: A perspective on lethal reperfusion injury. Journal of Cardiovascular Pharmacology. 2017;**6**(5):216

[24] Karila-Cohen D, Czitrom D, Brochet E, et al. Decreased no-reflow in patients with anterior myocardial infarction and pre-infarction angina. European Heart Journal. 1999;**20**(23):1724-1730

[25] Olivetti G, Quaini F, et al. Acute myocardial infarction in humans is associated with activation of programmed myocyte cell death in the surviving portion of the heart. Journal of Molecular and Cellular Cardiology. 1996;**28**(9):2005-2016

[26] Erlebacher JA, Weiss JL, Myron L, et al. Early dilation of the infarcted segment in acute transmural myocardial infarction: Role of infarct expansion in acute left ventricular enlargement. Journal of the American College of Cardiology. 1984;**4**(2):201-208

[27] Teringova E, Tousek P, et al. Apoptosis in ischemic heart disease. Journal of Translational Medicine. 2017;**15**:87

[28] Derek J. Hausenloy, et al. Inflammation following acute myocardial infarction: Multiple players, dynamic roles, and novel therapeutic opportunities. Pharmacology & Therapeutics. 2018;**186**:73-87

[29] Zhao ZQ, Nakamura M, Wang NP, Wilcox JN, Shearer S, Ronson RS, et al. Reperfusion induces myocardial apoptotic cell death. Cardiovascular Research. 2000;**45**:651-660

[30] Zhao ZQ, Velez DA, Wang NP, Hewan-Lowe KO, Nakamura M, Guyton RA, et al. Progressively developed myocardial apoptotic cell death during late phase of reperfusion. Apoptosis. 2001;**6**:279-290

[31] Yellon DM, Hausenloy DJ, et al. Myocardial reperfusion injury. The New England Journal of Medicine. 2007;**357**(11):1121-1135

[32] Hausenloy DJ, Yellon DM, et al. Targeting myocardial reperfusion injury—The search continues. The New England Journal of Medicine. 2015;**373**(11):1073-1075

[33] Braunwald E, Kloner RA, et al. Myocardial reperfusion: A double-edged sword? The Journal of Clinical Investigation. 1985;**76**(5):1713-1719

[34] Collet JP, Montalescot G, et al. The acute reperfusion management of STEMI in patients with impaired glucose tolerance and type 2 diabetes. Diabetes & Vascular Disease Research. 2005;**2**(3):136-143

[35] Iwakura K, Ito H, Kawano S, et al. Predictive factors for development of the no-reflow phenomenon in patients with reperfused anterior wall acute myocardial infarction. Journal of the American College of Cardiology. 2001;**38**(2):472-477

[36] Campo G, Valgimigli M, Gemmati D, et al. Value of platelet reactivity in predicting response to treatment and clinical outcome in patients undergoing primary coronary intervention: Insights into the STRATEGY Study. Journal of the American College of Cardiology. 2006;**48**(11):2178-2185

[37] Niccoli G, Giubilato S, Russo E, et al. Plasma levels of thromboxane A2 on admission are associated with no-reflow after primary percutaneous coronary intervention. European Heart Journal. 2008;**29**(15):1843-1850

[38] Niccoli G, Lanza GA, Shaw S, et al. Endothelin-1 and acute myocardial infarction: A no-reflow mediator after successful percutaneous myocardial revascularization. European Heart Journal. 2006;**27**(15):1793-1798

[39] Karila-Cohen D, Czitrom D, Brochet E, et al. Decreased no-reflow in patients with anterior myocardial infarction and pre-infarction angina. European Heart Journal. 1999;**20**(23):1724-1730

[40] Komamura K, Kitakaze M, Nishida K, et al. Progressive decreases in coronary vein flow during reperfusion in acute myocardial infarction: Clinical documentation of the no reflow phenomenon after successful thrombolysis. Journal of the American College of Cardiology. 1994;**24**(2):370-377

[41] Nallamothu BK, Bradley EH, Krumholz HM, et al. Time to treatment in primary percutaneous coronary intervention. The New England Journal of Medicine. 2007;**357**(16):1631-1638

[42] Turschner O, D'hooge J, Dommke C, et al. The sequential changes in myocardial thickness and thickening which occur during acute transmural infarction, infarct reperfusion and the resultant expression of reperfusion injury. European Heart Journal. 2004;**25**(9):794-803

[43] Uyarel H, Cam N, Okmen E, et al. Level of Selvester QRS score is predictive of ST-segment resolution and 30-day outcomes in patients with acute myocardial infarction undergoing primary coronary intervention. The American Heart Journal. 2006;**151**(6):1239.e1-1239.e7

[44] de Lemos JA, Braunwald E, et al. ST segment resolution as a tool for

assessing the efficacy of reperfusion therapy. Journal of the American College of Cardiology. 2001;**38**(5):1283-1294

[45] Buller CE, Fu Y, Mahaffey KW, et al. ST-segment recovery and outcome after primary percutaneous coronary intervention for ST-elevation myocardial infarction: Insights from the Assessment of Pexelizumab in Acute Myocardial Infarction (APEX-AMI) trial. Circulation. 2008;**118**(13):1335-1346

[46] Zweier JL, Talukder MA, et al. The role of oxidants and free radicals in reperfusion injury. Cardiovascular Research. 2006;**70**(2):181-190

[47] Barber AM, Maizel JV Jr, et al. Sequence EditingAligner: A multiple sequence editor and aligner. Genetic Analysis, Techniques and Applications. 1990;7(2):39-45

[48] Kalogeris T, Baines CP, Krenz M, et al. Cell biology of ischemia/ reperfusion injury. International Review of Cell and Molecular Biology. 2012;**298**:229-317

[49] Hoffman JW Jr, Gilbert TB, Poston RS, et al. Myocardial reperfusion injury: Etiology, mechanisms, and therapies. The Journal of Extra-Corporeal Technology. 2004;**36**(4):391-411

[50] Verma S, Fedak PW, Weisel RD, et al. Fundamentals of reperfusion injury for the clinical cardiologist. Circulation. 2002;**105**(20):2332-2336

[51] Reffelmann T, Hale SL, Dow JS, et al. No-reflow phenomenon persists long-term after ischemia/reperfusion in the rat and predicts infarct expansion. Circulation. 2003;**108**(23):2911-2917

[52] Farah A, Barbagelata A. Unmet goals in the treatment of acute myocardial infarction: Review. F1000Research. 2017;**6**(F1000 Faculty Rev):1243

[53] Farah A. Pereira JM, Infarto agudo de miocardio: Factores relacionados con la falta de resolución del segmento ST luego de una angioplastia primaria angiograficamente exitosa. Revista de la Federación Argentina de Cardiología. 2008;**37**:154-158

[54] ISIS-4 (Fourth International Study of Infarct Survival) Collaborative Group. ISIS-4: A randomised factorial trial assessing early oral captopril, oral mononitrate, and intravenous magnesium sulphate in 58,050 patients with suspected acute myocardial infarction. Lancet. 1995;**345**:669-685

[55] Yusuf S, Peto R, Lewis J, Collins R, Sleight. Beta blockade during and after myocardial infarction: An overview of the randomized trials. Progress in Cardiovascular Diseases. 1985;**27**:335-371

[56] ISIS-1. First International Study of Infarct Survival Collaborative Group. Randomised trial of intravenous atenolol among 16 027 cases of suspected acute myocardial infarction. Lancet. 1986;**2**:57-66

[57] The MIAMI Trial Research Group. Metoprolol in acute myocardial infarction: Patient population. The American Journal of Cardiology. 1985;**56**:10G-14G

[58] van der Horst IC, Zijlstra F, van't Hof AW, et al. Glucose-insulin-potassium infusion in patients treated with primary angioplasty for acute myocardial infarction: The glucose-insulin-potassium study: A randomized trial. Journal of the American College of Cardiology. 2003;**42**:784-791

[59] Finney SJ, Zekveld C, Elia A, Evans TW. Glucose control and mortality in critically ill patients. Journal of the American Medical Association. 2003;**290**:2041-2047

[60] Clement S, Braithwaite SS, Magee MF, et al. Management of diabetes and hyperglycemia in hospitals. Diabetes Care. 2004;**27**:553-597

[61] van den Berghe G, Wouters P, Weekers F, et al. Intensive insulin therapy in the critically ill patients. The New England Journal of Medicine. 2001;**345**:1359-1367

[62] O'Gara PT, Kushner FG, Ascheim DD, CaseyJr DE, Chung MK, de Lemos JA, et al. ACCF/AHA guideline for the management of ST-elevation myocardial infarction. Circulation. 2013;**127**:e362-e425

[63] Ibanez B, James S, et al. 2017 ESC guidelines for the management of acute myocardial infarction in patients presenting with ST-segment elevation. European Heart Journal. 2018;**39**:119-177

Chapter 14

Management of Ascending Aorta Calcification in Coronary Artery Bypass Grafting

Chuan Wang, Yang Yu, Chengxiong Gu and Jingxing Li

Abstract

Neurological complications are one of the most common complications after coronary artery bypass grafting. With the development of off-pump coronary artery bypass grafting (OPCABG), the incidence of postoperative neurological complications caused by aortic intubation decreased significantly; however, the continuous suture of the great saphenous vein-aortic anastomosis in the coronary artery bypass grafting requires the operation of surgical clamp and perforation on the ascending aorta, which may lead to potential plaque detachment. Calcification of ascending aorta is an independent risk factor for cerebrovascular events after OPCABG. Therefore, it is crucial to explore and operate on the ascending aorta. There are three main methods of proximal anastomosis in OPCABG: (1) partial blocking of ascending aorta with side wall clamp for anastomosis; (2) application of proximal anastomosis auxiliary device (Enclose, Heartstring, etc.) for proximal anastomosis; and (3) original auxiliary device (urethra catheter-water sac) or no-clamp surgical techniques for proximal anastomosis.

Keywords: neurological complications, coronary artery bypass grafting, ascending aorta, stroke, clamp, proximal anastomosis, auxiliary device

1. Introduction

Neurological complications are the most common complications after coronary artery bypass grafting (CABG) with high mortality rate [1]. With the advantages of off-pump coronary artery bypass grafting (OPCABG), the proportion of OPCABG in CABG is increasing continuously. The use of OPCABG procedures peaked in 2002 (23%) and in 2008 (21%), followed by a progressive decline in OPCABG frequency to 17% by 2012 [2].OPCABG is regarded as a milestone in the development of CABG and the most effective minimally invasive surgery as it avoids the injury of multiple organ malfunction caused by cardiopulmonary bypass [3–4]. With the widespread of OPCABG, the incidence of postoperative neurological complications caused by aortic intubation decreased significantly [5–6]. Nevertheless, great saphenous vein is still the main material for most CABG. It has been nearly half a century since the continuous suture of the great saphenous vein-aortic anastomosis in the coronary artery bypass grafting required the operation of surgical clamping and perforation on the ascending aorta, which may lead to potential plaque detachment and cause postoperative neurological complications [4]. Calcification of ascending aorta is an independent risk factor for cerebrovascular events after OPCABG, especially for postoperative stroke [3]. Therefore, careful exploration and accurate management of the ascending aorta are important. Traditional proximal anastomosis in OPCABG requires partial blocking of ascending aorta with side wall clamp; however, for patients with ascending aortic disease (e.g., serious ascending aorta atherosclerosis), connective tissue disease-related arteritis and syphilitic arteritis, the mechanical damage of aortic intima may be caused by the lateral cutting force produced by side wall clamp, which may lead to the rupture, dissection of aorta, rupture and detachment of atherosclerotic plaque and other serious perioperative complications. In recent years, a large number of auxiliary devices for proximal anastomosis of grafts have emerged, which can complete great saphenous vein-aortic anastomosis safely, simply, reliably and quickly without clamping ascending aorta, including commercial proximal anastomosis auxiliary device (Enclose, Heartstring, etc.) [7–9], original auxiliary device (urethra catheter-water sac) or no-clamp surgical techniques for proximal anastomosis [10–12]. This chapter will mainly introduce the anastomotic method of the auxiliary device of proximal anastomose.

2. Enclose technique

Proximal anastomosis auxiliary device was introduced to resolve the disadvantage of side wall clamping [13]. These devices were designed to avoid clamping the lateral wall of the aorta and to reduce complications of the ascending aorta and the nervous system. For patients undergoing CABG, OPCABG is recommended to reduce the risk of cerebral complications caused by side wall clamping. Selective use of Enclose proximal anastomotic device in patients with severe ascending aorta atherosclerosis will be discussed in this section.

2.1 Composition and principle of Enclose II anastomotic device

The device is composed of upper and lower rhombic mechanical jaws. The upper knob can adjust the vertical movement of the upper jaw, and it can make the upper and the lower jaws match at the anastomosis position of the ascending aorta to form a low-pressure cavity. The lower knob controls the opening and closing of the rhombic membrane at the end of the lower jaw, which makes the proximal anastomose area form a bloodless field of vision.

2.2 Method of application

2.2.1 Position selection

The ascending aorta should be explored routinely to avoid the atherosclerotic area on the aortic wall. Puncture site should be selected in the softest part of anterior wall of ascending aorta. The diameter of anastomosis area is about 1 cm.

2.2.2 Placement

- First, a purse suture with 2–0 polypropylene suture and rubber sleeve is used at the insertion point, and then mean arterial pressure is maintained at 100 mmHg (1 mmHg = 0.133 kPa) by medical management. The aorta wall is punctured at the central position of the purse suture with the puncture needle provided by Enclose.

- The lower jaw of Enclose is inserted into the aorta through the above-mentioned puncture point and placed at the pre-selected anastomotic position, and then the sleeve is tightened to limit the bleeding.

- Unscrew the membrane at the end of the lower jaw with the self-contained rotary rod of Enclose.

- Adjust the knob of the upper jaw to move the upper arm vertically downward and then attach the aortic adventitia and tighten the fixator. When no blood flows out of the suction tube of the lower arm, a blood-free environment is formed between the intima and the arterial wall. Behind the suction tube, a 50 ml syringe can be connected to absorb a small amount of blood oozing from the anastomosis area.

- Use a circular knife to cut the aortic wall at the preselected anastomosis position perpendicular to the metal rod of the lower jaw.

- Use Enclose' s own perforator to drill through the aortic incision. The perforator shall be close to the metal rod of the lower jaw to ensure full layer drilling (**Figure 1**).

2.2.3 Anastomosis

Anastomosis of saphenous vein (A) to ascending aorta (B) is performed with 6–0 polypropylene suture. The local bleeding that affects the suture field can be removed by suction. At the same time, maintain systolic blood pressure of systemic circulation at 90–100 mmHg level to reduce bleeding and ensure full layer suture of aortic wall and then exhaust and knot (**Figure 2**).

2.2.4 Remove

Close membrane after anastomosis and then release and remove Enclose. Knot the purse suture and use 2–0 polypropylene suture with felt pad to mattress suture for reinforcement.

2.3 Key points of Enclose using technique

2.3.1 Position selection

A considerable proportion of patients with coronary disease has ascending atherosclerosis. Many soft atherosclerotic plaques similar to "toothpastes" exist in the middle layer of ascending aorta, whereas obvious calcification can be identified by finger touch on the surface of aorta. Therefore, the plaques are prone to break and fall off after the application of side wall clamp and lead to organ embolism along with blood flow. In addition, except for the requirement of healthy aortic tissue at the puncture insertion point and anastomotic site, healthy tissue should also be selected between the two points as much as possible to avoid excessive bleeding due to atherosclerosis or calcification of the arterial wall between the two points, or plaque falling off due to extrusion.

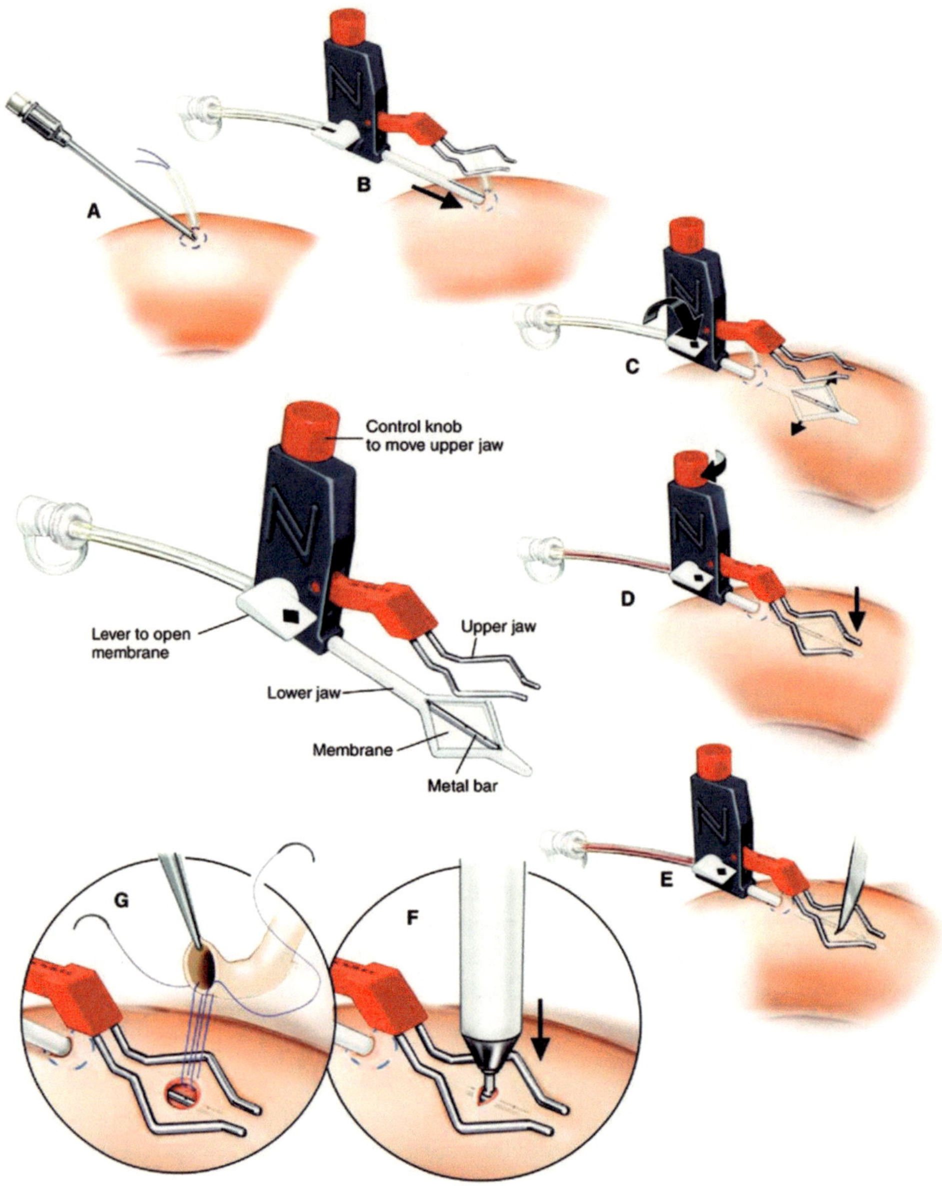

Figure 1.
Enclose device demonstration. (A) Needle puncture; (B) Enclose insertion; (C) Membrane unscrewed; (D) Upper jaw downward; (E) Circular knife cut; (F) Perforation; (G) Anastomosis.

2.3.2 Avoid damage to Enclose membrane

Most of the damage occurred in the process of aortic wall incision with circular knife and suturing. The aortic wall should be cut perpendicular to the connecting rod as much as possible to avoid cutting the diaphragm. When suturing, the needle should be carefully pressed against the inner wall of the aorta from internal to external, to avoid massive hemorrhage caused by deep penetration of Enclose diaphragm or vertical needle insertion. Slight injury of diaphragm may lead to increased bleeding risk in the operation area. In most cases, operations can be continued under the control of blood pressure and sufficient suction. If the diaphragm's damage is too serious, most of the surgeons will have to use other methods to avoid massive blood loss.

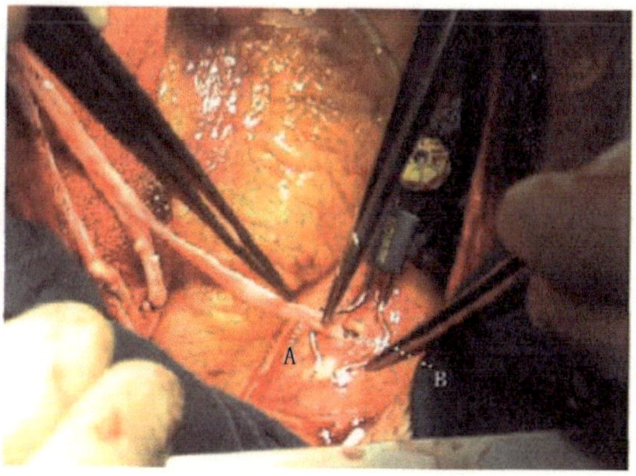

Figure 2.
Application of Enclose: (A) the great saphenous vein; (B) aortic anastomosis.

2.3.3 Puncture point reinforcement

Although we use 2–0 polypropylene suture to reinforce the puncture points during the operation for the Enclose cases, there are still a few patients in intensive care unit (ICU) with pericardial drainage fluid increase sharply and in bright red color. This is found to be blood leakage at the puncture point during emergency thoracotomy and hemostasis. The secondary suture for reinforcement with 2–0 polypropylene and felt pad can effectively stop bleeding. The reason for bleeding may be attributable to the inaccurate suture during the process. When the blood pressure is stable without obvious bleeding under anesthesia, the huge postoperative blood pressure fluctuation may increase the arterial pressure and lead to suture avulsion.

2.3.4 Mechanical failure

We have met several cases where the Enclose membrane could not be opened and the equipment was replaced. It is considered to be related to the technology and process in the production process. Therefore, it is necessary to test whether the membrane can open and close smoothly before each aortic implantation.

2.3.5 Aortic wall injury

Implantation and use of Enclose may also lead to injury, rupture and even aneurysm formation of the aortic wall. It may be due to the insertion of Enclose's lower jaw into the wall of ascending aorta, or due to the damage of aortic intima caused by overcompression, which is easy to form aneurysm when the blood pressure rises. Therefore, it is very important to control blood pressure during the operation and, at the same time, on the premise of no blood environment in the operation area, to loosen the knob as much as possible to reduce the excessive pressure on the aortic wall.

2.3.6 Re-implantation

It is often the case that the intimal dissection of the internal mammary artery (IMA) has to be replaced by the total vein coronary artery bypass grafting. Thus, Enclose was re-implanted after the injury of the IMA or when the flow of the IMA graft is poor. The distance between the suture and the punch hole should not be too wide (≤5 cm); otherwise, the hemostasis effect of membrane will be affected. The suction tube of the stabilizer should be connected with the suction device or 50 ml syringe to eliminate possible blood accumulation and keep the operation field clean.

2.4 Advantages and limitations of Enclose technology

2.4.1 Advantages

- The Enclose greatly reduces the risk of plaque falling off due to the clamping of ascending aorta, and it has fewer requirements for anastomotic area, which merely concerns a relatively soft and healthy area with a diameter about 1 cm.

- Compared with the disposable aortic proximal anastomotic device such as Heartstring, Enclose can support the operation of two or more anastomoses, especially for the aged patients undergoing total vein CABG with severe aortic atherosclerosis.

- Compared with the first generation of products, Enclose II improved the way of opening the internal aortic diaphragm umbrella: from the hand push knob to the rotary rod operation. This facilitates the operation in the narrow pericardial cavity. Meanwhile, the design of hexagon suture ring is more reasonable than the rhombic suture ring from the previous generation.

2.4.2 Limitations

- Enclose requires at least two healthy areas of the aorta: one is the insertion point, and the other is the anastomosis point. Its application is limited to patients with large-area diffuse calcification aorta.

- A completely bloodless operation field could not be guaranteed. When the suture is too tight, there will be different degrees of bleeding.

- Due to the technology in the production process, Enclose's membrane might fail to open and need to be replaced. However, the incidence of mechanical failure is very low.

- Enclose II is relatively expensive, which to some extent increases the medical expenses of patients.

2.5 Clinical significance of Enclose technology

Cerebrovascular complications are one of the most common complications after CABG. The main reasons could be mainly attributable to the atherosclerotic plaque or new thrombus falling off and embolism of ascending aorta or carotid artery during and after operation [14]. Other possible causes might be the excessive anticoagulation, or the sudden rise of blood pressure, causing the rupture and hemorrhage of cerebral vessels [15]. Atherosclerosis is a group of systemic diseases, and vascular endothelial dysfunction has been widely considered as the most important initiating link in its process and exists in the whole process of atherosclerosis. Atherosclerosis is a chronic, progressive and multiple endovascular disease, involving many large and medium-sized arteries. For patients with severe coronary atherosclerosis, especially those over 70 years old, the incidence of aortic atherosclerosis or calcification is higher. Therefore, the use of no-clamp aortic proximal anastomotic device can reduce the cerebrovascular complications caused by aortic atherosclerosis.

3. Heartstring technique

The Heartstring proximal anastomosis system is suitable for the proximal anastomosis of the graft and the aorta without the use of aortic clamp in CABG [16–17]. The first generation of Heartstring proximal anastomosis system was launched by Guidant Company in 2002 and the most commonly used Heartstring III was launched by MAQUET after continuous technical improvement. The American Thoracic Surgery study [18] of 1380 patients with aortic calcification found that the predicted risk of stroke in patients using Heartstring was reduced by 44%, especially in patients with aortic calcification above grade II (**Figure 3**).

3.1 Device composition of Heartstring proximal anastomosis system

Heartstring proximal anastomotic system consists of proximal anastomotic device, conveying device, loading device and aortic perforator device. The Heartstring anastomotic device enters the aorta through the aortic incision established by the aortic drilling device and provides an anastomotic area for proximal anastomosis. The conveyor is a syringe-like tube with a piston, which is used to place the Heartstring anastomosis device into the aorta. The loading device is used to roll up the Heartstring anastomosis device and load the Heartstring anastomosis device into the conveyor. The aortic perforator device is a disposable device, which consists of a handle, a drilling device, an aortic block, a cover, a needle, a safety lock and an action button, which is used to establish an aortic incision for anastomosis.

3.2 Indications and contraindications of Heartstring technology

3.2.1 Indications

For patients with high risks of atherosclerosis, the possibility of ascending aortosclerosis is increased, and the operation of aorta needs to be reduced or avoided. A strict aortic non-touch technique can most effectively reduce the occurrence of plaque embolism. This requires the use of an auxiliary device for proximal aortic anastomosis. The Heartstring proximal anastomotic system is adopted in CABG to

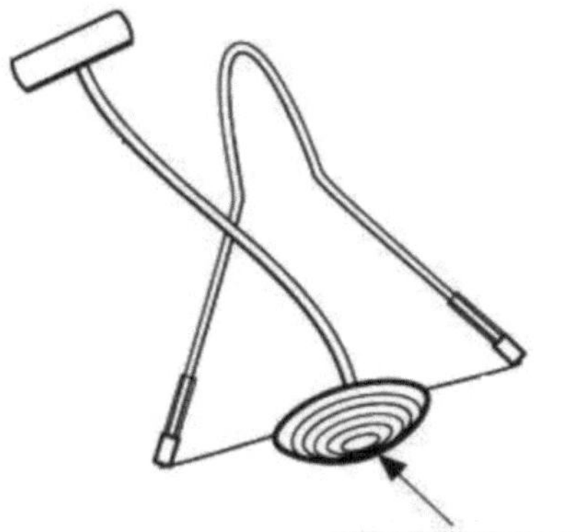

Figure 3.
The Heartstring device.

maintain hemostasis during operation and to complete the proximal anastomotic operation without the use of arterial side wall clamp.

3.2.2 Contraindications

- If conventional anastomosis is impossible due to a significant disease in an aortic region, do not use the Heartstring proximal anastomosis system in that region. It can also be judged by echocardiography.
- Do not use the Heartstring proximal anastomosis system in patients with aortic diameter less than 2.5 cm.

3.3 Method of application

- Heparin was used according to CABG standard procedure.
- Remove the device from the sterile packaging and make sure that the safety lock is locked.
- Load the Heartstring proximal anastomosis device into the conveyor tube. Avoid triggering the conveyor when loading.
- Take the conveyor out of the loader then unlock the Heartstring.
- Establish soft and safe aortic anastomosis area with aortic perforator device.
- Deliver the Heartstring device to the anastomose point. The presence of blood in the conveyor indicates the correct insertion. Use carefully when inserting the conveyor to reduce the risk of aortic posterior wall penetration (**Figure 4**).
- Heartstring anastomose after the proximal anastomose device is in position. During suturing, it is necessary to be careful and avoid movement of the proximal anastomotic device of Heartstring or winding of the suture around the rod of the anastomotic device. If the above-mentioned happens, please return the needle and ensure the hemostasis. If hemostasis is insufficient, use a partial occlusal clamp, remove the Heartstring proximal anastomotic device and use the aortic clamp to complete the anastomosis.
- Remove the Heartstring proximal anastomotic device after the anastomosis is completed. Do not continue to pull the anastomotic rod if resistance is constantly remains when pulling out the Heartstring, or the non-invasive anastomotic device is not pulled out successfully.
- The aortic perforator is a disposable device. If multiple proximal anastomoses are needed on the ascending aorta, select a location at least 1.5 cm from the previous anastomotic position.

3.4 Consideration of Heartstring technology

- Surgeons should be properly trained before using the Heartstring proximal anastomosis system.
- For disposable use. Do not re-sterilize.

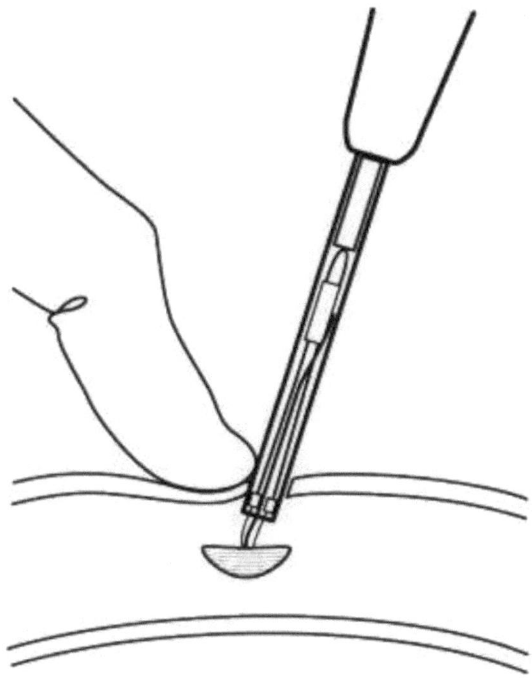

Figure 4.
Place the Heartstring proximal anastomotic device into the aortic incision and extract the conveyor.

- Do not use the Heartstring proximal anastomotic system in the aorta that cannot be partially clamped, to prevent patients from being at risk from bleeding.
- To ensure effective hemostasis, make sure that the anastomoses are at least 1.5 cm apart before performing multiple anastomoses.
- Check the unit to guarantee that it is not damaged during transportation.
- Aortic perforator should only be used on the unmodified aortic tissue. Use on altered tissue, such as the presence of a cardiologic orifice and/or an aortotomy incision, may result in an unblocked aortic incision and the embolus may enter in the aorta.

3.5 Advantages and limitations of Heartstring technology

3.5.1 Advantages

Heartstring is also a proximal anastomotic device that can effectively reduce the probability of aortic atherosclerotic plaque shedding or dissection. Its advantages are as follows:

- Low requirements for anastomotic area. A relatively healthy area with a diameter of around 1 cm available for suture will be sufficient, especially for those with multiple plaques in the ascending aorta.
- Heartstring is easy to operate and does not need to be punched or sutured in other positions of the ascending aorta.

- The sealing membrane of Heartstring is composed of a line-type concave disc with good adhesion. At the end of anastomosis, "hat" shaped membrane can be pulled out directly through the anastomosis position, avoiding the risk of aortic wall damage when other devices are pulled out through the anastomosis position.

3.5.2 Limitations

When using Heartstring for proximal anastomosis, the uneven calcified aortic inner wall may lead to a loose fit between the plug-like membrane and the inner wall of the ascending aorta, causing continuous bleeding of the anastomosis and affecting the operation.

3.6 Heartstring technology and stroke

Stroke is one of the most serious complications of coronary revascularization, with high morbidity, mortality and cost. High-risk factors include peripheral vascular disease, left main artery disease, diabetes mellitus, atherosclerosis and calcification of arterial wall. After OPCABG, the risk of both stroke and mortality has been reduced, especially for high-risk groups and elderly patients [3]. However, the causes of stroke are various, not a single technology (including OPCABG) can completely avoid the occurrence of postoperative stroke. The off-pump total artery CABG provides a relatively "non-touch" way for revascularization and is effective to reduce the complications of nervous system. Although non-touch technology may be the best clinical option, it cannot be applied to every patient, nor can it be carried out routinely in most medical centers. When high-risk patients do need proximal anastomosis, Heartstring can assist to complete the proximal anastomosis with minimum aortic contact.

In the past few years, more evidences have shown that Heartstring technology could significantly minimize atherosclerotic embolism and neurological complications compared with side wall clamp, but those researches did not classify aortic lesions [19–20]. Another randomized controlled trial from Emory University showed that the use of Heartstring technology in patients with low risk of atherosclerotic embolism can significantly reduce cerebral embolic events. For patients with aortosclerosis of grade I or II, Heartstring technique can reduce solid emboli by 35% [21]. Emmert et al. took the total arterial CABG as the gold standard for clinical trial [22]. It is demonstrated that the incidence of stroke and major adverse cardiovascular and cerebrovascular event (MACCE) was 0.7 and 6.7% in the OPCABG with Heartstring group, 2.3 and 10.8% in the OPCABG with side wall clamp group, and 0.8 and 7.9% in the total arterial CABG group [22]. Hilker et al. performed 542 proximal anastomoses in 412 consecutive patients with Heartstring technique [23]. The incidence of postoperative stroke in this series was 0.48%, whereas the prediction of preoperative stroke was 1.3%. It indicated that the Heartstring technology could reduce the risk of stroke prediction by 44% [23]. This technology might not be as beneficial for patients with aortosclerosis I, as for patients with aortosclerosis II or above, among which there is no stroke incidence that occurred even in patients with aortosclerosis. More importantly, there was no significant difference in the incidence of stroke between the clampless off-pump CABG and the no-touch technique [24], which indicated that the clamp per se was an independent risk factor for the stroke. The combination of OPCABG and Heartstring technology not only achieves the revascularization but also has a relatively low incidence of neurological complications compared with percutaneous coronary intervention (PCI) [25–26]. In comparison with the traditional CABG with cardiopulmonary bypass, OPCABG is indeed a step forward.

4. Urethra catheter-water sac technique

When the great saphenous vein anastomosis with the ascending aorta, the ascending aorta should be clamped with side wall clamp, which may cause the atherosclerotic plaque of the ascending aorta to fall off and, thus, increase the risk of cerebral infarction. Further, the falling-off plaque may also block the great saphenous vein graft and reduce its patency rate. We applied the self-made water sac blocking method for the patients with severe ascending aortic calcification upon OPCABG and achieved satisfying results.

4.1 The birth of water sac technique

Patients with severe calcification in the ascending aorta are more likely to have stroke after anastomosis of ascending aorta and great saphenous vein in OPCABG. The most common reason is the loose or detached atherosclerotic plaque on the inner wall of ascending aorta, or detached thrombus due to clamp damage. Multivariable analysis revealed that the use of aortic wall clamp was the most important independent risk factor for postoperative stroke, resulting in a sixfold increase of postoperative stroke rate. It is suggested that the indicators of serious calcification of ascending aorta include carotid stenosis, hypertension, peripheral vascular disease or abdominal aortic aneurysm, male gender, renal insufficiency and left main artery disease in patients over 65 years old.

There are two main methods hitherto to solve the problem of proximal anastomosis in patients with calcification of ascending aorta, including using proximal anastomotic device and using non-touch ascending aorta of CABG. The former mainly includes the application of Enclose, Heartstring and other devices, while the latter mainly refers to the methods of CABG without ascending aorta operation, such as bilateral internal mammary artery and other forms of total arterial CABG.

The indications of non-touch technique of ascending aorta are limited to some extent, and the requirements to operation are relatively high. Moreover, collection of bilateral internal mammary artery will reduce the blood supply of sternum, affect the healing of sternum, and may cause complications such as loosening of sternum, delayed healing and infection of incision. Radial artery is also commonly used in total arterial CABG; however, when comparing with internal mammary artery, it is more prone to produce spasm and affect surgical effect.

There are some limitations in the use of proximal anastomotic devices. For example, when using Heartstring for proximal anastomosis, the internal umbrella cap may not fit tightly with the uneven calcified aortic inner wall, causing continuous bleeding at the anastomosis and affecting the operation. When using Enclose for proximal anastomosis, at least two holes are needed to be drilled in the ascending aorta, increasing the chance of atherosclerotic plaque falling off. Further, the needle tip may puncture the diaphragm with hemostatic effect and lead to uncontrollable bleeding. In addition, the cost of proximal anastomotic device is high and will increase the medical burden for patients in developing countries and remote areas.

Given the above situation, we have figured out the method of water sac blocking proximal anastomosis method in clinical practice. Its short-term and medium-term effects were similar to those of patients without ascending aortic calcification who used side wall clamp, and no patients had complications such as stroke or proximal anastomotic stenosis. It is well demonstrated that OPCABG combined with water sac blocking anastomotic method can further reduce the incidence of postoperative stroke.

4.2 Operation process

"Water sac blocking" refers to the method of proximal anastomosis without using side wall clamp when anastomosing great saphenous vein or radial artery with ascending aorta (**Figure 5**).

The specific processes are as follows:

- Left internal thoracic artery and great saphenous vein are harvested routinely. In OPCABG, the internal thoracic artery is usually anastomosed to the left anterior descending branch, and the rest are treated by sequential CABG of great saphenous vein.
- When the saphenous vein is anastomosed with the ascending aorta, the adventitia of the artery is cut off at the perforating position.
- After purse string is anastomosed, use a sharp knife to prick a small incision, and press to stop bleeding.
- Use an aortic perforator to make a hole.
- Quickly insert a 12–14F urethra catheter into the aorta, inject 8–10 ml sterile normal saline through the water injection hole, make the water sac inflate, fix the distal end, and make the water sac tightly close to the anastomosis position for hemostasis.
- The saphenous vein was anastomosed with ascending aorta by 6–0 polypropylene suture while removing the pre-sutured purse string. The direction of the needle entering the aortic wall was from the internal to the external, without penetrating the whole layer of the arterial wall. The total number of needles was 8–10.
- Use a syringe to suck out the normal saline in the water sac, quickly remove the urethra catheter, pull down the great saphenous vein, and tighten the suture and knot.
- Lastly, another 6–0 polypropylene suture was used to full-layer suture the aortic wall along the previous anastomosis position. (**Figure 6**).

4.3 Considerations in the use of water sac blocking method

- Since the needle tip of the anastomosis is easy to puncture the water sac, polypropylene suture for the first time in non-full-layer type, and then another

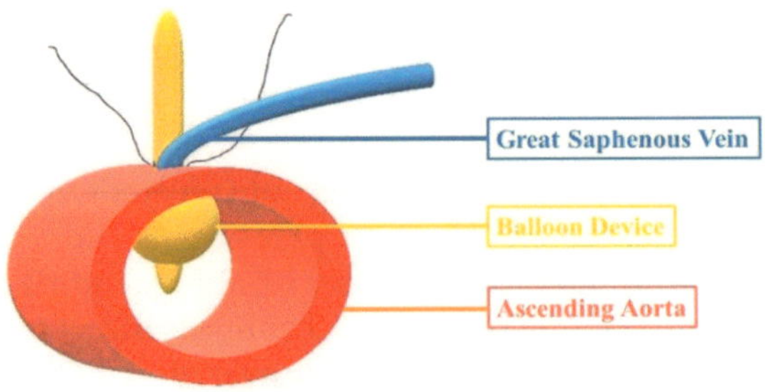

Figure 5.
Composition of the water sac device.

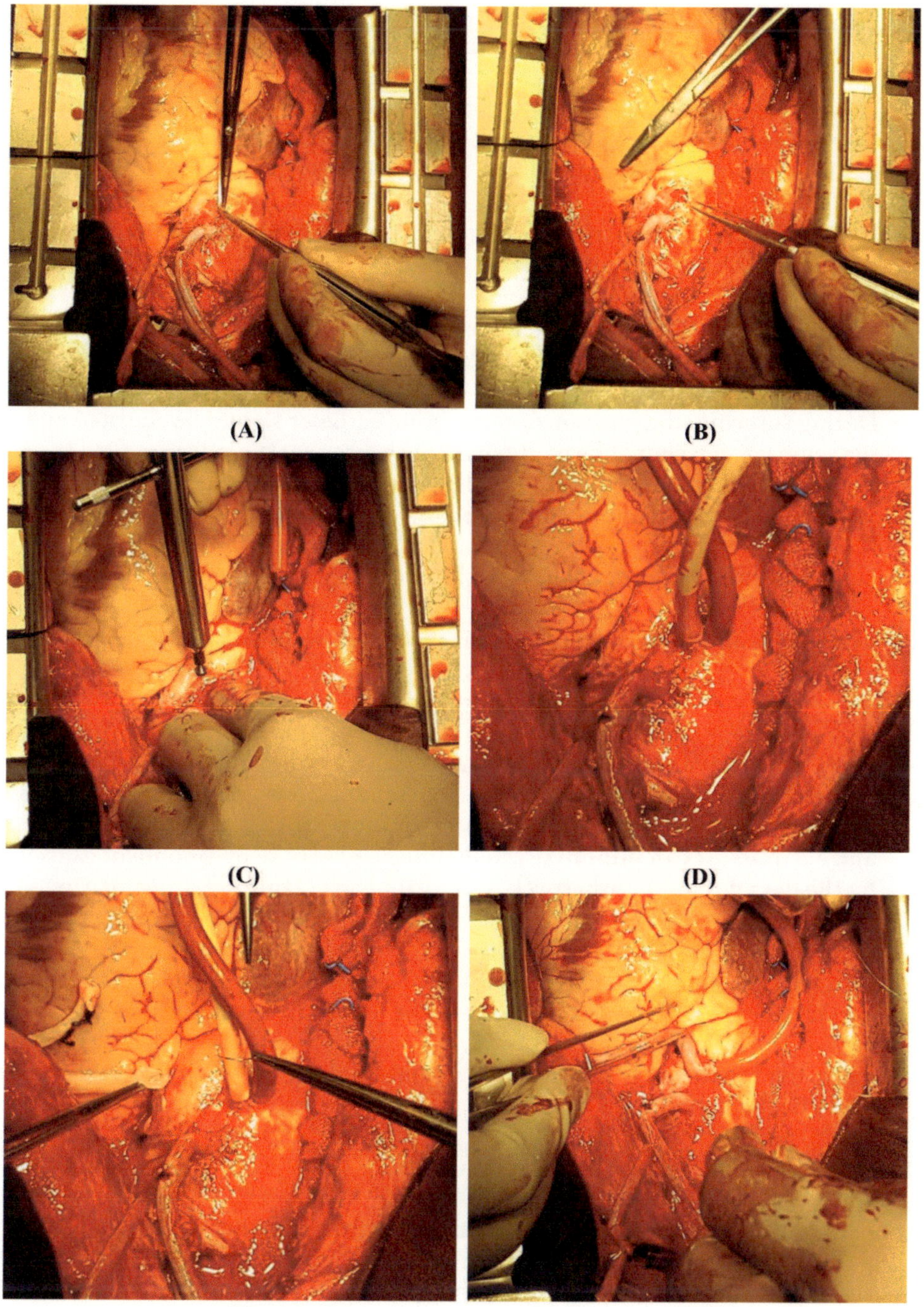

(A) **(B)**

(C) **(D)**

(E) **(F)**

Figure 6.
Procedures: (A) cutting off the adventitia; (B) purse string suture; (C) perforation and finger hemostasis; (D) urinary catheter insert and sterile normal saline injection; (E) great saphenous vein anastomosis (non-full layer); (F) balloon suction and removing for secondary anastomosis (full layer).

polypropylene suture can be performed for full layer suture after knotting to ensure the accuracy of the anastomosis.

- The change of arterial pressure should be observed when injecting water into water sacs, and the circulation index should not be affected as much as possible. The amount of water injected into the water sac is usually less than 10 ml; otherwise, it may cause bursting or affect the left ventricular blood flow.

- When the distal end of the urethra catheter is fixed after the water injection, the rubber tube should keep a certain tension to make the water sac stay closed to the inner wall of the aorta.

- During the drill, anesthesiologists should control blood pressure and slow down heart rate to minimize bleeding.

- When inserting the catheter, it is necessary to press the anastomose with the help of fingers and inject water quickly to avoid excessive bleeding.

- During suturing, the position of the urethra catheter should be adjusted and the same tension should be maintained to ensure that the suturing field is exposed. Avoid the bleeding caused by the needle penetrating the water sac or pulling out the urethra catheter-water sac.

- Surgeons should be properly trained before using water sac blocking method.

4.4 Advantages and limitations of urethra catheter-water sac technology

4.4.1 Advantages

- As an innovative suture method, "water sac blocking" method has the advantages of both OPCABG and proximal anastomosis device. It requires no additional medical costs, and the operation process is simple, effective and accurate. It can minimize the incidence of stroke or embolism caused by the detachment of atherosclerotic plaque via clamping or intubating on the aorta.

- This method is very safe. Due to the softness of the water sac, it is rare that the aortic wall will be damaged, even when the water sac is broken.

- For patients who fail to use Heartstring and Enclose, the water sac method could be the remedy.

4.4.2 Limitations

- During the first suture, it is possible that the urethra catheter could not be pulled out when the needle caught the outer membrane of the water sac. In this case, it may be necessary to cut the suture and pull out the urethra catheter, and then repeat the operation.

- It is relatively time-consuming due to the requirement for secondary suture. Moreover, the operation around the aortic incision is more frequent, which increases the risk of bleeding.

4.5 Clinical significance of urethra catheter-water sac technology

For patients with severe aortic atherosclerosis, avoiding the use of side wall clamp is one of the important methods to reduce postoperative neurological complications [27]. The water sac blocking method is simple, effective, accurate and cost-efficient (the cost of the catheter is negligible), with minimized risk of stroke or cerebral infarction caused by the detachment of atherosclerotic plaque due to the clamping of the aortic wall. When proximal anastomosis is performed in patients with severe ascending aortic calcification, the water sac method is a feasible option and has a wide range of clinical application and dissemination value.

5. No clamp anastomosis technique

When using great saphenous vein to anastomose with ascending aorta during OPCABG, it is necessary to clamp part of ascending aorta wall and may cause ascending aorta atherosclerotic plaques to fall off, leading to cerebral embolism. Meanwhile, it may also induce great saphenous vein graft obstruction and influence its patency rate. We applied "no clamp" suture method in OPCABG for patients with severe aortic calcification and achieved satisfying results.

5.1 The birth of no clamp technique

Although OPCABG avoids cardiopulmonary bypass and greatly reduces brain damage caused by cerebral air embolism and insufficient perfusion, the incidence of neurological complications (including stroke, transient ischemic attack, coma, postoperative delirium or epileptic attack, etc.) remains one of the most common postoperative complications [28]. Cerebral infarction is mostly related to atheromatous plaque or calcification breaking and detachment in the aorta caused by operating on it, and cerebral hemorrhage may also be related to post infarction hemorrhage [29–30]. Patients often show delayed awake or coma for longer time as this kind of disease often occurs in the operation or the early postoperative period. However, patients could hardly move and remain in the state of respiratory assistance; as a result, computed tomography (CT) or magnetic resonance imaging (MRI) diagnose and further treatment are often delayed with more serious consequences. Among all the risk factors, calcification plaque shedding caused by clamping the ascending aorta is the most important risk factor [31]. Thus, using proximal anastomotic device to assist or complete proximal aortic anastomosis without side wall clamp can effectively avoid the complications caused by clamping ascending aorta during traditional proximal aortic root anastomoses, such as the damage of the aortic wall and the detachment of atheromatous plaque. Therefore, avoiding the ascending aorta clamping is the key to reduce the incidence of aortic dissection and nervous system complications in OPCABG, and thus improving the postoperative survival rate. Indicators of severe ascending aortic calcification include carotid stenosis, hypertension, peripheral vascular disease or abdominal aortic aneurysm, male gender, renal insufficiency and being over 65 years old. As an innovative suture method, the no clamp suture method can minimize the incidence rate of systemic infarction caused by the detachment of atherosclerotic plaques. The operation process is simple, effective, accurate and cost-efficient. Therefore, in the OPCABG for patients with severe ascending aortic calcification, the method without clamp has its practical and generalization value.

5.2 Operation process

The method without clamp refers to that when the great saphenous vein is anastomosed with ascending aorta, and the aortic wall is not clamped with side wall clamp. The specific operation process is as follows:

- Use 6–0 polypropylene suture to perform end to side anastomosis in anticlockwise direction before perforating ascending aorta. The direction of the needle entering the aortic wall is from the internal to the external through the whole layer of the arterial wall.

- The polypropylene suture is divided into two clusters, and two thick sutures for traction are used to pull it in the opposite direction respectively to fully expose the position of the anastomosis.

- Use a sharp knife to pierce the artery wall in the middle of the anastomotic position, press with fingers for hemostasis, and then use an aortic perforator to perforate (**Figure** 7).

- Remove the traction suture, pull down the great saphenous vein, tighten the polypropylene suture and knot.

- Finally, another 6–0 polypropylene suture was used to suture the aortic wall along the previous anastomosis position.

5.3 Considerations of no clamp technique

- Before aortic wall suture with polypropylene, ascending aorta palpation should be carried out in order to avoid atherosclerotic plaques and local thickening part and prevent plaques detachment.
- The two traction sutures should be pressed as close to the aortic surface as possible for maximum expose of anastomotic position.
- The perforator shall be positioned accurately before drilling to prevent damage to the polypropylene suture.
- During drilling, anesthesiologists should reduce blood pressure and slow down heart rate to minimize bleeding.
- As the polypropylene suture requires a long distance in the aortic wall, it may be astringent when tightening, and as a result, it should be tightened one by one with a nerve hook.

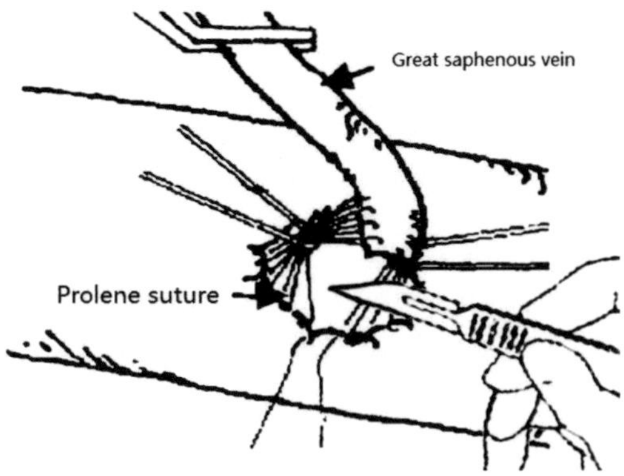

Figure 7.
Puncture the artery wall and press it with fingers to stop bleeding.

5.4 Advantages and limitations of no clamp technology

5.4.1 Advantages

- As an original suture method, "no clamp" method has the advantages of both OPCABG and proximal anastomosis device. It requires no additional medical costs, not even tiny cost of urethra catheter. The operation process is simple, effective and accurate, with minimum risk of neurological complications from clamping or intubating on the aorta.
- Compared with the water sac method, no clamp method avoids the possible risks associated with water sac. Direct suture is fast and effective. This technique is the alternative if the water sac technique is unavailable because of the severe uneven aortic inner wall.
- For patients who fail to use Heartstring and Enclose, no clamp method could be also considered as remedy.

5.4.2 Limitations

- Both the piercing and perforating operation could damage or even cut off the suture, causing severe hemorrhage or suture failure. In this case, repeated suture is required.
- This operation is also relatively time-consuming due to the secondary suture. Moreover, the piercing and perforating operation is under no cover of any inner aortic device, such as diaphragm umbrella of Enclose, spiral coil shape umbrella of Heartstring and water sac, which increases the possibility of bleeding and operative time.
- Because the great saphenous vein is closed to the anastomotic position after the first suture and blood vortex exists during the secondary suture, a high accuracy of the suture is required to avoid thrombosis.
- Surgeons should be properly trained before using no clamp method.

5.5 Clinical significance of no clamp technology

The most common cause of stroke after OPCABG is the detachment of embolus, which is closely related to the progressive arteriosclerosis of ascending aorta. "No clamp" method is simple and effective, with minimum risk of the infarction induced by the detachment of atherosclerotic plaques through clamping operation.

6. Conclusions

When OPCABG is performed in patients with severe ascending aortic calcification, the above methods of proximal anastomosis are of practical and dissemination value. Based on decades of clinical experience, when encountering atherosclerotic plaque of ascending aorta, proximal anastomosis devices can be used to anastomose proximal aorta as priority, in order to maximally avoid the detachment of aortic atherosclerotic plaque or the damage of aortic dissection. When the proximal anastomosis device or the suture fails, the water sac or no clamp method could also be applied for remedy. For well-trained surgeons, they will be able to use water sac or no clamp method for proximal anastomosis directly, saving huge costs while achieving the same outcomes. The two original techniques are of great significance for patients in developing countries and remote areas. All these surgical applications aim to avoid complications of nervous system and embolism caused by plaque detachment due to partial blocking of ascending aorta with side wall clamp for proximal anastomosis.

Conflict of interest

The authors declare no conflict of interest.

Author details

Chuan Wang, Yang Yu, Chengxiong Gu and Jingxing Li*
Department of Cardiac Surgery, Beijing Anzhen Hospital, Capital Medical University, Beijing, China

*Address all correspondence to: sci4vv@hotmail.com

References

[1] Davila-roman VG, Barzilai B, Wareing TH. Atherosclerosis of the ascending aorta. Prevalence and role as an independent predictor of cerebrovascular events in cardiac patients. Stroke. 1994;**109**(11):1637-1643

[2] Bakaeen FG, Shroyer AL, Gammie JS, et al. Trends in use of off-pump coronary artery bypass grafting: Results from the Society of Thoracic Surgeons adult cardiac surgery database. The Journal of Thoracic and Cardiovascular Surgery. 2014;**148**(3):856-853

[3] Goto T, Baba T, Matsuyama K, et al. Aortic atherosclerosis and postoperative neurological dysfunction in elderly coronary surgical patients. The Annals of Thoracic Surgery. 2003;7(5):556-563

[4] Wang B, Jia M, Jia S, et al. Influencing factors for early acute cerebrovascular accidents in patients with stroke history following off-pump coronary artery bypass grafting. Heart, Lung & Circulation. 2014;**23**(6):560-565

[5] Sylivris S, Levi C, Matalanis G, et al. Pattern and significance of cerebral microemboli during coronary artery bypass grafting. The Annals of Thoracic Surgery. 2013;**9**(6):1062-1070

[6] Chavanon O, Carrier M, Cartier R, et al. Increased incidence of acute ascending aortic dissection with off-pump aortocoronary bypass surgery? The Annals of Thoracic Surgery. 2001;**71**:117-121

[7] Patel NC, Hemli JM. Anastomotic devices in coronary artery surgery: It is about the anastomosis? Multimedia Manual of Cardiothoracic Surgery. 2013;**2013**:mmt019

[8] Akpinar B, Guden M, Sagbas E, et al. Clinical experience with the novare enclose ii manual proximal anastomotic device during off-pump coronary artery surgery. European Journal of Cardio-Thoracic Surgery. 2005;**27**(6):1070-1073

[9] Wang S, Zhao T, Liu D, et al. Enclose-without blocking the proximal anastomosis system in the application of OPCAB in elder patients. Chinese Journal of Cardiology. 2011;**9**(6):426-428

[10] Lev-Ran O, Braunstein R, Sharony R, et al. No-touch aorta off-pump coronary surgery: The effect on stroke. The Journal of Thoracic and Cardiovascular Surgery. 2011;**129**(2):307-313

[11] Fukuda I, Daitoku K, Minakawa M, et al. Shaggy and calcified aorta: Surgical implications. General Thoracic and Cardiovascular Surgery. 2013;**61**(6):301-313

[12] Wolf LG, Abu-Omar Y, Choudhary BP, et al. Gaseous and solid cerebral microembolization during proximal aortic anastomoses in off-pump coronary surgery: The effect of an aortic side-biting clamp and two clampless devices. The Journal of Thoracic and Cardiovascular Surgery. 2007;**133**(2):485-493

[13] Aranki SF, Shekar PS, Ehsan A, et al. Evaluation of the enclose proximal anastomosis device in coronary artery bypass grafting. The Annals of Thoracic Surgery. 2005;**80**(3):1091-1095

[14] Abu-Omar Y, Balacumaraswami L, Pigott D, et al. Solid and gaseous microembolization during off-pump, on-pump, and open cardiac surgery procedures. The Journal of Thoracic and Cardiovascular Surgery. 1994;**109**(11):1637-1643

[15] Barbut D, Hinton RB, Szatrowski TP. Cerebral emboli detected during bypass surgery are associated with clamp removal. Stroke. 1994;**28**(3):266-278

[16] Medalion B, Meirson D, Hauptman E, et al. Initial experience with the heartstring proximal anastomotic system. The Journal of Thoracic and Cardiovascular Surgery. 2012;**164**(3):402-409

[17] Vicol C, Oberhoffer M, Nollert G, et al. First clinical experience with the heartstring a device for proximal anastomoses in coronary surgery. The Annals of Thoracic Surgery. 2012;**109**(5): 724-728

[18] Thourani VH, Razavi SA, Nguyen TC, et al. Incidence of postoperative stroke using the heartstring device in 1,380 coronary artery bypass graft patients with mild to severe atherosclerosis of the ascending aorta. The Annals of Thoracic Surgery. 2014;**97**(6):2066-2072

[19] Kim DJ, Lee SH, Joo HC, et al. Effects of a proximal seal system on neurologic outcomes of off-pump coronary artery bypass grafting. International Heart Journal. 2019;**60**(3):593-600

[20] Lamm P, Eifert S, Kilian E, et al. Preventing blood loss during application of the HEARTSTRING proximal seal system. The Annals of Thoracic Surgery. 2009;**88**(1):310-312

[21] El Zayat H, Puskas JD, Hwang S, et al. Avoiding the clamp during off-pump coronary artery bypass reduces cerebral embolic events: Results of a prospective randomized trial. Interactive Cardiovascular and Thoracic Surgery. 2012;**14**(1):12-16

[22] Emmert MY, Seifert B, Wilhelm M, et al. Aortic no-touch technique makes the difference in off-pump coronary artery bypass grafting. The Journal of Thoracic and Cardiovascular Surgery. 2011;**142**(6):1499-1506

[23] Hilker M, Arlt M, Keyser A, et al. Minimizing the risk of perioperative stroke by clampless off-pump bypass surgery: A retrospective observational analysis. Journal of Cardiothoracic Surgery. 2010;**5**:14

[24] Formica F, Tata G, Singh G, et al. Incidence of perioperative stroke in clampless aortic anastomosis during off-pump coronary artery bypass grafting. Heart and Vessels. 2018;**33**(6):595-604

[25] Emmert MY, Grunenfelder J, Scherman J, et al. HEARTSTRING enabled no-touch proximal anastomosis for off-pump coronary artery bypass grafting: Current evidence and technique. Interactive Cardiovascular and Thoracic Surgery. 2013;**17**(3):538-541

[26] Liu R, Gu C, Chen C, et al. Application of heartstring in non-blocking proximal anastomosis system in OPCAB. Chinese Journal of Thoracic and Cardiovascular Surgery. 2006;**22**(5):347

[27] Yu Y, Gu CX, Wei H, et al. Evaluation of the early and medium-term curative effect of water sac blocking used in the proximal anastomosis during off-pump coronary artery bypass. Zhonghua Wai Ke Za Zhi. 2010;**48**(24):1864-1867

[28] Manabe S, Fukui T, Miyajima K, et al. Impact of proximal anastomosis procedures on stroke in off-pump coronary artery bypass grafting. Journal of Cardiac Surgery. 2009;**24**(6):644-649

[29] Tabas I, Garcia-Cardena G, Owens GK. The cell biology of disease: Recent insights into the cellular biology of atherosclerosis. Journal of Cell Biology. 2015;**209**(1):13-22

[30] Vassiliades TA Jr, Nielsen JL, Lonquist JL. Hemodynamic collapse during off-pump coronary artery bypass grafting. The Annals of Thoracic Surgery. 2002;**73**(10):1874-1879

[31] Neumann FJ. Sousa-Uva M, Ahlsson a, et al; ESC scientific document group. 2018 ESC/EACTS guidelines on myocardial revascularization. European Heart Journal. 2019;**40**:87-165

Chapter 15

Methods of Reconstruction for Distal Aortic Dissection

Mark Alekseevich Soborov

Abstract

The modern approach to the correction of aortic dissection involves the most complete reconstruction of the entire pathologically altered segment of the vessel, which is often impossible due to the vastness of the lesion and the associated severity of surgery. Reduction of intraoperative trauma can improve survival in the immediate postoperative period, and the completeness of reconstruction to reduce the number of complications and relapses in the long term. In this chapter, the methods of reconstruction of the aorta in case of distal dissection from a conventional open surgery to endovascular techniques, or usage of their combination for minimization of surgical trauma, are reviewed.

Keywords: aortic dissection, hemodynamic, surgical approach, aortic surgery, EVAR, hybrid

1. Introduction

Aortic dissection is defined as the penetration of blood masses between the inner and middle layers of the aortic wall, with the formation of a rupture of the inner layer of the aortic wall, intima. In this case, a flap is formed that divides the aortic lumen into true and false [1, 2].

The aortic wall consists of three layers: the inner tunica intima, the middle tunica media, and the outer tunic of adventitia. Despite the fact that different components and special types of cells form each of these layers, they all represent a single structure that can withstand high variable loads. The inner layer, tunica intima, has a thickness of 130 microns. Its first shell is the endothelium, a single-row layer of cells that directly contact the blood. Endothelial cells are oriented in accordance with the direction of blood flow [3]. The endothelium prevents thrombosis, has selective permeability to liquids and nutrients, participates in maintaining vascular tone, regulates blood pressure, has immunomodulatory and barrier functions, and plays an important role in regulating vasculoangiogenesis and remodeling the cardiovascular system [4]. A thin subendothelial shell, consisting of a small number of collagen-synthesizing fibroblasts and collagen fibers, attaches to the endothelium. The processes of endothelial cells connect the intima with the middle layer.

Tunica media is the thickest and most durable layer of the aortic wall that converts the pulsating blood flow, so it is most susceptible to variable loads. The average thickness of the media is up to 1.2 mm. Elastic plates separated by thin layers of connective tissue, collagen fibers, and smooth muscle cells form the structure of the media tunic. Elastic and collagen fibers make up 20–30% of the total volume of the aortic wall separately, and smooth muscle cells make up 5% [5]. Elastic plates are concentrically arranged fenestrated membranes (lamellae), the fibers of which are intertwined. The media tunic has 45–60 elastic plates covering 1/3–3/4 of the circumference of the aortic diameter. As a rule, these are oppositely twisted, cross-linked spiral structures arranged in a staggered order, which are held together by interlamellar connecting fibers. A network of fine collagen fibers surrounds both lamellar and connective elastic fibers. In addition, the elastic plates are supported by muscle fibers connected through points of contact with the mucoid membrane of the elastic plates. Interstitium contains colloidal mixtures of proteoglycans. The outermost elastic lamellar plates separate the aortic media from the thin adventitial layer [6, 7].

The adventitia tunic consists of loose connective tissue with a small number of elastic fibers, muscle cells, and macrophages. Through it from the outside, the vessels that feed the wall of the aorta vasa vasorum and nerve endings pass. Vasa vasorum, originated from the network of vessels located in adventitia, penetrate the outer third of the media and branch between the outer and middle layers, penetrating no deeper than the inner third of the media of the aorta. Thus, the outer third of the aorta receives nutrition through the vasa vasorum, while the inner layers are fed by diffusion from its lumen, which will support the structure of the aortic flow [8] (**Figure 1**).

Despite a long history of studying the pathogenesis of aortic dissection, it is still not clear enough. When studying the morphology of the aortic wall in patients with dissection, changes in the middle tunic of the media were most often detected. Gsell (1928) described damage to smooth muscle fibers during aortic dissection, Erdheim (1929) described damage to elastic fibers, and Cellina (1931) described a combination of these processes [6]. Currently, the media damage is, described as damage and loss of smooth muscle fibers, destruction and fragmentation of elastic plates, and filling of the resulting voids with proteoglycans [9] (**Figures 2** and **3**).

Such changes may occur in patients with inherited syndromes accompanied by connective tissue dysplasia, such as Marfan, Loeys-Dietz, Ehlers-Danlos, Turner, and others, or in their absence.

The same changes along with atherosclerosis are found in the aortic wall in elderly patients and with increased variable loads, in particular with arterial hypertension. It is, believed that due to the loss of elastic properties of the aortic wall, the vasa vasorum network is traumatized, which leads to the formation of lacunae

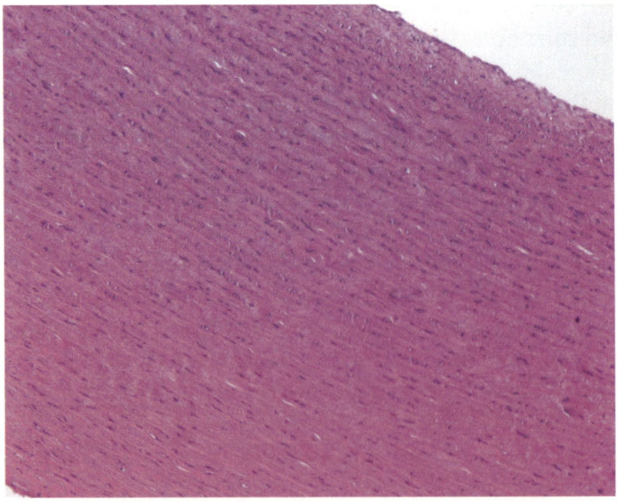

Figure 1.
Aortic sections from a normal subject. Panel is oriented with the intima at the top and the adventitia at the bottom; hematoxylin and eosin (H&E) staining.

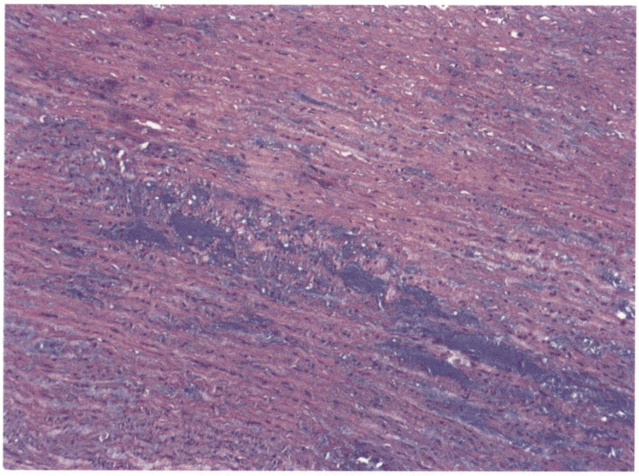

Figure 2.
Aortic sections from a patient with aortic dissection. Fragmentation of elastic fibers, loss of smooth muscle cells, and accumulation of proteoglycans (stained blue) in the medial layer.

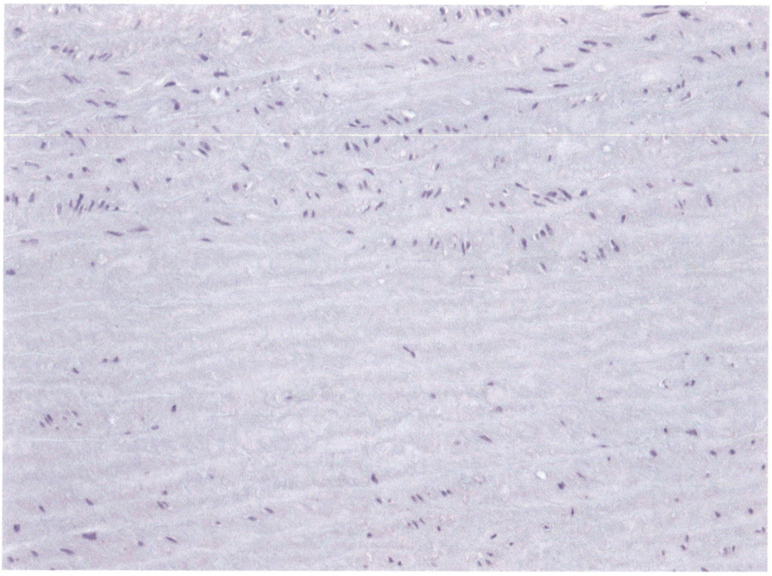

Figure 3.
Necrosis of the aortic media tunic, chaotic arrangement of smooth muscle and elastic fibers.

filled with blood, and subsequently an intramural hematoma. The beginning of the stratification is the rupture of the intima due to the impact of the peak load [6, 7] (**Figures 4** and **5**). However, this concept does not explain the mechanism of dissection in acute trauma in young patients with noncompromised aortic wall. In all likelihood, with excessive loads or due to degenerative changes within it, the aortic wall ceases to function as a whole and is divided into separate fragments with different mechanical properties (**Figure 6**).

The exact number of cases of distal aortic dissection is very difficult to determine, since this disease refers to various conditions due to different causes. It is important to divide the distal dissection into primary and secondary. Primary dissection is a firstly appeared dissection, and secondary distal dissection can be called the presence of active false lumen of the descending aorta, after correction of the proximal dissection.

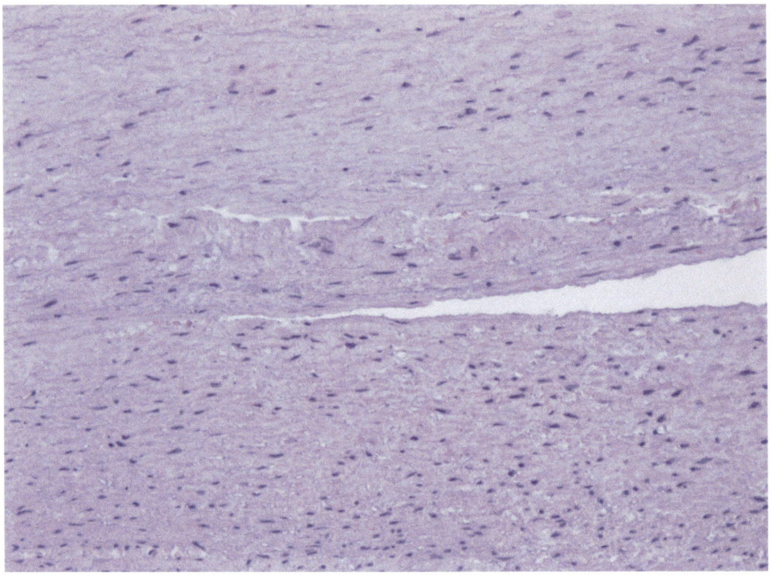

Figure 4.
Dissection in the middle layer of the aorta, tunic media. On the left are the nuclei of single erythrocytes.

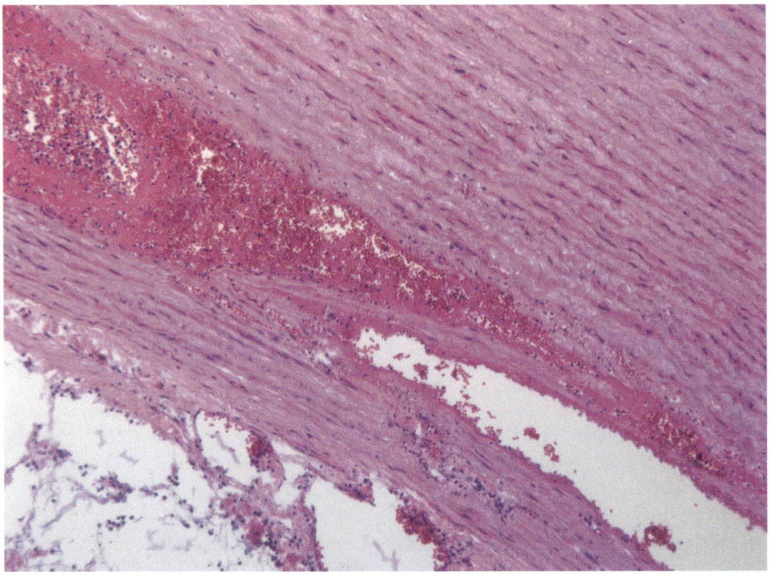

Figure 5.
Extensive acute aortic dissection. Areas of tearing are localized in the distal third of the media tunic closer to the adventitia. A large number of red blood cells are observed inside the false lumen.

Primary dissection may be associated with dysplasia of connective tissue due to congenital genetic syndromes such as Marfan, Loeys-Dietz, Ehlers-Danlos, Turner, and others. Connective tissue dysplasia in distal dissection can also occur without the presence of hereditary syndromes. Distal dissection occurs in patients without connective tissue dysplasia, for example, after trauma.

Recently, acute aortic syndrome has been isolated, which, in addition to aortic dissection, includes a penetrating ulcer and an intramural hematoma; these conditions are predictors of dissection and require exactly the same approach as the dissection itself.

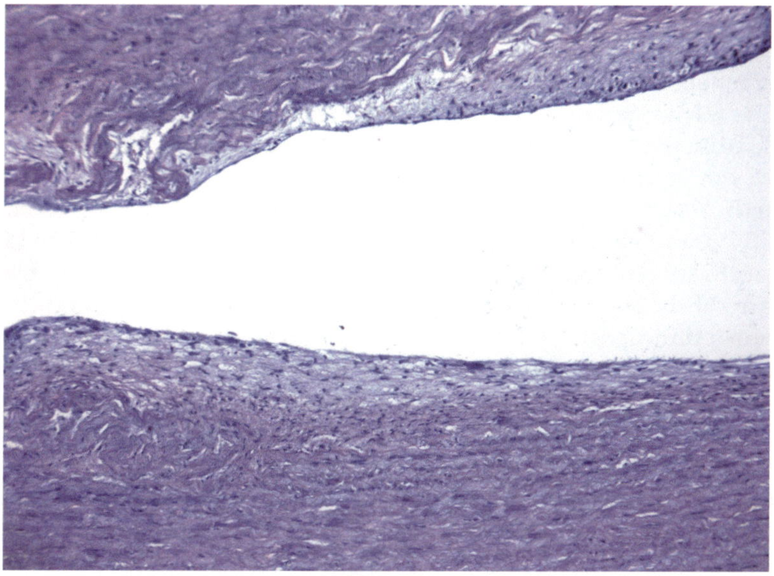

Figure 6.
Chronic aortic dissection. The formation of a pseudo-intima is observed along the edges of the false lumen.

Distal dissection or aortic dissection of type B most often affects male patients and has an incidence between 2.9 and 4.0 per 100,000 people per year [10]. The number of cases of distal dissection is increasing, with improved diagnostic capabilities and an aging population being put forward as reasons. A recent prospective analysis of 30,412 middle-aged men and women over a 20-year follow-up period showed the incidence of acute aortic dissection in 15 patients per 100,000 population per year [11]. The number of penetrating aortic ulcers has also increased. In symptomatic patients considered as candidates for invasive intervention, the prevalence of penetrating ulcer is from 2.3 to 7.6%, while in 90% of patients, the lesion is localized in the descending thoracic aorta [12]. The prevalence of intramural hematoma is from 5 to 20% of patients with acute aortic syndrome;, in 60% of cases, the descending thoracic aorta is involved in the process [13]. Blunt aortic trauma occurs in less than 1% of all road accidents. However, it is the second most common cause of death among trauma patients and accounts for 16% of all traumatic deaths [14]. Rupture of an aneurysm of the descending thoracic aorta occurs in 5 persons per 100,000 population per year. The average age of patients in this cohort is 70 years for men and 72 years for women [15]. Mortality in aneurysms and aortic dissection has recently increased from 2.49 per 100,000 to 2.78 per 100,000 of the population per year from 1990 to 2010, with a predominance of males [16].

Most clinical classifications of aortic dissection, including the first and most common, proposed by DeBakey, are based on the identification of the localization of the initial rupture of intima, since most of this largely depends on the severity of the patient's condition, further treatment tactics, and prognosis of his life. According to DeBakey, the aortic dissection is divided into three types: type I—primary rupture of intima is localized in the ascending aorta, and the dissection extends below the source of the left subclavian artery; type II—primary rupture of intima is localized in the ascending aorta, and the dissection extends no further than the source of the brachycephalic trunk; and type III—primary rupture of intima is localized below the source of the left subclavian artery and extends to the distal aorta, up to its bifurcation [17]. Subsequently, types I and II were combined into one type A, and type III was separated into type B, and this classification was called Standford [18].

Some authors began to call the type A dissection (types I and II by DeBakey) proximal, and type B (type III by DeBakey) distal, since apparently these terms most fully reflect the essence of pathological processes occurring inside the aorta [19, 20]. For forms where the dissection is limited to the aortic arch or extends retrograde from the descending aorta to the arch and ends before the ascending aorta, the term "non A non B" is proposed [21, 22].

Currently, new classifications that are more modern are proposed, in particular DISSECT classification, which considers six key parameters: duration of the disease, localization of intimal rupture, size of the stratified aorta, length of the affected area of the aorta, clinical complications of stratification, and the presence of false lumen thrombosis [23]. In the surgical treatment of distal dissection (type III DeBakey) within 30 days mortality surgery ranges from 10 to 24%, while at carrying out of conservative therapy, this index varies within 10%. Therefore, the distal dissection (type III DeBakey) is adopted a conservative wait-and-see tactic. Long-term results demonstrate the need for intervention in 20% of patients treated conservatively within 3 years from the beginning symptoms of the dissection [24].

The strategy and tactics of treatment of distal widespread aortic dissection are still the subject of discussion [25]. A majority of authors agree that invasive intervention is indicated by increasing the diameter of the aorta to 5.5 cm, with the combined diameter of the true and false lumen to 4.5 cm, or with complicated forms of dissection [22]. Complicated forms of aortic dissection type B are considered to be a rapid increase in the diameter of the aorta; rupture of the aorta and/or hypotension or shock; ischemia of internal organs, kidneys or lower limbs; paraplegia/paraparesis; periaortic hematoma; re-emerged or untreatable pain syndrome; and refractory to drug therapy hypertension. At the same time, with conservative treatment of complicated forms of distal aortic dissection, mortality is about 50% [26–29].

Consequently, most interventions in distal aortic dissection are carried out for emergency indications. Methods of reconstruction in distal aortic dissection can be divided into traditional open, video-assisted, X-ray endovascular, and hybrid.

2. Methods

Methods of reconstruction of distal aortic dissection: 1. thrombosis of false lumen by foreign bodies; 2. the creation of an artificial distal fenestration; 3. extraanatomical bypass surgery; 4. prosthetics between the two clamps; 5. prosthetics between the two clamps with the use of an extraanatomical bypass shunt; 6. prosthetics between the two clamps with the use of methods of extracorporal blood circulation; 7. prosthesis without the use of clamps by circulatory arrest; 8. endoprosthetics (stent grafts); 9. stenting; and 10. hybrid methods in the form of a combination of these techniques using different types of access.

Initially, the reconstruction of the descending aorta during dissection was carried out in nonradical ways, such as initiation of thrombosis of the false lumen by means of foreign elements or reduction of the diameter of the aorta outside by suture or exoprosthesis. In the future, methods of simple clamping of the aorta and its replacement were performed. Frozen arterial homografts and then synthetic vascular prostheses were used [30].

Despite such disadvantages as limiting the time of anastomosis not more than 30 min and the formation of tissue hypertension, in the areas above and below the imposition of clamps, the supporters of this method think because there is no need for systemic heparinization of the patient and the use of perfusion support. All these significantly reduce blood loss and surgery time [31]. In the early stages of surgery for rupture of the descending part of the thoracic aorta, the technique of bypass grafting was also used: ascending aorta—abdominal aorta. At the same time, a homograft was used as a shunt. However, this technique was not ideal due to the technical complexity of the shunt, its bulkiness, and insufficient reliability [32].

In 1955, based on the work of DeBakey et al., the first experience of reconstructive interventions on thoracic aorta with dissection in 6 patients was published [33]. In 1965, they analyzed 10-year results of treatment of thoracic aortic dissection, including T III. Two surgical techniques were described. Earlier, it was the formation of artificial distal fenestration in the thoracic aorta and reconstruction of the true lumen below its level. The authors themselves recognize this technique does not correspond to the concept of restoring integrity and normal function of the aorta, but rather palliative. Another technique was the imposition of the left-femoral bypass, the intersection of the aorta between the two clips superimposed directly at the ostium of the left subclavian artery and near the diaphragmatic opening, and the restoration of the integrity of the true lumen of the aorta and its replacement with a synthetic vascular prosthesis. At the same time, according to the authors, in the case of spreading the dissection proximal to the left subclavian artery, it could be sacrificed by ligation, or reimplanting its origin into a vascular prosthesis [34].

The use of cardiopulmonary bypass increased the safe time for anastomosis, but did not solve the problems associated with the imposition of clamps on the aorta, since in most patients with distal aortic dissection, the inlet of the false canal is located directly at the origin of the left carotid artery. In addition, the clamp applied at the level of the diaphragm to the aorta makes it difficult to form a qualitative distal anastomosis, and damage to the altered tissues of the aorta can cause its insolvency. Moreover, the problem of residual dissection below the diaphragm level remains unsolved.

DeBakey et al. in 1966 established the principles of the surgical technique of treatment of aortic dissection, including excision of the dissected intimal flaps, overlapping the proximal enter in false lumen and reconstruction of the aorta by the implantation of synthetic tubular prosthesis. Based on this, techniques for reconstruction of distal aortic dissection were further developed [35].

In 1974, Stanley Crawford reported on his experience with thoracoabdominal aneurysms and dissections. In earlier observations, the implantation of a synthetic Dacron graft was undertaken as an extraanatomical shunt with subsequent overlapping of the aortic lumen and serial reimplantation of the aortic branches by vascular prostheses in the wall of the aortic graft. In later cases, the vascular graft was placed inside the aneurysm with reimplantation of the origin of visceral vessels directly into the wall of the graft [36].

Currently, this technique is the basis for the open correction of extensive thoracoabdominal aortic dissection. However, the technical details of the operation are controversial.

1. Method of extracorporeal blood circulation:

    a. left-femoral bypass with or without oxygenation (left atrium eyelet or pulmonary vein-femoral artery);

    b. full bypass femoral artery—femoral vein.

2. Ways of protection of internal organs: normothermic perfusion with the perfusion of visceral vessels; hypothermia; and total circulatory arrest without the use of clamps on the aorta.

3. Method of implantation of vertebral arteries in the prosthesis for the prevention of spinal complications.

4. Method of implantation of the visceral branches.

There are various options to use this technology. In particular, in the conditions of left-femoral bypass and normothermal perfusion, the procedure is performed from thoracophrenolumbotomy access in stages. In the beginning, the clamping of a proximal segment of the aorta is done, the formation of a proximal anastomosis with a vascular graft to the descending thoracic aorta is carried out, and the mobilization of the thoracic aorta is produced. The clamp on the distal portion of the aorta is placed, producing distal anastomosis, dissecting aneurysm, and lumbar arteries are stitched, producing temporary occlusion of the visceral arteries with balloons catheters. Produce perfusion of the renal arteries to protect against ischemia; the intercostal arteries are implanted to the prosthetic aorta at the site Th8-L1 to restore adequate blood supply to the spinal cord, and renal arteries and visceral branches are implanted [37].

Further improvement of this technique was carried out by sewing visceral branches into the vascular prosthesis of the aorta on separate islands or using an aortic vascular prosthesis originally made with branches for the implantation of visceral arteries [38, 39]. The difference between the methods lies in the fact that the implantation of the origin of the vessels on a single island reduces the time of the procedure, but there is a risk of relapse in the long term, as in the bloodstream there are large areas of altered aortic tissue with untreated arterial origins. When using the technique of Coselli, the origins of the visceral vessels are filed separately to those already present in the aortic graft that prevents recurrence of the aneurysm, but does not allow avoiding the complications associated with the tension and kinking of the vessels and extends the duration of the procedure.

To prevent these complications, a modified technique of visceral arteries reimplantation was proposed. Its essence lies in the fact that used graft with four prestitched lateral branches. After applying the proximal and distal anastomoses, each lateral branch is wrapped around the main graft, forming a slightly curved loop around it. The opening of each visceral artery is sutured to the lateral branch. This method prevents bending of the lateral branches and allows for hemostasis with a good overview of all suture lines [40]. Estrera et al. describe a modification of the classical technique used by them in the correction of chronic complicated aortic dissection type B. The procedure is performed by bypass of the left ventricle on the scheme of the lower left pulmonary vein—distal aorta, through a vascular prosthesis attached to the aortic prosthesis. Is drainage of the cerebrospinal fluid, and neuromonitoring. After clamping the distal portion of the aorta and forming a wedge-shaped hole in the membrane between the true and false lumens, a distal anastomosis is formed to adequately supply them with blood. Then the clamp is shifted higher on the aortic prosthesis and the vascular prosthesis starts blood flow to the distal aorta, and then the aorta is clamped at the level of the left subclavian artery. The aorta is incised, intercostal arteries or clipped or made their temporary occlusion using a Fogarty catheter. A reversed elephant trunk is formed, then a proximal anastomosis is made. If necessary, intercostal arteries are drained into the vascular prosthesis on a single site, and prestitched to the aortic prosthesis with both ends. According to the authors of their more than 20 years of experience, it is shown that when using this technique, hospital mortality is 8.3%. Persistent neurological disorders occur in 1.3%, strokes 2.9%, the need for dialysis in 6%. 5-, 10-, 15-, and 20-year survival rates are 72%, 60%, 45%, and 39%, respectively [41].

At the same time, the technique of complete shutdown of the descending aorta from the systemic circulation using the methods of deep hypothermia without applying clamps to it has not lost its relevance [42]. According to some authors, this technique has significant advantages since it allows you to do without applying a clamp to the proximal portion of the descending thoracic aorta, as close as possible to impose anastomoses to the origin of the left subclavian artery and the aperture of the diaphragm, as well as in the case of retrograde dissection, if necessary, move to the distal portion of the aortic arch. The advantages of the technique include a bloodless surgical field, the return of a large amount of blood to the contour of the apparatus and hypothermic protection of the central nervous system, heart, and visceral organs. In addition, there is no need to use the drainage of cerebrospinal fluid, monitoring of evoked potentials, separate perfusion of renal and visceral arteries, and the insertion of epidural catheter [43].

Its main drawback is the need to protect the brain and spinal cord, as well as internal organs from hypoxia and a limited time of safe duration of circulatory arrest, no more than 90 min at a body temperature of 18°C [44]. The cooling phase of the patient takes quite a long time since the decrease in body temperature should be uniform, complete, and prolonged [45]. The time to reach the optimum temperature can take from 30 to 50 min [46]. The method of warming the patient should also be done slowly and in compliance with a number of different conditions. In conditions of complicated distal aortic dissection, the technique of circulatory arrest with deep hypothermia may not always be effective enough.

The influence of different approaches to revascularization of intercostal and lumbar arteries during reconstructive interventions on the distal aorta on the prevention of paraplegia has not been studied enough. One hundred consecutively operated patients were performed open reconstruction of the distal lesions of the aorta with a consistent overlap of the segmental arteries. Early mortality was 6%. The average length of stay in the intensive care unit was 2.5 days, and the average length of stay in the hospital was 10.0 days. On average, 8.0 ± 2.6 pairs of segmental arteries were closed, with an average of 4.5 ± 2.1 covered segment pairs being in the area between T7 and L1, where is the artery of Adamkewicz. Postoperative paraplegia occurred in 2 patients. The authors conclude that the overlap without reimplantation of 15 pairs of intercostal and lumbar arteries during the reconstruction of the distal aorta is safe, and is accompanied by a moderate number of paraplegia in the early and late postoperative period [47].

Radical surgery shows good immediate and long-term results in patients with hereditary connective tissue syndrome. In particular, in patients with Marfan syndrome, total replacement of the entire thoracoabdominal aorta and reconstruction of all visceral branches are recommended to avoid relapses in the long term, even if dilation in some segments is not expressed. In a study by Omura et al., a series of observations was reported in 20 patients with Marfan syndrome who underwent total replacement of the thoracoabdominal aorta for a dissecting aneurysm. All patients during the surgical intervention were performed cerebrospinal fluid drainage, distal perfusion of the aorta and selective perfusion of the internal organs. Deep hypothermia was used in 13 patients.

In the 30-day postoperative period, no fatal outcomes were observed. The average follow-up period was 54 months. One patient died of interstitial pneumonia 38 months after surgery. The survival rate for 8 years was 91.2 ± 9.0%. Two patients required additional interventions on the aorta. Actuarial index of freedom from operations on the aorta for 8 years was 83.9% ± 10.5%; no patient needed a rethoracotomy. During follow-up, neither false nor asymptomatic aneurysms by computed tomography (CT) were noted [48].

Even though the results of surgical treatment of distal aortic dissection have improved over the last decade, they are still not optimal, and hospital mortality is 25–50% [49, 50]. Complications associated with the open method of surgical intervention are the following: spinal cord ischemia (6.8%), cerebral circulation disorders (9%), abdominal ischemia or intestinal infarction (4.9%), and acute renal failure (19%) [51, 52].

The widespread use of open radical operations is limited by the severity of the patient's condition, the presence of concomitant diseases, and its physiological reserve. A significant disadvantage of this technology is a very low possibility of its replication. Such operations with a low level of mortality can be carried out only in specialized aortic centers with 20–30 years of experience in such operations and close-knit teams of highly qualified specialists. In conditions of acute complicated DeBakey type III dissection, this is not always possible and requires simpler and no less reliable solutions.

The need for their search and the beginning of the era of percutaneous transcatheter interventions on the coronary arteries prompted researchers to create a vascular prosthesis that could be placed inside the lumen of the aorta to block the entrance opening of the false canal and isolate its wall without performing extensive surgical access. In 1988, Volodos reported on the first percutaneous endoprosthesis of the thoracic aorta with a self-fixing synthetic prosthesis for a large posttraumatic aneurysm [53].

With significant advantages due to the reduction of intraoperative trauma and no need to protect the brain and spinal cord, as well as internal organs, the methods of transcatheter reconstruction of the distal aortic dissection initially had a number of limitations and did not immediately gain a leading position in the treatment of complicated distal aortic dissection [54].

Stent graphs are ideal for implantation in straight areas of the aorta, where there are no large hemodynamic values of arterial trunks; such in the reconstruction of the distal dissection can only be a portion of the descending thoracic aorta, from the ostium of the left common carotid artery and ending with the level of renal arteries. Despite the fact that during the period from the left subclavian artery to the renal from the descending aorta does not depart large arterial branches, overlapping its area for more than 20 cm at this level can lead to the development of pronounced spinal disorders [55–57]. The wall of the aorta is constantly shrinking, conducting a pulse wave, and violation of its elastic properties during dissection creates a tendency to irreversible dilation of the aorta and its thinning up to rupture [58].

To prevent spontaneous dislocation of the stent graft, two proximal landing zones of at least 1.5 cm and a distal zone of at least 2 cm in length are required [59].

For successful fixation of the stent graft in the landing zones, it is necessary to overestimate the pressure on the aortic wall in the places of fixation, which is achieved by increasing its landing size by 2–3 mm or more. In this regard, one of the most dangerous complications associated with the implantation of a stent graft is the retrograde progression of the dissection [60, 61].

In addition, the number of complications included caudal migration of the prosthesis under the influence of the pulse wave; the collapse of a stent graft; and lack of precision of its positioning, because this process performed distantly is not under direct visual, and under angiographic control, which may lead to the implantation of stent graft in the false lumen of the aorta [62].

Specific complications of implantation of stent graft also considered para prosthesis leakage (endoleaks) [55–57]. Endoleak type Ia is a frequent complication in the reconstruction of TEVAR for distal aortic dissection and is caused by inadequate sealing of the endograft's in the proximal area [63]. This endoleak that occurred immediately after TEVAR for acute dissection of type B may indicate the unstable condition of the aorta [64].

In most cases, proximal intimal fenestration in distal dissection is located near the ostium of the left subclavian artery, due to the formation of reverse blood flow in the aorta in this area [58]. Thus, in 20–30% of cases, stent graft implantation requires closure of the left subclavian artery ostium [65]. Intentional overlapping of the left subclavian artery of the stent graft leads to a statistically significant increase in the risk of stroke [66] and the frequency of spinal cord ischemia [67]. In this regard, current recommendations include revascularization of the left subclavian artery (LSA) [65]. In one retrospective comparative study, there was a statistically significant increase in the number of strokes and upper limb ischemia in patients who did not undergo revascularization of LSA in comparison with patients who underwent revascularization of LSA by reimplantation of its ostium or bypass surgery [68].

In order to reduce the aggressiveness of the intervention and increase the landing zone, the endovascular technique of parallel stent grafts is used, that is, implantation of a separate stent graft into the left subclavian artery, its placement parallel to the main stent graft, and removal of its orifice beyond the proximal landing zone of the main stent graft, the so-called chimney or snorkel technique [69]. Chimney is the method of choice in patients with complex aortic arch anatomy to extend the proximal landing zone and provide perfusion of the aortic arch branches [70]. This technique can be used in patients with aberrant right subclavian artery in the case of acute type B aortic dissection [71]. In addition, this endovascular technique can be used for revascularization of all branches of the aortic arch [72].

The technique of chimneys has a number of limitations, such as entanglement and bending of branches, but the most significant of them is the aggravation of the danger of the formation of endoleaks of type I, due to the loose fit of the main stent graft to the wall of the aorta in the landing zone [73].

To solve these problems for the purpose of endo prosthesis of the aortic arch, a number of commercially available endografts with preattached branches are produced; endoprostheses have a wide size range and do not need individual manufacture. Despite the shown good results in relation to the early postoperative mortality, the number of strokes, and the frequency of repeated interventions in patients with increased surgical risk, this procedure requires detailed preliminary calculations, is difficult to perform, and is more suitable for patients with residual dissection after reconstruction of the proximal aorta for type A dissection [74, 75].

The procedure of implantation of scalloped or fenestered stent grafts is less complicated; stent-graft with a half-opening on the edge or opening for the mouths of brachiocephalic vessels well adheres to the altered aortic wall, is easier to manufacture, and is more accessible than branched stent graft. However, fenestrated stent grafts are more prone to dislocation and show the worst results for the number of strokes and 30-day mortality [76].

All of the above techniques are also successfully used for revascularization of visceral branches. In addition, they have the same advantages and disadvantages as in the application of the aortic arch, as fenestrated stent grafts and the periscope technique, are well suited for the treatment of patients with complex anatomy in the region of the visceral branches of the aorta [77]. Technology chimney and periscopes are also used for the relief of endoleaks type I after EVAR prior to increase in the proximal and distal landing zones for endografts [78] . However, according to some authors, the application of chimney technology for revascularization of the visceral branches of the aorta in the late postoperative period increases the risk of violations of the patency of visceral implants and development of endoleaks [79].

Recently, for the revascularization of the visceral and iliac arteries, the sandwich technique has become widespread, which is a later modification of the chimney or periscope technique and is used to stop extended aortic lesions. In this case, the origin of the visceral branches prostheses is opened into the lumen of another stent graft, implanted on top of the first and overlapping it in a certain area. The feature of this technique is that there is a greater risk of developing "gutter" endoleaks, aorta overlap for a much longer distance, visceral arteries requires stent graft greater length. Nevertheless, this technique gives good results both in the near and in the long term and is not accompanied by a high frequency of spinal complications [80, 81].

According to a meta-analysis of the results of repeated open interventions after TEVAR in the aortic dissection, which consisted of 2029 cases in the TEVAR 2403 cases of aortic dissection, with an average follow-up period of 34 months, the most common reasons for reintervention was endoleak type I (35.2%), redo dissection (14.4%), and perfusion of the false lumen (9.3%) [82].

In another study of 2531 patients who had TEVAR performed for acute complicated aortic dissection type B, mortality within 30 days after the intervention was noted in 7.3% of cases; in comparison with the 2347 patients treated with conservative treatment for acute uncomplicated aortic dissection type B, where the mortality rate was 2.4%. In the group of 1276 patients where open surgery was performed, the mortality rate was 19%. Patients who were performed TEVAR had more favorable results in relation to remodeling of the aorta and survival associated with lesions of the aorta than patients treated with medical therapy [83].

Given the presence of a large number of endoleaks after TEVAR, it is suggested that this technique is not quite suitable for the treatment of aortic dissection since most patients do not have a suitable anatomy [84].

However, one study showed that TEVAR is safe to perform in chronic distal aortic dissection, but there are limitations due to the complex anatomy of the dissection. Unfavorable factors are the departure of less than two vessels from the true lumen of the aorta, the large diameter of the aorta before surgery and the location of the primary rupture at a greater curvature [85].

In addition, infrequent (0.4%) but quite a formidable complication is infection of stent grafts, developing mainly in weakened patients with immunosuppression. In this case, open intervention with complete excision of the infected material and extraanatomic revascularization or revascularization in situ is required [86].

In order to avoid many of these complications, the use of a bare metal balloon expandable stent was proposed for decompression of the false aortic lumen [87–89].

The stent can be opened to the required diameter, but not more than 4.5 cm, which is one of the significant limitations. It can also be used on any part of the aorta, since the opening of the stent cells has an area of at least 1 cm^2, which allows for unhindered perfusion of the branches of the aorta in any zone. The main disadvantage of the bare metal stent is that it does not completely cover the perfusion along the false lumen, since, as a rule, when dissection, there are a large number of small gaps along the false channel. However, in conservative treatment of type B dissection, there is also a valid false channel, and patients do without surgery for years. During implantation of the stent, the main task is the stabilization of the lumen of the aorta due to the redirection of the main mass of blood in the true lumen rather than achieving a perfect angiographic effect. The principal negative points are also considered that the bare metal stent is balloon expandable and this can lead to the progression of the dissection [90].

Nevertheless, if certain techniques are followed, such as controlled hypotension and gradual slow opening of the balloon, it is possible to achieve adequate stent adherence to the aortic wall even at the level of the aortic arch and brachiocephalic branches. The high degree of replication of the technique and the absence and versatility of bare metal stents are undeniable advantages. The combination of stenting with implantation of stent graft also gives good results in the implantation of the stent in the area of origin of the artery of Adamkewicz Th8-L1, as well as visceral and brachiocephalic branches. As a monomethod, the implantation of a bare metal stent gives good results in posttraumatic aortic dissection [91–93].

There is another more common technique of false lumen decompression, which is an endovascular balloon fenestration of the false lumen of the aorta in the distal region and a stent implantation in visceral branches. This technique improves patient outcomes in the long term, especially in relation to be aortospecifically complications [94].

As hybrid interventions for aortic dissection, two methods are described in the literature; one of them is the implantation of combined prostheses where a vascular prosthesis with preprepared one or several branches for implantation of brachiocephalic arteries is made together with a stent graft, which is implanted in the upper and middle portion of the descending aorta. This method is called "frozen elephant trunk" by analogy with the two-stage operation proposed by Borst in 1982. The technique is used in patients with proximal dissection passing to the descending thoracic aorta in order to reduce Borst procedure to one stage [95].

Another hybrid technique is debranching or a technique of open switching the branches of the aorta with subsequent implantation of a stent graft. This technique is widely used to increase the landing zone for stent graft, both in the area of the aortic arch and visceral branches [96, 97]. The advantages are less intraoperative trauma and no need for circulatory arrest, brain perfusion, and spinal cord protection. The disadvantages include the availability of open access and the interval between stages, which are not always acceptable with urgent intervention about the progression of distal dissection. In addition, a large number of complications at the stage of vascular switching accompany the technique of visceral debranching [98].

In the literature, for some reason, little attention is paid to the description of methods of prosthetics of the descending thoracic aorta and simultaneous implantation of bare metal stents in the visceral zone or on the contrary in the region of large spinal branches, in particular the Adamkewicz artery, under video or X-ray control with extensive distal aortic dissection. This technique significantly reduces operating access, limiting it to a thoracotomy, thus allowing for simultaneous intervention, for example, revascularization of the myocardium provides a good quality of anastomosis of the aorta, and significantly it reduces the time of circulatory arrest and at the same time provides good permeability of all visceral branches [99].

According to the 17-year follow-up of the International Registry of Acute Aortic Dissection (IRAD), most patients are treated conservatively; however, in recent years, the frequency of this treatment has decreased from 75 to 57%. The number of endovascular interventions performed has increased from 7 to 31%, the frequency of open surgical operations has decreased from 17 to 8%, and hybrid techniques were widely introduced (5%) [100].

3. Conclusion

Thus, it can be stated that transcatheter methods of treatment are first-line methods with complicated distal aortic dissection and suitable for this anatomy of the dissection. In case of impossibility of performance, transcatheter intervention should consider the implementation of an open or hybrid repair. Conservative management of patients is preferable in uncomplicated distal dissection. Improving knowledge in the field of brain and spinal cord physiology, as well as transcatheter and hybrid techniques, will allow safe interventions in stable patients with type B dissection to improve their survival and quality of life. Further progress in the treatment of distal aortic dissection depends not on the juxtaposition of different reconstructive techniques, but on their carefully thought-out choice and combination.

Author details

Mark Alekseevich Soborov
Federal State Autonomous Educational Institution of Higher Education, I.M. Sechenov First Moscow State Medical University of the Ministry of Health of the Russian Federation (Sechenov University), Russia

*Address all correspondence to: msoborov@mail.ru

References

[1] Hiratzka LF, Bakris GL, Beckman JA, et al. ACCF/AHA/AATS/ACR/ASA/SCA/SCAI/SIR/STS/ SVM guidelines for the diagnosis and management of patients with thoracic aortic disease: Executive summary. Journal of the American College of Cardiology. 2010, 2010;**55**(14):1509-1544. DOI: 10.1016/j.jacc.2010.02.010

[2] Riambau V, Böckler D, Brunkwall J, et al. ESVS guidelines descending thoracic aorta. European Journal of Vascular and Endovascular Surgery. 2017;**53**:4-52

[3] Davies PF. How do vascular endothelial cells respond to flow? NIPS. 1989;**4**:22

[4] Gerritsen ME. Physiological functions of normal endothelial cells. In: Loscalzo J, Creager MA, Dzau VJ, editors. Vascular Medicine. Vol. 3. New York: Little Brown; 1996

[5] Caro CG, Pedley TJ, Schroter RC, Seed WA. The Mechanics of the Circulation. Moscow; 1981. pp. 289-291. [in Russian]

[6] Doerr W. Thoracic aortic aneurysms. The Thoracic and Cardiovascular Surgeon. 1987;**35**(Special Issue):111-121

[7] Stone C, Borst H. Dissecting aortic aneurysm. In: Edmunds LH Jr, editor. Cardiac Surgery in the Adult. New York: McGraw-Hill; 1997. pp. 1153-1157

[8] Maiellaro K, Taylor WR. The role of the adventitia in vascular inflammation. Cardiovascular Research. 2007;**1**: 75:4:640-648

[9] Milewicz DM, Guo DC, Tran-Fadulu V, et al. Genetic basis of thoracic aortic aneurysms and dissections: Focus on smooth muscle cell contractile dysfunction. Annual Review of Genomics and Human Genetics. 2008;**9**:283-302

[10] Clouse WD, Hallet JW Jr, Shaff HV, Spittell PC, Rowland CM, Ilstrup CM, et al. Acute aortic dissection: Population-based incidence compared with degenerative aortic aneurysm rupture. Mayo Clinic Proceedings. 2004;**79**:176-180

[11] Landenhed M, Engstrom G, Gottsater A, Caulfield MP, Hedblad B, Newton-Cheh C, et al. Risk profiles for aortic dissection and ruptured or surgically treated aneurysms: A prospective cohort study. Journal of the American Heart Association. 2015;**4**(1):e001513

[12] Eggebrecht H, Nienaber CA, Neuhauser M, Baumgart D, Kische S, Schmermund A, et al. Endovascular stent graft placement in aortic dissection: A meta-analysis. European Heart Journal. 2006;**27**:489-498

[13] Evangelista A, Mukherjee D, Mehta RH, O'Gara PT, Fattori R, Cooper JV, et al. Acute intramural hematoma of the aorta: A mystery in evolution. Circulation. 2005;**111**:1063-1070

[14] European Commission. Mobility and Transport. Road safety. Available from: http://ec.europa.eu/transport/road_safety/specialist/statistics/

[15] Johansson G, Markström U, Swedenborg J. Ruptured thoracic aortic aneurysms: A study of incidence and mortality rates. Journal of Vascular Surgery. 1995;**21**:985-988

[16] Sampson UKA, Norman PE, Fowkes GR, Aboyans V, Song Y, Harrell FE, et al. Global and regional burden of aortic dissection and aneurysms. Global Heart. 2014;**8**:171-180

[17] Debakey ME, Henly WS, Cooley DA, Morris GC Jr, Crawford ES, Beall AC Jr. Surgical management of dissecting aneurysms of the aorta. The Journal of Thoracic and Cardiovascular Surgery. 1965;**49**:130-149. [PubMed: 14261867]

[18] Daily PO, Trueblood HW, Stinson EB, Wuerflein RD, Shumway NE. Management of acute aortic dissections. The Annals of Thoracic Surgery. 1970;**10**(3):237-247. [PubMed: 5458238]

[19] Cambria RP. Surgical treatment of complicated distal aortic dissection. Seminars in Vascular Surgery. 2002;**15**(2):97-107

[20] Bhamidipati C, Ailawadi G. Acute complicated and uncomplicated type III aortic dissection: An endovascular perspective. Seminars in Thoracic and Cardiovascular Surgery. 2009;**21**(4):373-386. DOI: 10.1053/j.semtcvs.2009.11.008

[21] Von Segesser LK, Killer I, Ziswiler M, Linka A, Ritter M, Jenni R, et al. Dissection of the descending thoracic aorta extending into the ascendingaorta. The Journal of Thoracic and Cardiovascular Surgery. 1994;**108**:755-761

[22] Urbanski PP, Wagner M. Acute non-A–non-B aortic dissection: Surgical or conservative approach? European Journal of Cardio-Thoracic Surgery. 2016;**49**:1249-1254. DOI: 10.1093/ejcts/ezv301

[23] Dake MD, Thompson M, van Sambeek M, Vermassen F, Morales JP. DISSECT: A new mnemonic-based approach to the categorization of aortic dissection. European Journal of Vascular and Endovascular Surgery. 2013;**46**(2):175-190

[24] Coady MA, Ikonomidis JS, Cheung AT, et al. Surgical management of descending thoracic aortic disease: Open and endovascular approaches: A scientific statement from the American Heart Association. Circulation. 2010;**121**:2780-2804

[25] Erbel R, Alfonso F, Boileau C, et al. Diagnosis and management of aortic dissection. European Heart Journal. 2001;**22**(18):1642-1681

[26] Hagan PG, Nienaber CA, Isselbacher EM, Bruckman D, Karavite DJ, Russman PL, et al. The International Registry of Acute Aortic Dissection (IRAD): New insights into an old disease. Journal of the American Medical Association. 2000;**283**:897e903

[27] Tsai TT, Trimarchi S, Nienaber CA. Acute aortic dissection: Perspectives from the International Registry of Acute Aortic Dissection (IRAD). European Journal of Vascular and Endovascular Surgery. 2009;**37**:149e59

[28] Suzuki T, Mehta RH, Ince H, Nagai R, Sakomura Y, Weber F, et al. Clinical profiles and outcomes of acute type B aortic dissection in the current era: Lessons from the International Registry of Aortic Dissection (IRAD). Circulation. 2003;**108**(Suppl 1): II312e7

[29] Elefteriades JA. Natural history of thoracic aortic aneurysms: Indications for surgery, and surgical versus nonsurgical risks. The Annals of Thoracic Surgery. 2002;**74**:S1877e80

[30] Thompson JE. Early history of aortic surgery. Journal of Vascular Surgery. 1998;**28**:746-752

[31] Cambria RP, Davison JK, Zannetti S, et al. Thoracoabdominal aneurysm repair: Perspectives over a decade with the clamp-and-sew technique. Annals of Surgery. 1997;**226**:294-303; discussion 303-5

[32] Shumacker HB Jr. Innovation in the operative management of the thoracoabdominal aneurysms.

Surgery, Gynecology & Obstetrics. 1973;**136**:793-794

[33] DeBakey ME, Cooley DA, Creech O. Surgical considerations of dissecting aneurysms of the aorta. Annals of Surgery. 1955;**142**:586-610

[34] DeBakey ME, Henly WS, Cooley DA, Morris GC Jr, Crawford ES, Beall AC Jr. Surgical management of dissecting aneurysms of the aorta. The Journal of Thoracic and Cardiovascular Surgery. 1965;**49**:130-149. PMID 14261867

[35] DeBakey ME, Beall AC Jr, Cooley DA, Crawford ES, Morris GC Jr, Garrett HE, et al. Dissecting aneurysms of the aorta. The Surgical Clinics of North America. 1966;**46**:1045-1055

[36] Crawford ES. Thoraco-abdominal aortic aneurysms involving renal, superior mesenteric and celiac arteries. Annals of Surgery. 1974;**179**:763-772

[37] Svensson LG, Crawford ES. Cardiovascular and Vascular Disease of the Aorta. Philadelphia, Pennsylvania: W.B. Saunders Company; 1997. p. 472

[38] Crawford ES, Crawford JL. Diseases of the Aorta: Including an Atlas of Angiographic Pathology and Surgical Technique. Vol. 401. Baltimore, USA: Williams & Wilkins; 1984

[39] Coselli JS, LeMaire SA. Open surgery for type I and II thoracoabdominal aortic aneurysms with the branched Coselli graft. In: Chiesa R, Melissano G, Alfred O, editors. Aortic Surgery «How to Do It» II. Italy: Arti Grafiche Colombo s.r.l.; 2006. pp. 80-81

[40] Kondoh H, Funatsu T, Taniguchi K. Modified technique for reconstructing the visceral arteries in thoracoabdominal aortic repair. Journal of Cardiac Surgery. 2013;**28**(1):56-58. DOI: 10.1111/jocs.12042. Epub: 10 December 2012

[41] Estrera AL, Sandhu H, Afifi RO, Azizzadeh A, Charlton-Ouw K, Miller CC, et al. Open repair of chronic complicated type B aortic dissection using the open distal technique. Annals of Cardiothoracic Surgery. 2014;**3**(4):375-384. DOI: 10.3978/j.issn.2225-319X.2014.07.07

[42] Kouchoukos NT, Daily BB, Rokkas CK, et al. Hypothermic bypass and circulatory arrest for operations on the descending thoracic and thoracoabdominal aorta. The Annals of Thoracic Surgery. 1995;**60**(1):67-76; discussion 76-7

[43] Kouchoukos NT, Masetti P, Rokkas CK, Murphy SF, Blackstone EH. Safety and efficacy of hypothermic cardiopulmonarybypass and circulatory arrest for operationson the descending thoracic and thoracoabdominal aorta. The Annals of Thoracic Surgery. 2001;**72**:699-707

[44] Mavroudis CD, Karlsson M, Ko T, et al. Cerebral mitochondrial dysfunction associated with deep hypotermic circulatory arrest in neonatal swine. European Journal of Cardio-Thoracic Surgery. 2018

[45] Harrington DK, Fragomeni F, Bonser RS. Cerebral perfusion. The Annals of Thoracic Surgery. 2007;**83**:799-804

[46] Gripper RB. Cerebral protection during aortic arch surgery. The Journal of Thoracic and Cardiovascular Surgery. 2001;**121**:425-427

[47] Etz CD, Halstead JC, Spielvogel D, et al. Thoracic and thoracoabdominal aneurysm repair: Is reimplantation of spinal cord arteries a waste of time? The Annals of Thoracic Surgery. 2006;**82**:1670-1678

[48] Omura A, Tanaka A, Miyahara S, Sakamoto T, Nomura Y, Inoue T, et al. Early and late results of graft replacement for dissecting aneurysm of thoracoabdominal aorta in patients with Marfan syndrome. The Annals of Thoracic Surgery. 2012;**94**(3):759-765. DOI: 10.1016/j.athoracsur.2012.04.061. Epub: 20 July 2012

[49] Umana JP, Miller DC, Mitchell RS. What is the best treatment for patients with acute type B aortic dissections—Medical, surgical, or endovascular stent-grafting? The Annals of Thoracic Surgery. 2002;**74**(5):S1840-3; discussion S57-63

[50] Estrera AL, Miller CC, Goodrick J, Porat EE, Achouh PE, Dhareshwar J, et al. Update on outcomes of acute type B aortic dissection. The Annals of Thoracic Surgery. 2007;**83**:S842e5

[51] Bozinovski J, Coselli JS. Outcomes and survival in surgical treatment of descending thoracic aorta with acute dissection. The Annals of Thoracic Surgery. 2008;**85**:965e70

[52] Trimarchi S, Nienaber CA, Rampoldi V, Myrmel T, Suzuki T, Bossone E, et al. Role and results of surgery in acute type B aortic dissection: Insights from the International Registry of Acute Aortic Dissection (IRAD). Circulation. 2006;**114**(Suppl 1):I357e64

[53] Volodos NL, Karpovich IP, Troyan VI, Kalashnikova Y, Shekhanin VE, Ternyuk NE, et al. Clinical experience of the use of self-fixing synthetic prostheses for remote endoprosthetics of the thoracic and the abdominal aorta and iliac arteries through the femoral artery and as intraoperative endoprosthesis for aorta reconstruction. VASA. Supplementum. 1991;**33**:939

[54] Fattori R, Cao P, De Rango P, Czerny M, Evangelista A, Nienaber C, et al. Interdisciplinary expert consensus document on management of type B aortic dissection. Journal of the American College of Cardiology. 2013;**61**:1661-1678. DOI: 10.1016/j.jacc.2012.11.072

[55] Eggebrecht H, Nienaber CA, Neuhäuser M, et al. Endovascular stent-graft placement in aortic dissection: A meta-analysis. The Journal of Thoracic and Cardiovascular Surgery. 2009;**138**(4):865-872. Epub: 08 April 2009

[56] Grabenwoger M, Alfonso F, Bachet J, et al. Thoracic endovascular aortic repair (TEVAR) for the treatment of aortic diseases: A position statement from the European Association for Cardio-Thoracic Surgery (EACTS) and the European Society of Cardiology (ESC), in collaboration with the European Association of Percutaneous Cardiovascular Interventions (EAPCI). European Heart Journal. 2012;**33**(13):1558-1563. DOI: 10.1093/eurheartj/ehs074

[57] Leurs LJ, Bell R, Degrieck Y, et al. Endovascular treatment of thoracic aortic diseases: Combined experience from the EUROSTAR and United Kingdom Thoracic Endograft registries. Journal of Vascular Surgery. 2004;**40**(4):670-679; discussion 9-80

[58] Zhorzholiani Sh. T, Talygin EA, Krasheninnikov SV, Tsigankov Yu M, Agafonov AV, Gorodkov AY, et al. Elasticity change along the aorta is a mechanism for supporting the physiological self-organization of tornado-like blood flow. I. SSN 0362-1197. Human Physiology. 2018;**44**(5):532-540

[59] Koschyk DH, Nienaber CA, Knap M, Hofmann T, Kodolitsch YV, Skriabina V, et al. How to guide stent-graft implantation in type B aortic dissection? Comparison of angiography, transesophageal echocardiography, and

intravascular ultrasound. Circulation. 2005;**112**:I260-I264

[60] Dong ZH, Fu WG, Wang YQ, et al. Retrograde type A aortic dissection after endovascular stent graft placement for treatment of type B dissection. Circulation. 2009;**119**:735-741

[61] Eggebrecht H, Thompson M, Rousseau H, Czerny M. Lönn L, Mehta RH et al.; European Registry on Endovascular Aortic Repair Complications. Retrograde ascending aortic dissection during or after thoracic aortic stent graft placement: Insight from the European registry on endovascular aortic repair complications. Circulation. 2009;**120**:S276-S281

[62] Sunder-Plassmann L, Orend KH. Stentgrafting of the thoracic aorta-complications. The Journal of Cardiovascular Surgery. 2005;**46**(2):121-130

[63] Millen AM, Osman K, Antoniou GA, McWilliams RG, Brennan JA, Fisher RK. Outcomes of persistent intraoperative type Ia endoleak after standard endovascular aneurysm repair. Journal of Vascular Surgery. 2015;**61**:1185-1191. DOI: 10.1016/ j.jvs.2014.12.041 3

[64] Huang W, Yang F, Luo J, Xie N, He P, Luo S, et al. Outcomes and morphologic changes of immediate type Ia endoleak following endovascular repair of acute type B aortic dissection. Annals of Vascular Surgery. 2014;**29**:174-182. DOI: 10.1016/ j.avsg.2014.10.015 4.

[65] Matsumura J, Lee W, Mitchell R, et al. The society for vascular surgeon practice guidelines: Management of the left subclavian artery with thoracic endovascular aortic repair. Journal of Vascular Surgery. 2009;**50**:1155-1158

[66] Fattorri R, Nienaber C, Rousseau H, et al. Result of endovascular repair of the thoracic aorta with the Talent thoracic stent graft: The Talent Thoracic Retrospective Registry. The Journal of Thoracic and Cardiovascular Surgery. 2006;**132**:332-339

[67] Freezor R, Lee W. Strategies for detection and prevention of spinal cord ischemia during TEVAR. Seminars in Vascular Surgery. 2009;**22**:187-192

[68] Zamor KC, Eskandari MK, Rodriguez HE, et al. Outcomes of thoracic endovascular aortic repair and subclavian revascularization techniques. Journal of the American College of Surgeons. 2015;**221**:93e101

[69] Mangialardi N, Ronchey S, Malaj A, et al. Value and limitations of chimney grafts to treat arch lesions. The Journal of Cardiovascular Surgery. 2015;**56**:503e511

[70] Hogendoorn W, Schlösser FJV, Moll FL, Sumpio BE, Muhs BE. Thoracic endovascular aortic repair with chimney graft technique. Journal of Vascular Surgery. 2013;**58**:502-511. DOI: 10.1016/j. jvs.2013.03.043

[71] Samura M, Zempo N, Ikeda Y, et al. Chimney technique for aortic dissection involving an aberrant right subclavian artery. The Annals of Thoracic Surgery. 2014;**97**(1):315-317. DOI: 10.1016/j. athoracsur. 2013.05.094

[72] Azevedo AI, Braga P, Rodrigues A, Ferreira N, Fonseca M, Dias A, et al. Persistent type I endoleak after endovascular treatment with chimney technique. Frontiers in Cardiovascular Medicine. 2016;**3**:32. DOI: 10.3389/fcvm.2016.00032

[73] Bosiersa MJ, Donas KP, Mangialardi N, Torsello G, Riambau V, Criado FJ, Veith FJ, Ronche S, Fazzini S, Lachat M.European Multicenter Registry for the Performance of the Chimney/ Snorkel Technique in the Treatment of Aortic Arch Pathologic Conditions. The Annals of Thoracic Surgery.

Volume 101, Issue 6, June 2016, Pages 2224-2230. https://doi.org/10.1016/j.athoracsur.2015.10.112

[74] Haulon S, Kratzberg J, Guihaire J. Fabre current status of Arch Branch Technology. Endovascular Today. 2018;**17**(11):71-76

[75] Haulon S, Greenberg RK, Spear R, et al. Global experience with an inner branched arch endograft. The Journal of Thoracic and Cardiovascular Surgery. 2014;**148**:1709-1716

[76] Tsilimparis N, Debus E, von Kodolitsch Y, et al. Branched versus fenestrated endografts for endovascular repair of aortic arch lesions. Journal of Vascular Surgery. 2016;**64**:592-599

[77] Lee JT, Lee GK, Chandra V, Dalman RL. Comparison of fenestrated endografts and the snorkel/chimney technique. Journal of Vascular Surgery. 2014;**60**:849-856

[78] Montelione N, Pecoraro F, Puippe G, et al. A 12 year experience with chimney and periscope grafts for treatment of type I endoleaks. Journal of Endovascular Therapy. 2015;**22**:568-574

[79] Scali ST, Feezor RJ, Chang CK, Waterman AL, Berceli SA, et al. Critical analysis of results after chimney endovascular aortic aneurysm repair raises cause for concern. Journal of Vascular Surgery. 2014;**60**:865-873

[80] Lobato AC, Camacho-Lobato L, Cury M. Applying sandwich techniques for complex aortoiliac and thoracoabdominal aortic aneurysms. Endovascular Today. 2016;**15**(3):82-87

[81] Lobato AC, Camacho-Lobato L. A new technique to enhance endovascular thoracoabdominal aortic aneurysm therapy: The sandwich procedure. Seminars in Vascular Surgery. 2012;**25**:153-160

[82] Zhang L, Zhao Z, Chen Y, Sun Y, Bao J, Jing Z, et al. Re-intervention after endovascular repair for aortic dissection: A systematic review and meta-analysis. The Journal of Thoracic and Cardiovascular Surgery. 2016;**152**:1279-1288.e3

[83] Moulakakis KG, Mylonas SN, Dalainas I, Kakisis J, Kotsis T, Liapis CD. Management of complicated and uncomplicated acute type B dissection. A systematic review and meta-analysis. Annals of Cardiothoracic Surgery. 2014;**3**:234-246

[84] Preventza O, Coselli JS. The solution is in the future, but hopefully it won't always be. The Journal of Thoracic and Cardiovascular Surgery. 2016;**152**: 1289-90 0022-5223/$36.00

[85] Sultan I, Siki MA, Bavaria JE, et al. Predicting distal aortic remodeling after endovascular repair for chronic DeBakey III aortic dissection. The Annals of Thoracic Surgery. 2018;**105**(6):1691-1696. DOI: 10.1016/j.athoracsur.2018.01.006. Epub 2018 Jan 31. PubMed PMID: 29391144

[86] Lichtenfels E, Frankini AD, Cardozo MA, et al. Stent graft infection. Jornal Vascular Brasileiro. 2011;**10**(1):50-54

[87] Trent MS, Parsonnet V, Shoenfeld R, et al. A balloon-expandable intravascular stent for obliterating experimental aortic dissection. Journal of Vascular Surgery. 1990;**11**(5):707-717

[88] Gherli T, Agostinelli A, Borrello B, et al. Combined treatment of acute type A aortic dissection with surgical and endovascular procedures. In: Aortic Surgery Symposium Materials. New York; 2006

[89] Roux D, Brouchet L, Ph C, et al. Type-A acute aortic dissection: Combined operation plus stent

management. The Annals of Thoracic Surgery. 2002;**73**:1616-1618

[90] Czerny M, Stöhr S, Aymard T, et al. Effect on false-lumen status of a combined vascular and endovascular approach for the treatment of acute type A aortic dissection. European Journal of Cardio-Thoracic Surgery. 2012;**41**(2):409-413. DOI: 10.1016/j.ejcts.2011.05.063

[91] Vazquez A, Garcia-Vivo R, Gil O, Gonzalez-Cruz A, et al. Combined use of covered and noncovered stent grafts for complete endovascular repair in complicated type B aortic dissection with visceral malperfusion. In: Aortic Symposium Materials. New York; 2012

[92] Kische S, D'Ancona G, Belu IC, et al. Perioperative and mid-term results of endovascular management of complicated type B aortic dissection using a proximal thoracic endoprosthesis and selective distal bare stenting. European Journal of Cardio-Thoracic Surgery. 2015;**48**:e77-e84

[93] Di Tommaso L, Giordano R, Di Tommaso E, Di Palo G, Iannelli G. Treatment with transfemoral bare-metal stent of residual aortic arch dissection after surgical repair of acute type an aortic dissection. Journal of Thoracic Disease. 2018;**10**(11):6097-6106. DOI: 10.21037/jtd.2018.10.51

[94] Midulla M, Renaud A, Martinelli T, Koussa M, Mounier-Vehier C, Prat A, et al. Endovascular fenestration in aortic dissection with acute malperfusion syndrome: Immediate and late follow up. The Journal of Thoracic and Cardiovascular Surgery. 2011;**142**(1):66e72

[95] Marco LD, Pantaleo A, Leone A, Murana G, Bartolomeo RD, Pacini D. The frozen elephant trunk technique: European Association for Cardio-Thoracic Surgery Position and Bologna Experience. Korean Journal of Thoracic and Cardiovascular Surgery. 2017;**50**:1-7

[96] Kuratani T. Best surgical option for arch extension of type B dissection: The endovascular approach. Annals of Cardiothoracic Surgery. 2014;**3**(3):292-299. DOI: 10.3978/j.issn.2225-319X.2014.04.04

[97] Chiesa R, Tshomba Y, Logaldo D, et al. Hybrid repair of aortic aneurysms and dissections: The European perspective. Texas Heart Institute Journal. 2011;**38**:687-690

[98] Chiesa R, Tshomba Y, Logaldo D, Kahlberg A, Baccellieri D, Apruzzi L. Possible graft-related complications in visceral debranching for hybrid B dissection repair. Annals of Cardiothoracic Surgery. 2014;**3**(4):393-399. DOI: 10.3978/j.issn.2225-319X.2014.05.06

[99] Belov Y, Charchan E, Soborov M. Reconstruction of distal aorta in case of thoraco-abdominal dissection. In: Aortic Symposium Materials. Houston; 2012. p. 11

[100] Pape LA et al. Presentation, diagnosis, and outcomes of acute aortic dissection: 17-year trends from the International Registry of Acute Aortic Dissection. Journal of the American College of Cardiology. 2015;**66**(4):350-358

Chapter 16

Nonresectional-Graded Neo Chordal Dynamic Repair of Mitral Valve: Stress Analysis Induced Surgical Innovation

Pradeep Kumar Radhakrishnan, Gayathri Ananyajyothi Ambat, Nihas Nazer and Nazer Yoosuf Abdul

Abstract

Drawbacks persist relating to irreversibility of leaflet resection, time-consuming leaflet reconstruction with sliding annuloplasty, monoleaflet function, and systolic anterior motion (SAM) risk. Graded neochordal reconstruction mitigates many of these but has the challenge of precise sizing and possibility of leaving excessive tissue, risking SAM. When this reconstruction is based on stress analysis and shear analysis methods the outcome gives the best results. Short term evaluation has been done with good outcomes.

Keywords: mitral valve repair, neochordal reconstruction, non resectional repair techniques, systolic anterior movement-SAM, MRI-Magnetic resonance Imaging Stress analysis, IVT –interventricular triangle, mitral regurgitation-MR, 3DECHO-3 dimensional echocardiography

1. Introduction

Evolution of repair techniques of mitral valve has taken a concurrent route along with that of cardiac surgery itself. From the concept of replacement to repair and now from respect rather than resect approach to the current non resectional method has been due to a better understanding of the dynamic nature of the valve. Stress pattern studies that have currently received a boost with technological advancements [1]. While "resection" techniques are associated with good results, reparability rates stood at around 60–70% for the last decade. We are presenting a new technique based on latest stress and dynamic updates on the valve, which would facilitate near to 100% reparability rates in future. All current studies support our view of adopting a completely nonresectional method in mitral valve repair – or the dynamic Indian Correction as we call it.

IntechOpen

2. Statistics

Mitral valve repair done via non resectional methods from January 2017 to November 2017 is included. Preoperative analysis included cardiac MRI and 3 D echocardiography. 25 patients who underwent non resectional methods during this period and techniques are discussed. Patients who underwent leaflet resection, LVEF less than 45%, reoperative mitral valve repairs, beating heart repairs or who underwent minimally invasive procedures during this period were excluded from the study. Intraop TEE was used in all cases. Approach to the mitral valve was through the superior septal approach with initial assessment done on beating heart. Repair was fashioned on arrested heart. After analysis of the valve artificial chordae were created with CV5 and CV6 e PTFE sutures (Gore-Tex R, WL Gore and associates Flagstaff AZ). Graded reconstruction with suture thickness simulating natural chordal stress patterns were used. The suture was first placed in the fibrous part of the papillary muscle. Pledgets and suture tie was avoided in the papillary muscle to minimize chances of ischemia, by taking a simple U stitch. The apposition points are marked on the anterior or posterior leaflets so that 1/3rd of the anterior leaflet enters the coapting zone (**Figure 1**). Slight billowing of anterior leaflet should be permitted as it reduces the stress. Intial position of neochordae can be fixed with a clip placed lightly 1.5 mm below the annular plane. Suture goes back through the leaflet edge from the atrial to the ventricular side placing knots on the ventricular side. The leaflet was drawn down into the ventricle so that the prolapse was eliminated and area of good zone of coaptation is ensured- usually 1/3rd. Peak height of coaptation point should be only up to the plane of annulus. Use the annular plane as a guide for fixing the neo chordal length. As many neochordae as deemed necessary is created following the natural line of attachment to papillary muscle. Avoid crossing the midline. Strut chordae are never excised. Repair methods are individualized as deemed necessary to shorten leaflet height of anterior leaflet or straightening of posterior leaflet margin. Plication of annulus at P2 and P3 needs to be done in ischemic lesions involving posterior wall. Pulling together of papillary muscles with Gore Tex sutures are done if more than 2 cm apart. Chordal shortening is avoided. In such cases leaflet folding by transferring tissue from atrial to coaptation zone is done. Coaptation zone along neochordae creation allows maximum coaptation at centre and less towards commissures as in the normal valve. Excess leaflet tissue may require plication. Sub commissural fusion has to be released. Chordal splitting

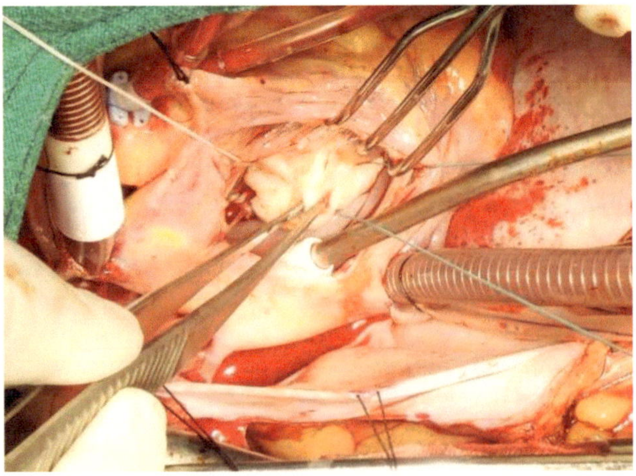

Figure 1.
Mitral valve non resectional graded chordal neoconstruction method.

is done in an individual fashion depending on the pathology. Leaflet thinning and open commissurotomy may be required in rheumatic lesions. Reduction annuloplasty ring is fashioned making allowance for a push up of the ring at the interventricular triangle region of the anterior leaflet to allow for the postero superior movement of the annulus. Keep the posterior leaflet height less than 2 cm. Diastolic and systolic assessment of repair is then done. Post bypass intraop TEE is done to confirm the results. Repair can be assessed in systole in beating heart before atrial septal closure or by simultaneous saline filling of aortic root and left ventricle. No residual mitral regurgitation is accepted. Repair success rate was 100%. No patients underwent mitral valve replacement. All repairs were successful on the first attempt.

3. Methodology

The data was analyzed using SPSS version 13.0 for windows XP. Descriptive statistics for continuous variables are expressed as median or mean as needed while qualitative variables expressed as percentage and $P < 0.05$ being considered significant.

4. Results

Demographic and clinical data was obtained from the hospital records. Mean age was 63 ± 7.7, 15 were male. All patients were in NYHA class III.2 patients required tricuspid valve repair and 4 patients needed coronary bypass surgery. Interpapillary distance in patients with inferior wall involvement was 31 ± 3 mm. One patient required LA myxoma removal. Median surgical risk based on Logistic Euroscore was 3.95% (2.38%). Median Total cross clamp time was 74 ± 7 min. Total extracorporeal time being a median of 120 (80 to 146) minutes. 4 neochordae were created in 10, 6 in 12, 2 in 3 patients. 28 sized annuloplasty ring was used in one patient, 30 in 12 patients, 32 in 11 patients and 34 in 1patient. Mean coaptation height achieved was 8 ± 3 mm. 25 patients had zero MR on post bypass TEE. No patients had SAM. Preoperative annular area was 19.2 ± 4 cm^2 and post op being 7.7 ± 2 cm^2 by 3D methods showing a reduction efficiency of 60%. The median ICU stay was 2 days (1–10) days and median total hospital stay was 7 days (5–17) days. One patient had atrial fibrillation which reverted with pharmacological therapy, 1 case of acute renal failure in a patient with chronic renal failure and type 1 neurological dysfunction in one patient. Preop ROA was median 9.10 (6.1–26.4) to post op of 1.10 (0.3–2.1) cm^2 $P = 0.001$. At follow up of 90 days the median ROA was −0.50 (0.9 cm^2) $P = 0.001$. LVEF was median of 63% (30–77) before surgery to 68% (55–80) post op $P = 0.14$. Clinical follow-up was 100%. 25 patients are alive, and all were free of MR signs and symptoms. No patient required reoperation for recurrent MR. Echocardiographic follow-up has been obtained at the discretion of the referring cardiologists. Echocardiograms have been obtained on all patients with a mean follow-up of 1 year. All cause mortality at 30 days, 60 days, 90 days; 1 year after surgery has been zero. No reoperations were needed due to recurrent mitral regurgitation, no new onset atrial fibrillation or embolism or endocarditis was noted. No death, reoperations, heart failure, endocarditis, thromboembolism or pacemaker implantations were needed in any of these patients on follow up until Dec 25th 2017 (median of 9 months). Follow-up was performed till Dec 25 2017 was 100% complete for survival. All patients are currently in NYHA class I.

5. Discussion

Mitral valve has stood the test for evolution and the extreme dynamic nature brings forth a great concept of engineering skills to repair and hold on to this precious tissue. Resection creates extreme stress and should be avoided at all costs. To replace when repair is feasible is a sin with our current understanding and technological evolution. Long term durability and SAM were intriguing concepts which made surgeons adopt technological modifications, but reparability rates remained constant in the last decade in most advanced cardiac centers around the world. The understanding of the intervalvular triangle as an important part of anterior leaflet and the concept of avoiding placing a horizontal stiff ring across it was emphasized by the American correction version of mitral repairs. Mitral valve stress analysis shows at the beginning of systole the marginal chordae carries the maximum stress. Stress increases now on the strut chordae in mid systole with more of leaflet coaptation with entire stress transfer to annulus during late systole with good leaflet coaptation [2, 3]. With annular dilatation stress is evenly distributed to all valvular structures and that is the reason why mitral regurgitation tends to be a progressive disease. Normal valve dynamics ensure optimal diastolic locking, proper zone of coaptation with excellent left ventricular outflow dynamics and smooth leaflet and chordal stress distribution. Of the various geometric, kinetic and structural factors that can lead to SAM, impaired aorto mitral coupling dynamics are most significant. It is important to avoid rigid and undersized rings which not only alter coupling dynamics but reduce the aorto mitral angle [4–7] also that lead to both LV inflow and outflow obstructions. Failures to recognize the interventricular component of anterior leaflet and aortomitral coupling dynamics are important reasons for failure of repair of this segment. Avoid resection and true sized annuloplasty rings that take the interventricular triangle are keys to success. Ischemic mitral regurgitation often with sagging P2 P3 areas require annuloplasty to correct this portion and then bringing the papillary muscles to within 2cm of each other before placing the ring – for which a true sized ring would be most effective. The goals of the Indian method of correction would be explained as follows

1. Eliminate mitral regurgitation

2. Ensure normal leaflet coaptation

3. Restore normal annular dynamics

4. Maintain normal left ventricular outflow dynamics

5. Restore stress ratios to normal thereby enhancing durability of repair.

6. Graded Neochordal reconstruction of the valve chordae for natural stress redistribution

It is an excellent reproducible and safe procedure with 0.2% mortality [8]. Failure with repair techniques to due to leaving behind areas of stress which has to be meticulously avoided by proper assessment and optimal repair [9].

6. Stress analysis

Current state of biomechanical and micro structural characterizations of the chordae tendineae, and shear stress areas are discussed in this with a new Indian surgical repair technique that takes advantage of this knowledge to repair the valve with better long term outcomes. This almost eliminates chordal failure in repairs making it durable. Customarily, finite element analysis (FEA) is used to predict material stress and strain fields rendered by applying a load on an initially unloaded model. MV leaflets are relatively non deformed during systolic loading. Leaflet strain in vivo is measured using sono micrometry in an ovine model, hybrid models of normal human MVs as constructed using transesophageal real-time 3-D echocardiography (rt-3DE) loaded repeatedly using FEA, and serial rt-3DE images of normal human MVs used to construct models at end diastole and end isovolumic contraction to detect any deformation during isovolumic contraction. Human MV deformed minimally during isovolumic contraction, as measured by the mean absolute difference calculated over the surfaces of both leaflets between serial MV models: 0.53 ± 0.19 mm. FEA modeling of MV models derived from in vivo high-resolution truly 3-D imaging is reasonable and useful for stress prediction in MV pathologies and repairs. Customarily, FEA is used to predict material stress and strain fields rendered by applying a load on an initially unloaded model. In general, the approach has been to use highly idealized and simplistic geometric models to analyze ex vivo or anatomically idealized MVs to assess physiology; to analyze standardized pathological valves to predict stress distribution and, potentially, the integrity and failure behavior of repair techniques; to "evaluate proposed surgical repairs" using idealized computational models, including models that attempt integration of fluid-structure interactions; or to evaluate pathological alterations on the function of idealized computational models. Superimposed tissue formation which is a main determinant of leaflet thickening in MVP, is related to increased stresses over the leaflets.

Chordae can be classified as true or false or as basal, marginal or strut chordae [8–10]. The commissural chordae also is a name that we have added to this as it is slightly thicker and helps to modify the surgical repair technique. Interestingly mitral valve (MV) anterior leaflet chordae are thicker than the MV posterior leaflet chordae [11]. Load or stress bearing is the strut chordae in the normal valve and it shifts to marginal chordae in leaftlet prolapse and makes this susceptible to rupture. On an average 25 chordae attached to an atrioventricular valve dissipates off the shear stress of systolic closure. The fact that stress and chordal thickness are linked can be understood by proper analysis of fetal hearts which shows thinner chordae.

Mitral chordae microstructure shows forms of collagen: (i) a mostly straight, dense, collagen fiber core (ii) widely spaced collagen fibers that wrap around the straight collagen fiber core with some angle of alignment on the primary axis. Fiber size and stress are again related. Tricuspid chordae have a greater collagen fiber density and a smaller fiber diameter, as these are subjected only to right heart pressures significantly lower than the right. From out in the arrangement is elastin sheath with fiber orientation at angles to longitudinal axis, straight fibers, undulated collagen fibers with circumferential orientation and a longitudinal structure in the centre. Diseases like myxomatous degeneration affect chordae more than the leaflets increasing its water and glycosaminoglycan contents. Proteoglycans contribute to calcification also. This promotes defective formation of elastin and collagen. In rheumatic involvement the collagen core is affected and fibrosis is an accompaniment.

Chordae even have blood supply and could be vehicles through which nutrient supply also reaches the leaflets. Distinct elastin layer and planar undulated collagen fibers are unique to human species showing some evolutionary advantage even in the micro structural design. Structure and mechanics decide on material properties in nature and emulating them could be the reason for success in surgical approaches to the valve too. Even while studying strut chordae the radial pattern of collagen fibers is seen for those inserted more anteriorly while circumferential pattern is noted in those inserting closer to annulus. Organized cross networking of collagen is noted at papillary muscle chordal junction also.

The microstructure of artificial chordae should also be looked into. The smooth micro porous structure which reduces thrombogenicity is the cause of calcification and rupture later.

Chordal biomechanics can be evaluated and demonstrated in labs using (i) uniaxial tensile testing; (ii) stress-relaxation testing; (iii) chordae-leaflet insertion region testing; and (iv) in vitro flow loop testing. Chordal ruptured at a strain of 21.4% and a stress of 3.1 × 108 dyne/cm^2. Tricuspid chordae are less extensible when compared with mitral chordae in uniaxial tensile testing. Aging causes the chordae to become stiffer. Interestingly rupture strains of myxomatous and normal chordae are similar. Here shifting of strain from basal to marginal chordae may be the precipitating factor for chordal rupture.

strut chordae to have the fastest and greatest relaxation behavior (49.1 ± 5.4%), followed by the basal chordae (42.4 ± 8.3%), and then the marginal chordae (33.2 ± 4.7%). Strut chordae are stiffer than the marginal and basal chordae; (ii) the basal chordae has greater extensibility than the marginal chordae; (iii) the mitral valve chordae were stiffer than their tricuspid valve counterparts; and (iv) the chordae attaching to the tricuspid valve septal leaflet are more extensible than the chordae attaching to the other two tricuspid valve leaflets. Studies using tensile testing devices have shown that marginal chordae ruptures at 68% less load and 28% less strain than the basal chordae. Posterior leaftlet chordae of mitral valve ruptures at 43% less load and 22% less strain compared with anterior leaftlet chordae. These factors clearly support the graded neochordal reconstruction of the mitral valve retaining the full advantages of the non resectional approach. Marginal chordae have the largest glycosaminoglycan concentrations and the smallest relaxation pattern while the strut chordae had the greatest relaxation pattern, but the lowest glycosaminoglycan content. Biaxial testing shows that the leaflet and papillary muscle insertions have a higher molecular strain than the rest of the chordae. Chordae experienced a strain rate of 75.3 ± 3.43% during systolic closure and a strain rate of −54.8 ± −56.6% during diastolic opening. Constant plateau of the chordal strain between 3.75% and 4.29% during valve closure is also noted in various studies. In this regard the greater compliance of e PTFE chordae could in fact be a surgical advantage [12, 13].

Knowledge is evolving about better understanding and importance of the chordae tendineae of the atrioventricular valves. Morphology and microstructure of the chordae and chordal subsets have been well-defined. There are no standard protocols for investigating chordae mechanics or microstructure as of now, though some investigators like us have ventured out into this area which will help future researchers as time progresses and better evaluation methods are available. Tissue mechanics of MV strut chordae have been well characterized, but future studies are warranted regarding the mechanics of TV chordae. These should be linked to stress analysis and microstructure changes for human chordae. Improved therapy and treatment outcomes with long term effects would result from such studies.

Chordae tendineae are critical to distributing shear stress during systolic movements of leaflets to the papillary muscles, preventing leaflet prolapse and regurgitation. Suboptimal outcomes with repair techniques are due to inability to understand [14–16]. Mechanics and microstructure of the chordae tendineae of these atrioventricular heart valves should be kept in mind and linked to the shear stress analysis on an individual patient basis and surgical repair techniques tailored according to it.

The chordae structures redistribute strain to the papillary muscles during systolic closure and prevent leaflet prolapse. The major stress occurs in the coapting leaftlet belly. In the case of chordae failure, such as elongation or chordal rupture with prolapse the shear stress points align along the tips of the leaflets. Uncontrolled regurgitation ends in cardiac failure. Leaftlet prolapse secondary to chordal rupture can be triggered by lower ventricular pressures. Major surgical approaches to counter chordal failure include shortening, transposition, and replacement. Shortening has been traditionally described to the superior to transposition in terms of freedom from late significant regurgitation [17]. Vulnerability to rupture is a concern which is overcome with the construction of neochordae. There is still a 13% incidence of recurrent regurgitation with such techniques [18]. Concerns include elongation of the synthetic chordae, rupture of the native chordae, calcification, or recurrent prolapse potentially caused by an elastic modulus higher than that of the native chordae still weigh in the mind of the surgeon [19–22]. Refinement of computational modelling methods and simulation tools may bring forth greater points that could be useful in the modification of surgical techniques and make treatment more individualized [23, 24]. Amalgamation of knowledge of morphology, microstructure and mechanics with material property knowledge of replacement materials will give surgical techniques the much needed support of durability in mitral valve repairs in the years to come [25–27].

7. Conclusion

The Indian Dynamic Correction of mitral valve differs from the French correction that there is no resection of the valve and from American correction in that a complete physio ring is used preserving the aorto mitral dynamics with graded Neochordal reconstruction which would simulate the natural stress redistribution dynamics. This would in future ensure 100% reparability and would increase the percentage of valve repairs in all centres. Stress dynamics enforce the need for proper surgical correction and the fallibility of the developing percutaneous concept in ignoring the aorto mitral dynamics..There is growing evidence showing that the "non-resection" technique has some potential advantages including: (I) preserved leaflet mobility; (II) larger surface of coaptation; (III) no changes in annular geometry; and (IV) implantation of larger prosthetic annuloplasty ring. The leaflet is the most precious part of the valve so preserve it. Mitraclips placed severely damage the valve and placing it has only options of replacing the valve if it fails. Current percutaneous methods fail to relieve the stress ratios and would certainly fail in the long run and surgery would remain the gold standard in future.

This paper was presented at the video Micro-symposium of Indian Association of Cardiothoracic Surgeons Held at Visakhapatanam India from Feb 1-5 -2018.

Author details

Pradeep Kumar Radhakrishnan[1*], Gayathri Ananyajyothi Ambat[2], Nihas Nazer[3] and Nazer Yoosuf Abdul[4]

1 Chief Division of Cardiothoracic and Vascular Surgery, Programme Coordinator Total Artificial Heart and Mechanical Circulatory Assist, GIMSR GITAM University India, Mentor Biovalley World Innovation Hub, India

2 Medical Student, GIMSR GITAM UNIVERSITY

3 Junior Resident Cardiac Surgery, Travancore Medical College Hospital, Kerala, India

4 Director and Chief Division of Cardiothoracic and Vascular Surgery, Travancore Medical College Hospital, Kerala, India

*Address all correspondence to: rpksai@hotmail.com

References

[1] Kobayashi J, Sasako Y, Bando K, Minatoya K, Niwaya K, Kitamura S. Ten-year experience of chordal replacement with expanded polytetrafluoroethylene in mitral valve repair. Circulation. 2000;**102**(Suppl 3):III30-III34

[2] Chiappini B, Sanchez A, Noirhomme P, Verhelst R, Rubay J, Poncelet A, et al. Replacement of chordae tendineae with polytetrafluoroethylene (PTFE) sutures in mitral valve repair: early and long-term results. *J Heart Valve Dis*. 2006;**15**:657-663

[3] Coutinho GF, Carvalho L, Antunes MJ. Acute mitral regurgitation due to ruptured e PTFE neo-chordae. *J Heart Valve Dis*. 2007;**16**:278-281

[4] Wendy, Tsang Massimiliano, Meineri Rebecca, T. Hahn Federico, Veronesi, Shah Mark, Sandeep Nathan Mark Russo Roberto M. Lang Eric M. Horlick. A three-dimensional Echocardiographic study on aortic–mitral coupling in transcatheter aortic valve replacement. *European Heart Journal - Cardiovascular Imaging*, 2013;10:1: 950-956

[5] Orszulak, T.A.; Schaff, H.V.; Danielson, G.K.; Piehler, J.M.; Pluth, J.R.; Frye, R.L.; McGoon, D.C.; Elveback, L.R. Mitral regurgitation due to ruptured chordae tendineae: Early and late results of valve repair. J. Thorac. Cardiovasc. Surg. 1985, 89, 491-498. [CrossRef]

[6] Jeresaty, R.M.; Edwards, J.E.; Chawla, S.K. Mitral valve prolapse and ruptured chordae tendineae. Am. J. Cardiol. 1985, 55, 138-142. [CrossRef] .

[7] Espino DM, Hukins DW, Shepherd DE, Buchan KG. Mitral valve repair: An in-vitro comparison of the effect of surgical repair on the pressure required to cause mitral valve regurgitation. J. Heart. Valve Dis. 2006;**15**:375

[8] Silver, M.D.; Lam, J.H.C.; Ranganathan, N.; Wigle, E.D. Morphology of the human tricuspid valve. Circulation 1971, 43, 333-348. [CrossRef]

[9] Lomholt M, Nielsen SL, Hansen SB, Andersen NT, Hasenkam JM. Differential tension between secondary and primary mitral chordae in an acute in-vivo porcine model. J. Heart. Valve Dis. 2002;**11**:337-345

[10] Lam, J.H.C.; Ranganathan, N.; Wigle, E.D.; Silver, M.D. Morphology of the human mitral valve: I. Chordae tendineae: A new classification. Circulation 1970, 41, 449-458. [CrossRef]

[11] Zuo, K.; Pham, T.; Li, K.; Martin, C.; He, Z.; Sun, W. Characterization of biomechanical properties of aged human and ovine mitral valve chordae tendineae. J. Mech. Behav. Biomed. Mater. 2016, 62, 607-618. [CrossRef]

[12] Revuelta, J.M.; Garcia-Rinaldi, R.; Gaite, L.; Val, F.; Garijo, F. Generation of chordae tendineae with polytetrafluoroethylene stents: Results of mitral valve chordal replacement in sheep. J. Thorac. Cardiovasc. Surg. 1989, 97, 98-103. [CrossRef]

[13] Gunnal, S.A.; Wabale, R.N.; Farooqui, M.S. Morphological study of chordae tendinae in human cadaveric hearts. Heart Views 2015, 16, 1-12. [CrossRef]

[14] Millington-Sanders, C.; Meir, A.; Lawrence, L.; Stolinski, C. Structure of chordae tendineae in the left ventricle of the human heart. J. Anat. 1998, 192, 573-581. [CrossRef] [PubMed]

[15] De Almeida MTB, Aragao ICSA, Aragao FMSA, Reis FP, Aragao JA. Morphological study on mitral valve chordae tendineae in the hearts of

human fetuses. Int. J. Anat. Var. 2019;**12**:17-20

[16] Jett, S.V.; Laurence, D.W.; Kunkel, R.P.; Babu, A.R.; Kramer, K.E.; Baumwart, R.; Towner, R.A.; Wu, Y.; Lee, C.-H. An investigation of the anisotropic mechanical properties and anatomical structure of porcine atrioventricular heart valves. J. Mech. Behav. Biomed. Mater. 2018, 87, 155-171. [CrossRef] [PubMed]

[17] Smedira, N.G.; Selman, R.; Cosgrove, D.M.; McCarthy, P.M.; Lytle, B.W.; Taylor, P.C.; Apperson-Hansen, C.; Stewart, R.W.; Loop, F.D. Repair of anterior leaflet prolapse: Chordal transfer is superior to chordal shortening. J. Thorac. Cardiovasc. Surg. 1996, 112, 287-292. [CrossRef]

[18] Khoiy, K.A.; Asgarian, K.T.; Loth, F.; Amini, R. Dilation of tricuspid valve annulus immediately after rupture of chordae tendineae in ex-vivo porcine hearts. PLoS ONE 2018, 13, e0206744. [CrossRef]

[19] Tabata, M.; Kasegawa, H.; Fukui, T.; Shimizu, A.; Sato, Y.; Takanashi, S. Long-term outcomes of artificial chordal replacement with tourniquet technique in mitral valve repair: A single-center experience of 700 cases. J. Thorac. Cardiovasc. Surg. 2014, 148, 2033-2038.e2031. [CrossRef] [PubMed]

[20] Cochran, R.P.; Kuzelman, K.S. Comparison of viscoelastic properties of suture versus porcine mitral valve chordae tendineae. J. Card. Surg. 1991, 6, 508-513. [CrossRef] [PubMed]

[21] Colli, A.; Manzan, E.; Rucinskas, K.; Janusauskas, V.; Zucchetta, F.; Zakarkaite, D.; Aidietis, A.; Gerosa, G. Acute safety and efficacy of the NeoChord procedure. Interact. Cardiovasc. Thorac. Surg. 2015, 20, 575-581. [CrossRef]

[22] Butany, J.; Collins, M.J.; David, T.E. Ruptured synthetic expanded polytetrafluoroethylene chordae tendinae. Cardiovasc. Pathol. 2004, 13, 182-184. [CrossRef]

[23] Carpentier A, Adams DH, Filsoufi F. Carpentier's Reconstructive Valve Surgery From Valve Analysis to Valve Reconstruction. Philadelphia, PA, USA: Saunders Elsevier Health Sciences; 2011

[24] Phillips, M.R.; Daly, R.C.; Schaff, H.V.; Dearani, J.A.; Mullany, C.J.; Orszulak, T.A. Repair of anterior leaflet mitral valve prolapse: Chordal replacement versus chordal shortening. Ann. Thorac. Surg. 2000, 69, 25-29. [CrossRef]

[25] McQueen, D.M.; Peskin, C.S.; Yellin, E.L. Fluid dynamics of the mitral valve: Physiological aspects of a mathematical model. Am. J. Physiol. Heart Circ. Physiol. 1982, 242, H1095–H1110. [CrossRef]

[26] Lim KH, Yeo JH, Duran C. Three-dimensional asymmetrical modeling of the mitral valve: A finite element study with dynamic boundaries. J. Heart. Valve Dis. 2005;**14**:386-392

[27] Wang, Q.; Sun, W. Finite element modeling of mitral valve dynamic deformation using patient-specific multi-slices computed tomography scans.

Chapter 17

Complications of Minimally Invasive Left Ventricular Assistance Device Implantation

Mleyhi Sobhi, Miri Rim and Denguir Raouf

Abstract

Indication of Ventricular assistance is advanced cardiac failure with maximal medical and surgical treatment has been used. The ventricular assistance has two main purposes: first, to maintain circulation by discharging the ventricle (s) untill to recovery, or to ensure patient survival by replacing cardiac function permanently or transitionally for patients waiting for heart Transplantation. The encouraging results of the partial or total artificial heart and the miniaturization of these devices allow their use in permanent implantation for patients with heart failure that is not eligible for heart transplantation. In left mono-ventricular assistance, blood is taken from the apex of the left ventricle (LV) and reinjected in the ascending aorta. The classic surgical approach is a total median sternotomy. Other minimally invasive approaches for the implantation or explanation of left ventricular assist devices have been published and have shown encouraging results. These alternatives currently play an important role in certain indications and in patients with heavy medical history. Nevertheless, the complications of the ventricular assistance even by minimally invasive approaches might be serious and represent a turning point in the life of the patients. In this chapter, we describe the implantation technique of left ventricular assistance device (LVAD) and we discuss its advantages and disadvantages including possible complications.

Keywords: minimally invasive, surgery, LVAD, implantation, complications

1. Introduction

End-stage heart failure has an increasing incidence and prevalence worldwide. In Germany, 1 to 2% of the population suffers from chronic heart failure, with approximately 80,000 new cases per year. Cardiac transplantation has been the therapy of choice for patients with drug-resistant heart failure, but the decreasing number of donor organs leads to a significant prolongation of the waiting time for cardiac transplantation, resulting in an increased mortality of these patients [1, 2]. Indication of ventricular assistance device is for patients with advanced heart failure in whom maximum medical and surgical treatment has been exhausted. The purpose of ventricular assistance is twofold: first, to maintain circulation by discharging the ventricle (s) untill to recovery, and second, to ensure the survival of the patient by replacing the cardiac function, permanently or while waiting for a heart transplantation [3, 4].

The encouraging results of the partial or total artificial heart and the miniaturization of these devices make it possible to consider their use in permanent implantation for patients with heart failure who are not eligible for heart transplantation.

In left mono-ventricular assistance, the blood is taken through a cannula placed at the apex of the left ventricule (LV) and re-injected to the patient by a vascular prosthesis anastomosed to the ascending aorta. The classic surgical approach is a total midline sternotomy. Alternative minimally invasive approaches for implantation or explantation of left ventricular assist devices have been published and have shown encouraging results [5]. These alternatives currently play an important role in certain precise indications and in the most complex patients. Nevertheless, the complications after the implantation of mechanical assistance, even by a minimally invasive route, are still serious and can be lethal.

The impact of heart failure on individuals and society in general continues to grow. Heart transplantation remains the gold standard for treating patients with end-stage heart failure. The development of artificial hearts, partial and total, was mainly inspired by the disproportion between the number of available grafts and the number of candidates for heart transplantation. The significant technological advances made since Kolff's first work in 1957 allow these patients to return to their homes while awaiting the transplant. The encouraging results of the artificial heart and the miniaturization of these devices now make it possible to consider their use in permanent implantation for patients with heart failure who are not eligible for transplantation [6].

The objectives can be divided into two categories:

- Support and optimization of hemodynamic constants while waiting for the replacement of an irreversibly damaged heart (bridge-to-transplantation). This attitude improves pulmonary hypertension and prevents multiorgan failure [7].

- Definitive implantation of a mechanical heart because the patient has a 1-year mortality greater than 50% but is not a candidate for a heart transplantation (destination therapy); survival then depends on the technical reliability of the system and on intercurrent complications. It is currently 60–86% at 1 year, more than double that of maximum medical treatment [8–11].

Implanted early enough in the course of the disease, ventricular assistance helps restore renal and hepatic functions, reduce pulmonary hypertension, mobilize excess interstitial fluid and prevent the onset of a multiorgan failure. Criteria for LVAD implantation are the persistence of the following settings despite maximum medical treatment:

- Cardiac index <2.0 L/ min/m^2

- Mean arterial pressure (MAP) <60 mmHg, systolic arterial pressure < 80 mmHg.

- Central venous pressure CVP and/or mean arterial pressure > 20 mmHg,

- systemic arterial resistance >2,000 dynes/s/cm-5.

- Lesft ventricular ejection function <0.25

- Venous saturation of oxygen <55%

- diuresis <20 mL/hour.
- Persistent metabolic acidosis.

Assistance is contraindicated in active systemic infection, irreversible neurological impairment, and end-stage renal or hepatic failure. Severe peripheral vascular disease and haematological disorders are relative contraindications [12]. The aortic valve must be continent, otherwise the flow of assistance will flow back into the LV and dilate it. Severe pulmonary hypertension or right heart failure are a contraindication to left monoventricular assistance; in this case, biventricular assistance must be performed (20% of cases).

Of course, ventricular assistance is an expensive therapy. Long-term implanted pumps (destination therapy) represent an expense of around € 220,000 [13]. Ventricular assist systems can be classified in three generations [3, 14]:

- 1st generation: extracorporeal pulsatile devices, often pneumatic, driven by an external console (Thoratec PVAD ™, Abiomed BVS 5000 ™); they are bulky and contain many moving parts, including valves.
- 2nd generation: implantable pulsatile systems, most often electric (HeartMate XVE ™, LionHeart ™, Thoratec IVAD ™).
- 3rd generation: implantable axial flow systems, designed for long periods (HeartMate II ™, Jarvik 2000 ™, BerlinHeart ™); the only moving part is the rotor, valves are unnecessary; the latest models operate by magnetic levitation which eliminates the axes of the rotor, sources of wear.

HEARTMATE LVAD device is a mechanical, continuous flow, electrical, intracorporeal, monoventricular left circulatory device. This system is indicated when the patient's body surface area is ≥1.2 m2 in the following situations:

- Indication in an acute situation: acute mono or biventricular failure in patients with heart failure, not controlled by optimal treatment, in the absence of a conventional therapeutic alternative (drug and / or intervention and/or surgery).
- Elective indication: advanced chronic heart failure with mono or biventricular failure, when life is threatened despite optimal treatment, and at the end of a multidisciplinary consultation.

The contraindications to HEARTMATE mechanical device are:

- severe pulmonary dysfunction and fixed pulmonary arterial hypertension.
- Severe hepatic insufficiency (cirrhosis, portal hypertension, ...).
- Major disorders of blood crass and uncontrolled bleeding.
- Uncontrolled systemic septic and inflammatory syndrome.
- Documented irreversible central nervous system damage, recent stroke and cachexia.

- Systemic diseases with involvement of several organs.
- Psychiatric disorders jeopardizing adherence to treatment and lack of cooperation.
- A condition with a bad prognosis when life expectancy is less than 2 years.
- An untreated septal rupture.
- A body surface area < 1.2 m2.

"HeartMate" is one of the continuous flow systems which are driven by an axial turbine (HeartMate ™ II, BerlinHeart ™, Jarvik 2000 ™, DeBakey MicroMed ™) or a centrifugal pump (HeartMate ™ III). They are implanted by sternotomy or thoracotomy. The blood is taken from the apex of the LV and returned to the ascending or descending aorta through a tubular prosthesis. The assured flow rate is 3 to 10 L/min. These simpler and quieter continuous flow systems are less prone to embolism and infections than pulsatile systems [14, 15]. In addition, they let the heart continue to eject which promotes its recovery.

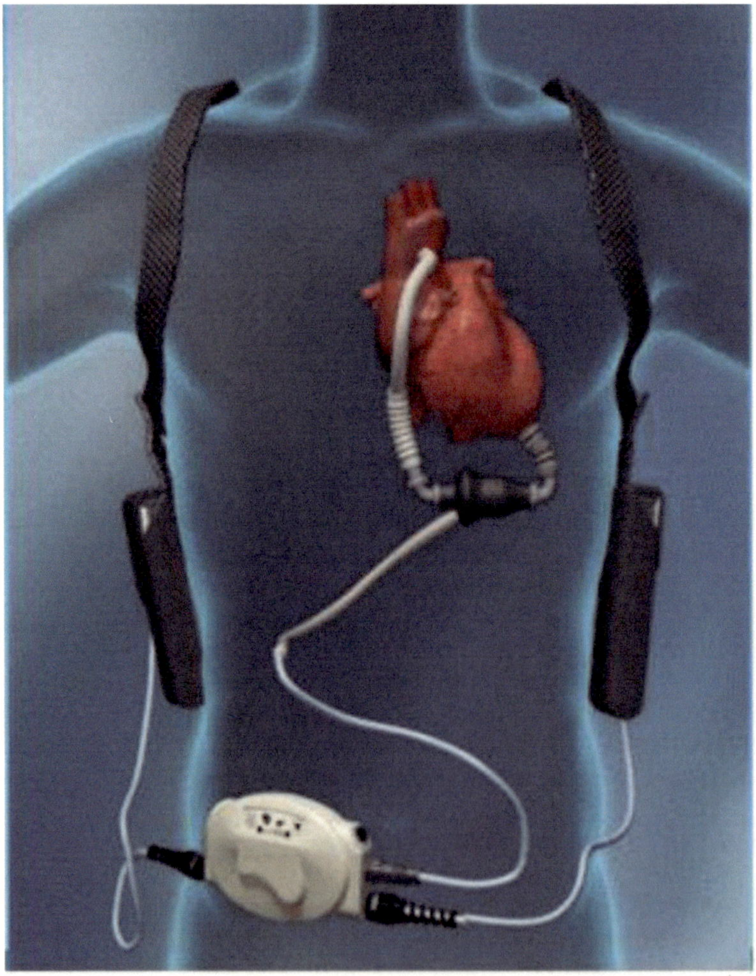

Figure 1.
LVAD device.

Their size is small, and they can be implanted in short patients. The arterial curve is practically flat, the systolic and diastolic blood pressure are the same as the Mean arteriel pressure. The functionality of the LV results in hooks added to this curve; these are all the more important as the LV performs better or the pump output decreases.

The smaller design of the pump and its intrapericardial location has allowed the development of less invasive alternatives and implantation techniques. The technique of left ventricular assistance by minimally invasive approach has been described in several publications [5, 16–19]. It consists of an upper J-shaped mini-sternotomy or an anterior thoracotomy in the 2nd right intercostal space for access to the ascending aorta (site of anastomosis of the ejection voice) as well as to the right atrium (if atriocaval cannulation) and a left subcostal approach or a left anterolateral thoracotomy of 8 to 10 Cm for access to the apex of the heart and implantation of the device (**Figure 1** and **2**).

According to Anson et al. [18], the use of small incisions allows exposure of the exact areas required for cannulation without the need for cardiac manipulation which is often poorly tolerated in these severe patients, and therefore implantation without cardiopulmonary bypass (CBP) becomes possible. In the study of Bantayehu Sileshi et al. [17] including 51 HeartWare implantations for patients waiting for heart transplantation, eighteen of them were with minimally invasive approach without CPB. The choice of the surgical technique was made by a multidisciplinary committee, taking into consideration the contraindications, in particular the respiratory one, for thoracotomy. Univariate analysis revealed a statistically significant reduction in the duration of treatment with inotropic drugs ($p = 0.04$), and reduced intraoperative

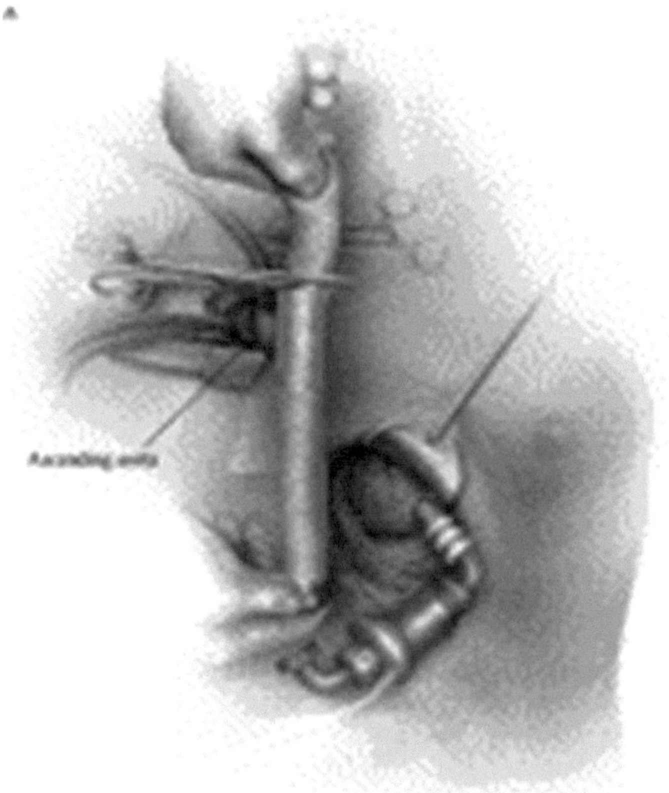

Figure 2.
Minimally invasive LVAD implantation approach.

blood transfusion (p = 0.08) in minimally invasive implantations. Conversly, there was no difference regarding the duration of intensive care stay (p = 0.5), the total intra-hospital saty (p = 0.76) and the total time of mechanical ventilation (p = 0.32). There were four in-hospital deaths and three stroke complications all were operated on by sternotomy under CBP. Authors showd also an increasing risk of infection, bleeding and redo-sternotomy complications at the time of heart transplantation [20].

Less invasive surgical approaches have been developed with the hope of reducing CPB time and operative trauma, minimizing perioperative blood loss, protecting cardiac structures from multiple re-entries, and preserving the heart geometry [21].

Haberl and al. recently described their clinical experience in minimally invasive implantation for HeartWare and HeartMate II [22]. Of the 27 patients in their study, 5 (19%) were performed without CPB. They had a reported in-hospital mortality of 14.8%, and an average hospital stay of 30 days. They concluded that minimally invasive LVAD implantation is feasible and safe. Moreover, Anelechi C [5] thinks that this technique is inadequate for patients who have previously had cardiac surgery without giving any arguments.

Minimally invasive approach was also recommended for the device remove or changing [23–27]. For example, the team of Igor D. Gregoric [23] showed the superiority of the subcostal route alone to change HeartMate XVE by HeratMate II compared to sternotomy with left subcostal approach in terms of transfusion, operative duration and postoperative stay. The same results were found in the study of John m. Stulak and his colleagues [26].

2. Complications

The complications related to the different assistance systems are numerous [11, 28, 29]:

- Infections in 32 to 45% of cases.
- Bleeding in 27% of cases.
- Arrhythmias in24% of cases.
- Thromboembolism and stroke (10–39% depending on the device type)
- Renal failure in 20% of cases.
- Systemic inflammation and lack of cellular immunity.
- Hemolysis: depending on the pump models.

infectious complications are the most serious with 41% of deaths linked to sepsis [30]. Continuous-flow turbine systems have a clearly lower complication rate (infections, thromboses, mechanical problems) than pulsatile systems [31].

There are basically three disadvantages of continuous flow systems:

- malfunction causes the equivalent of acute aortic insufficiency because there is no valve in the system.
- As they generate negative pressure in the LV, the ventricle can collapse with a sudden drop in preload and a risk of air embolism by aspiration of air at the sutures;

- The continuous flow causes stasis in the aortic valve if it no longer opens; this can give rise to thrombi, with the risk of systemic embolization.

Thrombosis of the ventricular assist device (VAD) is associated with significant morbidity and mortality, usually requiring device replacement. Since 2011, there has been a sharp increase in the incidence of VAD thrombosis, from 2.2% before 2011 to 8.4% in 2013 [32]. The exact reason for this increase is unknown and numerous studies aim to identify it [33]. Diagnostic markers, including increased plasma lactate dehydrogenase (LDH), free plasma hemoglobin, or abnormal responses to programmed increases in pump speed (ramp test) [34] should allow early and more accurate diagnosis. [35].

The formation of thrombi in the aortic root in patients implanted with HeartMate II has been previously reported in the literature [36, 37]. The flow in the root of the aorta in patients with continuous flow LVAD has been shown experimentally to be relatively stagnant, especially when the aortic valve does not open [38] and such stasis often involves the non-coronary sinus and can be an important risk factor for thrombosis. Sachin Shah and colleagues [39] report a case of occlusion of the left common coronary trunk by aortic root thrombus in a patient with HeartMate II.

The optimal strategy for the prevention of this complication is not yet well defined; however, special attention to anticoagulation and antiplatelet therapy in the postoperative period, as well as adjusting the pump speed to allow intermittent opening of the aortic valve may be important considerations. For those who develop an aortic root thrombus, but remain asymptomatic, intensification of anticoagulation and antiplatelet therapy alone may sometimes be sufficient [39].

3. Conclusion

In conclusion, with the limited number of organ donors, long-term ventricular support systems are slowly becoming an alternative to heart transplantation. Significant technical advances have allowed the development of small, space-saving ventricular assist devices with fewer complications.

Minimally invasive alternative approaches for implantation or explantation of left ventricular assist devices have become valid and reproducible. Nevertheless, complications, in particular thromboembolic still serious. Only multidisciplinary work associating surgeon, cardiologist and anesthetist with perfect knowledge of the management of these patients and these machines can prevent complications abd death.

Author details

Mleyhi Sobhi*, Miri Rim and Denguir Raouf
Cardiovascular Surgery Department, Faculty of Medicine of Tunis, La Rabta Hospital, University of Tunis el Manar, Tunisia

*Address all correspondence to: mleyhisobhi@yahoo.com

References

[1] Haeck ML, Beeres SL, Höke U, Palmen M, Couperus LE, Delgado V, Logeman EA, Maas JJ, Klautz RJ, Schalij MJ, Verwey HF. Left ventricular assist device for end-stage heart failure: results of the first LVAD destination program in the Netherlands. Neth Heart J. 2015 Feb;23(2):102-108. doi: 10.1007/s12471-014-0602-4.

[2] Christiansen S, Klocke A, Autschbach R. Past, present, and future of long-term mechanical cardiac support in adults. J Card Surg. 2008 Nov-Dec;23(6):664-676. doi: 10.1111/j.1540-8191.2008.00696.x.

[3] TERRACCIANO CM, MILLER LW, YACOUB MH. Contemporary use of ventricular assist devices. Annu Rev Med 2010; 61:255-270.

[4] VEGAS A. Assisting the failing heart. Anesthesiology Clin 2008; 26:539-564.

[5] Anelechi C Anyanwu. Nonsternotomy Approaches to Left Ventricular Assist Device placement: Combined Left Subcostal–Right Minithoracotomy Technique. Operative Techniques in Thoracic and Cardiovascular Surgery. Nov 2014; vol 19(3): 254-275.

[6] E. Flecher, T. Joudinaud, J.-M. Grinda. Histoire de l'assistance circulatoire mécanique et du cœur artificiel. Annales de chirurgie oct 2006; Vol 131(8): 473-478.

[7] CHRISTIANSEN S, KLOCKE A, AUTSCHBACH R. Past, present, and future of long term mechanical cardiac support in adults. J Card Surg 2008; 23:664-676.

[8] BADIWALA MV, RAO V. Left ventricular device as destination therapy: are we there yet ? Curr Opin Cardiol 2009; 24:184-189.

[9] BIRKS EJ, GEORGE RS, HEDGER M, et al. Reversal of heart failure with a continuous-flow left ventricular assistance device and pharmacological therapy. Circulation 2011; 123:381-390.

[10] LONG JW, KFOURY AG, SLAUGHTER MS, et al. Long term destination therapy with the HeartMate XVE left ventricular assist device: improved outcomes since the REMATCH study. Congest Heart Fail 2005; 11:133-138.

[11] ROSE EA, GELIJNS AC, MOSKOWITZ AJ, et al. REMATCH study group. Long-term mechanical left ventricular assistance for end-stage heart failure. N Engl J Med 2001; 345:1435-1443.

[12] EL-MAGHARBEL I. Ventricular assist devices and anesthesia. Semin Cardiothor Vasc Anesth 2005; 9:241-249.

[13] MOHACSI P, STALDER M, MARTINELLI M, et al. Transplantation cardiaque et assistance circulatoire mécanique. Situation actuelle et perspectives. 2ème partie. Forum Med Suisse 2011; 11:98-102.

[14] THUNBERG CA, GAITAN BD, ARABIA FA, et al. Ventricular assist devices today and tomorrow. J Cardiothorac Vasc Anesth 2010: 24:656-680.

[15] FRAZIER OH, GEMMATO C, MYERS TJ, et al. Initial clinical experience with the HeartMate II axial-flow left ventricular assist device. Tex Heart Inst J 2007; 34:275-281.

[16] Chad EW, Julien SB, Jason K, et al. Minimally invasive thoracic left ventricular assist device implantation: Case series demonstrating an integrate multidisciplinary strategy. Journal of

cardiothoracic and vascular anesthesia, avril 2015 vol 29(2):271-274.

[17] Bantayehu S, Nicholas AH, Mary ED et al.In-hospital outcomes of minimally invasive off-pump left thoracotomy approach using a centrifugal continuous-flow left ventricular assist device. J Heart lung Transplant 2015;34:107-112.

[18] Anson C, Yoan L, Annemarie K, et al. Off-pump implantation of the HeratWare HVAD left ventricular assist device through minimally invasive incisions. Ann Thorac Surg 2011; 91:1294-1296.

[19] Schmitto JD, Molitoris U, Haverich A, et al. Implantation of a centrifugal pump as a left ventricular assist device through a novel, minimized approach: upper hemisternotomy combined with antero-lateral thoracotomy. J Thorac Cardiovasc Surg 2012;143:511-513.

[20] Unsworth B, Casula RP, Kyriacou AA, et al. The right ventricular annular velocity reduction caused by coronary artery bypass graft surgery occurs at the moment of pericardial incision. Am Heart J 2010;159:314-322.

[21] Schmitto JD, Mokashi SA, Cohn LH. Minimally-invasive valve surgery. J Am Coll Cardiol 2010;56:455-462.

[22] Haberl T, Riebandt J, Mahr S, Laufer G, Rajek A, Schima H, Zimpfer D. Viennese approach to minimize the invasiveness of ventricular assist device implantation†. Eur J Cardiothorac Surg. 2014 Dec;46(6):991-996; discussion 996. doi: 10.1093/ejcts/ezu051.

[23] Igor D, Brian A, Leon J, et al. Clinical Experience With Sternotomy Versus Subcostal Approach for Exchange of the HeartMate XVE to the HeartMate II Ventricular Assist Device. Ann Thorac Surg 2008;85:1646-1650.

[24] Sajjad M, Butt T, Oezalp F, et al. An alternative approach to explantation and exchange of the HeartWare left ventricular assist device European Journal of Cardio-Thoracic Surgery 43 (2013) :1247-1250.

[25] Diana GS, Prashant NM, Bartlomiej Z, et al. Minimally invasive access for off-pump HeartWare left ventricular assist device explantation. Interactive cardiovascular and thoracic surgery 17 (2013):581-582.

[26] John MS, Jennifer C, Jonathon WH, et al. Device exchange after primary left ventricular assist device implantation: indications and outcomes. Ann Thorac Surg 2013;95:1262-1268.

[27] Rojas SV, Avsar M, Khalpey Z, et al. Minimally invasive pff_pump left ventricular assist device exchange: anterolateral thoracotomy. Artif Organs 2014;38(7):539-542.

[28] DENG MC, EDWARDS LB, HERRTZ MI, et al. Mechanical circulatory support data base of the international society for heart and lung transplantation: second annual report 2004. J Heart Lung Transplant 2004; 23:1027-1034.

[29] STONE ME. Current status of mechanical circulatory assistance. Semin Cardiothor Vasc Anesth 2007; 11:185-204.

[30] CHRISTIANSEN S, KLOCKE A, AUTSCHBACH R. Past, present, and future of long term mechanical cardiac support in adults. J Card Surg 2008; 23:664-676.

[31] MITTER N, SHEINBERG R. Update on ventricular assist devices. Curr Opin Anaesthesiol 2009; 23:57-66.

[32] Starling RC, Moazami N, Silvestry SC, et al. Unexpected abrupt increase in left ventricular assist device

thrombosis. N Engl J Med, 2014; 370:33-40.

[33] Edo Y. Birati MD, J. Eduardo Rame MD. Diagnosis and Management of LVAD Thrombosis. Curr Treat Options Cardio Med, February 2015, 17:2.

[34] Uriel N, Morrison KA, Garan AR, et al. Development of a novel echocardiography ramp test for speed optimization and diagnosis of device thrombosis in continuous-flow left ventricular assist devices: the Columbia Ramp Study. J Am Coll Cardiol, 2012; 60:1764-1765.

[35] Uriel N, Han J, Morrison KA, et al. Device thrombosis in HeartMate II continuous-flow left ventricular assist devices: a multifactorial phenomenon. J Heart Lung Transplant, 2014;33: 51-59.

[36] Freed BH, Jeevanandam V, Jolly N. Aortic root and valve thrombosis after implantation of a left ventricular assist device.J Invasive Cardiol, 2011; 23:63-65.

[37] Demirozu Z, Frazier O. Aortic valve noncoronary cusp thrombosis after implantation of a nonpulsatile, continuous-flow pump. Tex Heart Inst J, 2012, 39 (5):618-620.

[38] Kar B, Delgado R, Frazier O, et al. The effect of LVAD aortic outflow-graft placement on hemodynamics and flow. Implantation technique and computer flow modeling.Tex Heart Inst J, 2005;32: 294-298.

[39] Sachin S, Mehra M, Couper G, Desa A. Continuous flow left ventricular assist device related aortic root thrombosis complicated by left main coronary artery occlusion. The Journal of Heart and Lung Transplantation, 2014; 33 (1):119-120.

Chapter 18

Internal Flow Choking in Cardiovascular System: A Radical Theory in the Risk Assessment of Asymptomatic Cardiovascular Diseases

Valsalayam Raghavapanicker Sanal Kumar, Shiv Kumar Choudhary, Pradeep Kumar Radhakrishnan, Rajaghatta Sundararam Bharath, Nichith Chandrasekaran, Vigneshwaran Sankar, Ajith Sukumaran and Charlie Oommen

Abstract

The theoretical discovery of Sanal flow choking in the cardiovascular system (CVS) demands for interdisciplinary studies and universal actions to propose modern medications and to discover new drugs to annul the risk of flow-choking leading to shock-wave generation causing asymptomatic-cardiovascular-diseases. In this chapter we show that when blood-pressure-ratio (BPR) reaches the lower-critical-hemorrhage-index (LCHI) the flow-choking could occur in the CVS with and without stent. The flow-choking is uniquely regulated by the biofluid/blood-heat-capacity-ratio (BHCR). The BHCR is well correlated with BPR, blood-viscosity and ejection-fraction. The closed-form analytical models reveal that the relatively high and the low blood-viscosity are cardiovascular-risk factors. In vitro data shows that nitrogen, oxygen, and carbon dioxide gases are predominant in fresh blood samples of the human being/*Guinea-pig* at a temperature range of 37–40 °C (98.6–104 °F). In silico results demonstrate the occurrence of Sanal flow choking leading to shock wave generation and pressure-overshoot in CVS without any apparent occlusion. We could conclude authoritatively, without any *ex vivo* or *in vivo* studies, that the Sanal flow choking in CVS leads to asymptomatic-cardiovascular-diseases. The cardiovascular-risk could be diminished by concurrently lessening the viscosity of biofluid/blood and flow-turbulence by increasing the thermal-tolerance level in terms of BHCR and/or by decreasing the BPR.

Keywords: asymptomatic cardiovascular disease, biofluid choking, BHCR, risk factors, sanal flow choking

1. Introduction

The cardiovascular system (blood circulatory system) is an internal fluid flow loop with multiple branches, transport nutrients and oxygen to all cells in the body.

The center of the cardiovascular system (CVS) is the heart, which is accountable to pump blood through the complex network of viscoelastic vessels, viz., arteries, veins and capillaries. Blood flow in CVS is inherently an unsteady phenomenon experiencing with transient events. Blood flow begins when the heart relaxes between two heartbeats. Due to the cyclic nature of the heart the velocity and pressure of the internal fluid (blood/biofluid) circulating through the viscoelastic vessels varies with time. Blood flow in CVS is typically laminar but due to its pulsatile nature makes possible the flow transition to turbulent. Furthermore, the variations in the fluid flow properties and vessel geometry due to pathophysiological reasons, including the seasonal effects, contribute for the transition of laminar flow to turbulent.

Diseases of the CVS are manifold in gravity and microgravity environment (human spaceflight) and afflict millions of patients worldwide including cases of: coronary artery disease (CAD), ischemic gangrene, abdominal aortic aneurysms, moyamoya disease, and stroke. A few of these dysfunctions are reported to be the end result of atherosclerosis, characterized by plaque accumulation within the walls of the arteries. Atherosclerotic cardiovascular disease (CVD) is the leading cause of death for both men and women. There is no clear age cut point for defining the onset of risk for CVD, which is corroborated from the clinically detected elevated risk factor levels and subclinical abnormalities of adolescents as well as young adults. The hemodynamic characteristics of blood flow have long been thought to play an important role in the pathogenesis of atherosclerosis. In light of the discovery of internal flow choking in CVS [1, 2], the hemodynamic characteristics of blood flow need to be examined in detail for exploring the causes and effects of flow choking in gravity and microgravity environment for an authentic conclusion in the risk assessment of asymptomatic cardiovascular diseases.

Heart failure (HF) is the cardiovascular epidemic of the 21st century [2]. Although there has been significant advancement in the diagnosis, prognosis, treatment and prevention of HF with reduced ejection fraction (EF), the morbidity and mortality are still extensive. This is particularly true due to the Covid-19 pandemic (www.escardio.org). The EF is a blood flow measurement in percentage (%), specifying how much blood the left ventricle pumps out with each contraction. The EF measurement under 40% may be an indication of HF or cardiomyopathy. An EF from 41–49% may be considered as "borderline" cases having the history of stroke (memory effect). A normal heart's EF may be between 50–70%. An EF value higher than 75% generally indicates hypertrophic cardiomyopathy (HCM), which could affect people of any age [2]. HCM is reported as a cause of acute HF particularly in young people, including young athletes. Although all these percentage demarcations of the EF are meaningful for the diagnosis, until the discovery of the Sanal flow choking the EF estimations were not supported by any closed-form analytical model for taking brilliant clinical decisions case by case. The recent theoretical discovery of the Sanal flow choking [1, 2] provides an insight for the risk assessment of asymptomatic cardiovascular diseases. Moreover, the Sanal flow choking model could generate universal benchmark data for predicting the condition of internal flow choking in CVS for taking an authentic conclusion on the desirable EF in terms of blood flow percentage for healthy subjects for reducing the risk of acute-heart-failure. The European Society of Cardiology (ESC) reported (2020) that patients with cardiovascular risk factors and established cardiovascular disease (CVD) represent a vulnerable population when suffering from the Covid-19. It is important to note that patients with cardiac injury in the context of Covid-19 have an increased risk of morbidity and mortality.

The acute-heart-failure is an event rather than a disease [3, 4]. Therefore, many researchers argued for a radical change in thinking and in therapeutic drug development through multidisciplinary research [1–6]. Of late, Kumar et al. [2] reported conclusively that the transient event causing the acute-heart-failure is due to the phenomenon of internal flow choking (biofluid/Sanal flow choking) at a critical total-to-static pressure ratio. Internal flow choking is a compressible fluid flow effect caused by the blockage factor, which occurs at a critical blood-pressure-ratio (BPR), irrespective of the incoming flow velocity. In the CVS, the total pressure is considered as systolic blood pressure (SBP) and the static pressure is denoted as diastolic blood pressure (DBP). The physical situation of internal flow choking in the micro/nanoscale fluid flows in the circulatory system is more susceptible at microgravity condition due to altered variations of blood viscosity, turbulence and the BPR (SBP/DBP). During a long-term human spaceflight mission, the major factor that affects cardiovascular dysfunctions is the absence of gravity [6]. Cardiovascular changes in actual spaceflight differ from those in stimulations such as head-down bedrest or dry immersion [7]. The changes in the cardiovascular system begin solely with the fluid shift associated with microgravity, followed by the decreased circulatory blood volume, cardiac size, and aerobic capacity, and the most prominent symptom, postflight orthostatic intolerance. These symptoms are generically known as "cardiovascular deconditioning" [7–11]. Microgravity environment decreases plasma volume and increases the hematocrit compared with the situation on the earth surface, which increases the relative viscosity of blood. Since blood viscosity strongly depends on hematocrit there are possibilities of an early flow choking in microgravity environment due to an enhanced boundary layer blockage [6].

Human blood is a compressible fluid with different degrees of the compressibility percentage because the specific volume (or density) of blood does change with temperature and/or pressure [1, 2]. Therefore, the specific heat at the constant-pressure (C_p) is always higher than the specific heat at the constant-volume (C_v) of all human blood. The ratio of C_p and C_v is defined as the blood-heat-capacity-ratio (BHCR), which is an important parameter determining the thermal-tolerance level of blood [2]. The specific heat capacity depends on the number of degrees of freedom and each independent degree of freedom permits the particles to store thermal energy and as a result the BHCR will be always greater than one. It corroborates that blood is a compressible fluid and internal flow choking in CVS could occur at a critical BPR irrespective of hypertension or hypotension. Traditionally hypertension is considered as a cardiovascular-risk-factor in patients with systemic autoimmune and chronic inflammatory diseases. Until the theoretical discovery of the internal flow choking in CVS there were no authentic conclusions to support whether hypertension or hypotension is more risk with regards to the hemorrhagic stroke and acute myocardial infarction [1, 2]. The fact is that an acute-heart-failure could occur in both hypertension or hypotension patient because the controlling parameter of this event is the blood-pressure-ratio (BPR). In brevity, attaining the critical BPR is considered as the risk factor for asymptomatic cardiovascular diseases. At the threshold of the internal choking condition, a minor oscillation in BPR for both *hyper* and *hypo* subjects is likely to aggravate the cardiovascular risk. In light of the discovery of internal flow choking in CVS [1, 2], the classic definition of the hypertension causing cardiovascular risk is largely arbitrary [SBP ≥140 and/or DBP ≥90 mmHg]. The prevailing cardiovascular risk data remains challenging owing to the fact that the internal flow choking could occur in both hypertension or hypotension subjects once SBP/DBP reaches the critical BPR. The internal flow choking could happen anywhere in CVS including capillaries, vasa vasorum and/or nanoscale vessels. Capillaries are tiny blood vessels connecting arteries to veins. These blood vessels carry oxygen and nutrients to individual cells throughout the body. The vasa vasorum is a network of small blood vessels that are found in large veins (e.g., the venae cavae) and arteries such as the aorta and its branches. These small vessels serve to provide blood supply and nourishment for tunica adventitia and outer parts of tunica media of large vessels. Arteries deliver blood from the heart to the rest of the body and Veins return the blood back to the heart from the rest of the body. It is important to note that the pressure inside of arteries is very different from the pressure inside of veins. The pressure created by the heart pushes the blood through the arteries and the pressure inside the arteries is directly related to the blood pressure. The pressure in the veins is very low. Of late Kumar et al. [2, 3] reported that not the pressure but the magnitude of the blood-pressure-ratio (BPR) is the risk factor for acute-heart-failure and the brain hemorrhage because at the choked flow condition there are possibilities of the occurrence shock wave and pressure-overshoot in any vessel with divergent and/or bifurcation region causing aneurysm or wall tearing.

A brain hemorrhage is a type of stroke. It is caused by an artery in the brain bursting and causing localized bleeding in the surrounding tissues. Brain arteriovenous malformations (AVMs) are abnormal connections of arteries and veins [12]. An AVM can develop anywhere in the body, but occurs most often in the brain. Brain AVMs are a leading cause of the hemorrhage in children and young adults, although they can cause other morbidities such as seizures, focal neurological deficits, and headaches. There is usually high flow through the feeding arteries, nidus, and draining veins, which may result in rupture and intracranial hemorrhage, the most severe complication of an AVM. Clinically, brain AVMs are technically challenging and resource-intensive to manage with the available therapeutic modalities and often require multi-modal therapy. The factors influencing risk of hemorrhage associated with sporadic brain AVM is still poorly understood. It has already been established that blood/biofluid is a compressible viscous fluid and internal flow choking can occur anywhere in CVS at a critical BPR causing asymptomatic hemorrhage. In light of the theoretical discovery of the phenomenon of internal flow choking in nano scale fluid flows [1, 2], further studies on the pathogenesis of asymptomatic intracranial hemorrhage is envisaged [13]. Briefly, the concept of internal flow choking in blood circulatory system provides an insight for the diagnosis, prognosis, treatment and prevention of the asymptomatic coronary artery disease (CAD) and peripheral artery disease (PAD).

2. Internal flow choking

Internal flow is a flow for which the fluid is bounded by walls. Internal flow choking is a compressible fluid flow effect and a fluid dynamic condition in wall-bounded systems associated with the venturi effect. Admittedly, when a flowing fluid at a given pressure and temperature passes through a constriction (such as the throat of a convergent-divergent (CD) nozzle or a valve in a pipe) into a lower pressure environment the fluid velocity increases for meeting the continuity condition set by the law of nature, viz., the law of conservation of mass. The conservation of mass (continuity) is a fundamental concept of physics and it tells us that at the steady state condition the mass flow rate through a tube is a constant and equal to the product of local density, local velocity, and local cross-sectional area of the tube. The local cross-sectional area can alter due to the boundary layer blockage (i.e., boundary layer displacement thickness) as a result of the viscous flow effect. The cardiovascular system or hemodynamic process is said to be in a steady state if the state variables which define the behavior of the system or the process are unchanging in time.

All fluids in nature are viscous and compressible [1] and prone to create boundary layer over the bounding walls altering the effective geometric shape of the tube. The magnitude of boundary layer blockage depends up on the rheology of fluid and the type of flow featuring from laminar, transitional to turbulent flow characteristics. Boundary layer is the layer of fluid in the immediate vicinity of a bounding surface where the effects of viscosity are significant in the flow. Note that because of the greater velocity gradient at the wall the frictional shear stress in a turbulent boundary layer is greater than in a purely laminar boundary layer. And as a result, the turbulent boundary layer thickness will be higher than laminar boundary layer thickness. The main known parameter characterizing laminar–turbulent transition is the *Reynolds number*, which is defined as the ratio of inertial forces to viscous forces within a fluid which is subjected to the relative internal movement due to different fluid velocities. The transition to turbulence can occur over a range of *Reynolds numbers*, depending on many factors, including the wall surface roughness, heat transfer, vibration, noise, and other disturbances. The parameters influencing the local *Reynolds number* in a tube are local density, local viscosity, local velocity and the local diameter (a characteristic length). In fact, a decade before, blood was treated as a Newtonian fluid but later the established viscoelastic properties make human blood non- Newtonian [14, 15]. It depends on the elastic behavior of red blood cells. For compressible fluids, viscosity depends on temperature and varies very slowly with low pressure levels. It is an established fact that viscosity variations of fluids will be significant at high pressure levels and low temperature. The viscosity of water increases exponentially with decrease in temperature and is affected by the type and concentration of solutes. Although many empirical laws are available for predicting viscosity of gases, there is no established law for predicting the viscosity of blood in all directions as it possesses anisotropic characteristics. Anisotropy just refers to the properties of a material being directionally dependent. Many biological fluids have elements of anisotropy, because they are made of different cells and plasma that react differently to stresses. For example, blood has to flow in arteries and veins, which range in size from very large to extremely small under pressure pulses emanating from the heart. So the corpuscles in the blood vary in shape along the flow direction and in transverse directions. When they have to squeeze through a tiny vessel, they are extremely distorted and the "fluid" becomes highly anisotropic. Since Newton's law of viscosity is not a fundamental law of nature; and in light of the theoretical discovery of the Sanal flow choking in the CVS, it is desirable to establish a mathematical model to predict accurately the directionally dependent viscosity of blood at various patho-physiological ranges of pressure and temperature for a credible decision making on the possibilities of the occurrence of internal flow choking in the circulatory circuit *a priori*. Such a model will be useful for a credible risk assessment of asymptomatic cardiovascular diseases through in silico methodology with compressible viscous flow models.

The blood/biofluid compressibility effects on mass flow rate have some surprising results. At a particular total condition, there is a maximum limit of mass flow that occurs when the flow Mach number is equal to one (i.e., local flow velocity equal to the local velocity of sound). The limiting of the mass flow rate is called choking of the flow, which occurs at the sonic fluid flow condition (i.e., Mach number (M) equal to one). It is important to note that although the fluid velocity reaches sonic condition and becomes choked, the mass flow rate is not choked. The mass flow rate can still be increased if the upstream pressure is increased as this increases the density of the gas entering the orifice. Internal flow choking occurs when sonic velocity is reached at the constriction section. And the flow becomes independent from downstream conditions. In other words, internal flow choking occurs in CVS at a critical blood pressure ratio (SBP/DBP), which is governed by the biofluid/blood heat capacity ratio (BHCR).

$$BPR = \frac{SBP}{DBP} = \left(\frac{BHCR+1}{2}\right)^{BHCR/BHCR-1} \quad (1)$$

The analytical model (Eq. (1)) derived from the compressible flow theory [1, 5, 16, 17] dictates the exact condition of internal flow choking in CVS. It is pertinent to note that if the blood vessel is having the shape of a convergent-divergent (CD) nozzle due to occlusion, stenosis, vasospasm and/or the effect of boundary layer blockage (**Figure 1**) there are possibilities of the generation of shock waves and transient pressure-overshoot in the downstream region of the vessel after attaining the internal flow choking condition (Eq. (1)) as a result of supersonic flow development. Occlusion of the blood vessel causing internal flow choking may be due to atherosclerotic plaque, an embolised blood clot, necrosis or a foreign body presence. According to the law of nature, with a mathematical proof [5, 16], for a compressible fluid to expand isentropically from subsonic ($M < 1$) to supersonic ($M > 1$) speeds, it must flow through a convergent-divergent duct or a CD-shaped streamtube [5, 6, 16, 17] experiencing with a physical situation of internal flow choking at a critical BPR (**Figure 2**). The critical BPR for internal flow choking is governed by the BHCR as dictated by Eq. (1). There are two types of internal flow choking in CVS viz., biofluid choking and Sanal flow choking. Biofluid flow choking occurs in CVS due to the plaque induced CD nozzle flow effect and/or due to vasospasm (**Figure 1(a–d)**) or any other type of occlusion. A vasospasm is the narrowing of the arteries caused by a persistent contraction of the blood vessels, which is known as vasoconstriction. Vasospasms can affect any area of the body including the brain (cerebral vasospasm) and the coronary artery (coronary artery vasospasm). The Sanal flow choking phenomenon is established as the fluid-throat induced internal flow choking due to the boundary layer formation in the real world flows (continuum/non-continuum) owing to the compressible viscous flow effect [1, 2]. The Sanal flow choking creates a physical situation of boundary layer blockage persuaded biofluid flow choking of the circulatory circuit at a critical systolic-to-diastolic blood pressure ratio (BPR) in all the subjects with and without any plaque (**Figure 1(d–g)**) and/or apparent occlusion.

The internal flow choking is a new theoretical concept in biological science applicable to continuum and non-continuum biofluid flows. As the pressure of the nanoscale biofluid/non-continuum-flows rises, average-mean-free-path diminishes and thus, the *Knudsen number* lowers heading to a zero-slip wall-boundary condition with compressible viscous flow effect, which increases the risk of cardiovascular diseases. Eq. (1) tells us that low BPR, high BHCR or high thermal tolerance of blood reduces the risk of internal flow choking, which in turn reduces the possibilities of shock wave generation and pressure overshoot causing asymptomatic cardiovascular diseases. At a critical BPR, the Sanal flow choking occurs anywhere in the CVS, including micro/nanoscale vessels with sudden expansion/divergence or bifurcation regions. The Sanal flow choking leads to supersonic flow development heading to the shock wave generation in viscoelastic vessels creating memory effect (stroke history). It occurs due to the boundary layer persuaded convergent-divergent (CD) duct shape of the flow passage (**Figure 3**).

The shock wave can occur anywhere at any time in the supersonic flow when there is a flow compression due to streamtube effect or geometric effect or any

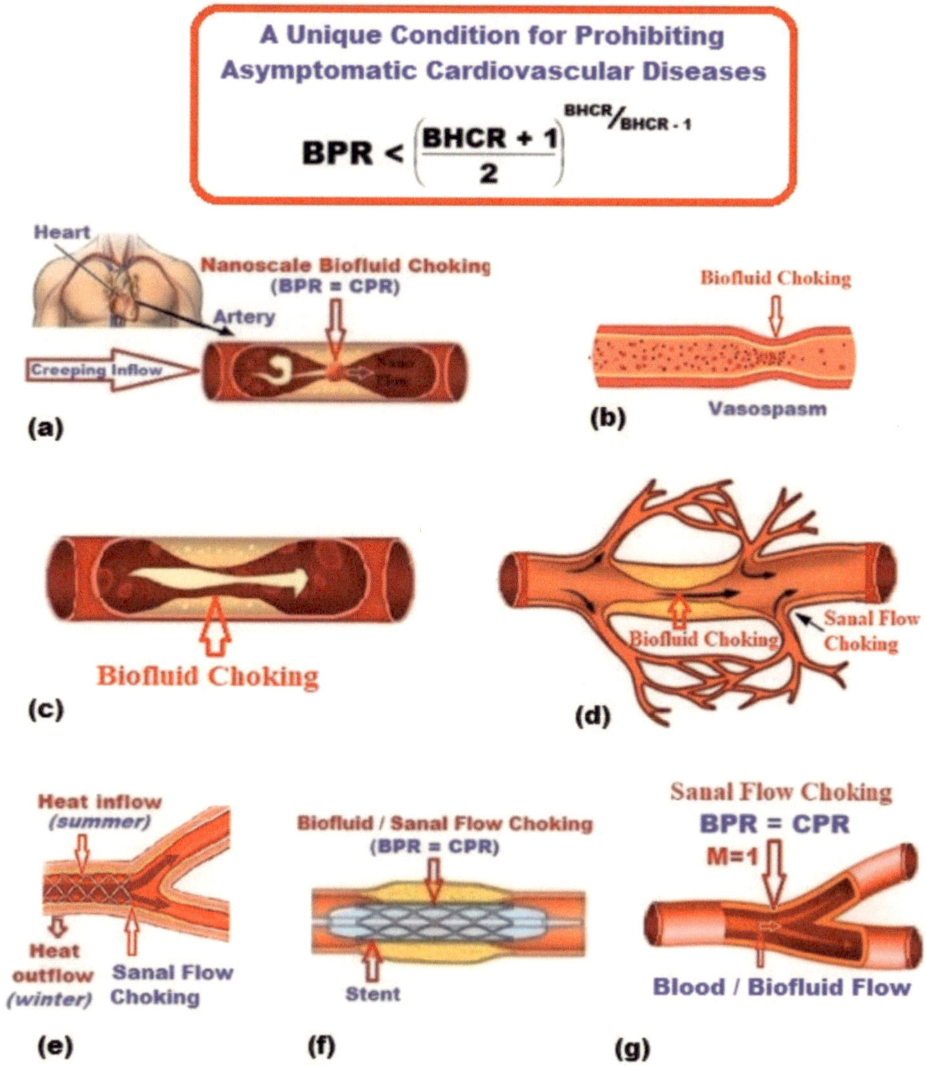

Figure 1.
Demonstrations of different physical situations of internal flow choking (biofluid/Sanal flow choking) at a critical blood-pressure-ratio (BPR) [1]. (a) physical situation of biofluid choking in an artery with plaque deposit similar to a CD nozzle flow passage, (b) demonstrating the possibilities of biofluid choking at a critical BPR due to vasospasm, (c) a partially blocked artery demonstrating the CD nozzle flow passage causing biofluid choking, (d) demonstrating the possibilities of biofluid choking and Sanal flow choking in an artery with plaque and collateral circulation, (e) demonstrating the physical situation of the Sanal flow choking at the presence of a stent in an artery with bifurcation, (f) a partially blocked artery with stent creating a situation of biofluid flow choking at a critical BPR due to CD nozzle shaped flow passage, (g) demonstrating the physical situation of the Sanal flow choking in a healthy subject having an artery with bifurcation.

other flow disturbance. Normal shock waves create very sharp transient pressure-overshoot in CVS, which leads to bulging or tearing of vessels. The tearing (hemorrhagic stroke) or bulging of vessels (aneurysm) depend on the memory effect (stroke history) and relaxation modulus of the viscoelastic vessels. Memory effect depends on the strength of the shock wave and the associated occurrence of the transient pressure-overshoot over the years due to the frequent fluctuations in BPR, due to various reasons, ranging from unchoked to choked biofluid flow conditions. Note that large oscillations in BPR leads to *arrhythmia*. Most heart valve problems

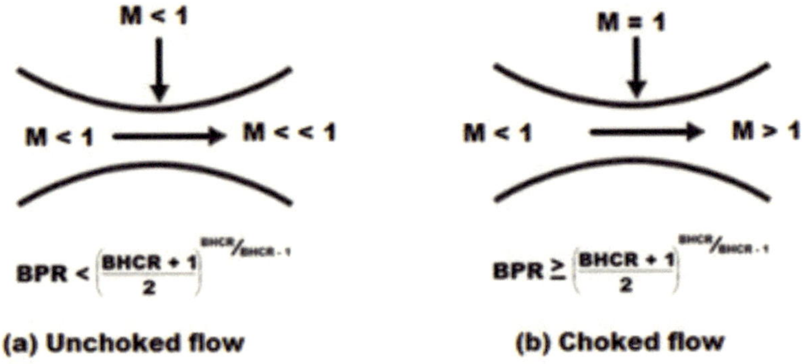

Figure 2.
Demonstrating the physical situation of the internal flow choking and unchoking condition in a CD duct or a CD shaped streamtube.

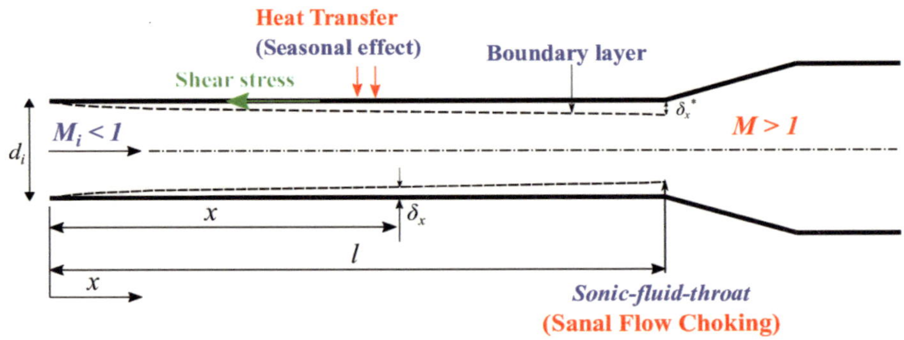

Figure 3.
Demonstrating the Sanal flow choking phenomenon in an idealized physical model of an artery with a divergent port.

involve the aortic and mitral valves, possibly because of its geometric shape similar to a convergent-divergent (CD) duct flow passage [2, 6]. All these deliberations lead to establish herein that the internal flow choking is an undesirable phenomenon in CVS as it leads aneurysm, hemorrhagic stroke, moyamoya disease, myocardial infarction. The significant clinical aspect is that; the internal flow choking is uniquely regulated by the biofluid/blood heat-capacity-ratio (BHCR). Of late V.R.S.Kumar et al. [2] correlate the BHCR with BPR, blood viscosity (BV) and ejection fraction (EF) for establishing the concept of internal flow choking causing asymptomatic cardiovascular diseases for taking brilliant clinical decisions in case by case manner [18–30].

3. Analytical methodology

The analytical prediction of the Sanal flow choking [1, 2] is a breakthrough in biological science, which creates a radical change in the diagnostic sciences of asymptomatic cardiovascular diseases because the various causes of the Sanal flow choking are complementing with all the established concepts in the medical sciences [2]. The concepts of Sanal flow choking is reviewed herein for highlighting pragmatic solutions for reducing the risk of internal flow choking leading to shock wave generation causing asymptomatic cardiovascular diseases. The whole blood viscosity is popularly the one of Virchow's triad, which is a recognized concept pronounces the three wide types of causes that are believed to interpose to thrombosis causing cardiovascular complications, viz., hypercoagulability, hemodynamic changes (stasis, turbulence), endothelial injury/dysfunction. Furthermore, it is well known that blood is a non Newtonian fluid [2] as blood viscosity changes due to fluid force, seasonal effects and blood thinning medications.

Viscosity variations are depending on the shear rate or shear rate history of the blood/biofluid, which could vary due to local effects too. Blood temperature decreases during the winter season resulting an increase in blood viscosity and the inverse effect happens during the summer season [5, 18]. It corroborates that the boundary-layer-blockage (BLB) factor causing the Sanal flow choking would alter due to the blood viscosity variations as a consequence of the blood-thinning medication and/or the seasonal effects [2, 18]. Indeed, boundary-layer-blockage induced internal flow choking is more prone during the winter season than the summer season due to the higher blood viscosity at the relatively low blood temperature. It leads to say that the risks of internal flow choking leading to asymptomatic cardiovascular diseases would be high during the winter than in the summer season [5, 18]. It is important to note that disproportionate blood-thinning medication will increase the Reynolds number, which produces the high-turbulence-level creating enhanced boundary-layer-blockage (BLB)-factor causing an early internal flow choking. Therefore, we can establish that relatively high blood viscosity and low blood viscosity are risk factors for an early internal flow choking in cardiovascular system (CVS) causing asymptomatic stroke/hemorrhage and acute heart failure, which is correlating with the established index, viz., International normalized ratio (INR). Therefore, the real effect of viscosity on internal flow choking in CVS needs to be established through randomized clinical trials for taking preventive strategies for reducing the risk of asymptomatic hemorrhage and acute heart failure. On this rationale, it is essential, rather needed, perhaps inevitable to declare an exact condition for prohibiting the internal flow choking in the CVS, in terms of viscosity, density, Reynolds number, biofluid/blood-heat-capacity-ratio (BHCR), blood-pressure-ratio (BPR), the ejection fraction in terms of biofluid/blood flow rate (BFR), and stenosis (vessel geometry), which are accomplished through the closed-form analytical models (Eqs (2), (3)). Eqs (2), (3) are declaring the unchoked flow condition in the CVS, which could predict the cardiovascular risk for taking a conclusive clinical decision on each and every subject in all seasons. Accurate estimation of the parameters highlighted in Eqs (2), (3) are absolutely required for the future health care management of all subjects aiming for prohibiting asymptomatic cardiovascular diseases.

$$\left[\frac{(BFR)_{local}\, V_{local}}{(BHCR)_{lowest}\,(DBP)\, A_{local}}\right]^{1/2} < 1 \tag{2}$$

$$\frac{(Reynolds\ number)(kinematic viscosity)}{Hydraulic diameter\ \ of\ \ the\ \ vessel}\left[\frac{Blood\, Density}{(BHCR)(DBR)}\right]^{1/2} < 1 \tag{3}$$

It is evident from Eq. (1), and Eqs (2), (3) that a decrease in BHCR, DBP and the vessel diameter increases the cardiovascular risk, which is correlating with the existing clinical findings [2, 18, 28, 29]. Eq. (1) also reveals that an increase in systolic blood pressure (SBP) increases the cardiovascular risk (CVR). Briefly, an increase in BPR increases the CVR. Eq. (1) and Eqs (2), (3) are two independent and complementing conditions set for prohibiting the internal flow choking in the CVS. Eq. (2) is an offshoot of Eq. (3), which highlights the coupled effect of thermo-fluid dynamics properties of biofluid/blood along with the vessel blockage in terms of the hydraulic diameter. Note that nanoscale fluid flow system with apparently high-risk blockage (**Figure 1(a)**) must always maintain the flow Mach number less than one as dictated by Eqs (2) and (3) for negating the undesirable internal flow choking causing shock wave generation and pressure-overshoot in the CVS leading to acute myocardial infarction. In such cases the flow Mach number can be retained always less than one by keeping BPR always less than the lower critical hemorrhage index (LCHI), which can be achieved by increasing the BHCR through drugs or otherwise. Analytical model (Eq. (2)) proves that the stents could reduce the risk of the heart attack but no better than drugs for increasing the BHCR owing to the fact that the Sanal flow choking could occur with and without stent. The impeccable analytical models presented herein as Eqs (2), (3) reveal that the usage of blood-thinners without increasing the BHCR create high risk of bleeding and stroke. The fact is that the blood-thinner decreases the viscosity and increases the *Reynolds number*, which augments the turbulence level causing an enhanced boundary layer blockage, which predisposes for an early flow choking. The flow turbulence enhances the deficit of energy in the type of friction, which increases the boundary layer blockage in the vessels and generates heat and augment the internal energy affecting a reduction in BHCR. Additionally, turbulence enhances the perfusion pressure essential to push the blood flow, which creates an early undesirable Sanal flow choking in the circulatory system.

3.1 Lower critical hemorrhage index

In order to avoid internal flow choking in CVS an unchoked–fluid-flow condition must be maintained throughout the circulatory system. It could be achieved by maintaining the BPR always lower than the lower-critical-hemorrhage-index (LCHI), which is dictated by the lowest value of the BHCR (Eq. (4)) of the evolved gases from blood or foreign gases entered in the CVS. Air can enter in veins and arteries during surgical procedures. It has been reported that non meticulous brain surgeries result in an air embolism. Significant venous air embolism may develop acutely during the perioperative period due to a number of causes such as during head and neck surgery, spinal surgery, improper central venous and hemodialysis catheter handling, etc. The trend of using self-collapsible intravenous (IV) infusion bags instead of the conventional glass or plastic bottles has several advantages, one of them being protection against air embolism [31].

$$BPR < LCHI = \left(\frac{(BHCR)_{evolved\ gases\ with\ the\ lowest\ BHCR} + 1}{2} \right)^{(BHCR)_{lowest}/(BHCR)_{lowest}-1} \tag{4}$$

$$UCHI = \left(\frac{(BHCR)_{blood} + 1}{2} \right)^{(BHCR)_{blood}/(BHCR)_{blood}-1} \tag{5}$$

Note that BHCR of CO_2 is lower than air, which creates an early internal flow choking. For instance, if CO_2 is the dominant gas in the CVS it is mandatory to maintain BPR lower than 1.82, within the pathophysiological range of human temperature, for creating an unchoked flow condition for prohibiting the shock wave generation [1] causing asymptomatic cardiovascular diseases due to transient pressure-overshoot. Note that BHCR of CO_2 decreases from 1.31 @ 0 °C to 1.281 @ 100 °C. Eq. (4) shows that the BHCR is having the bearing on all the parameters highlighted in Eqs (2), (3) for prohibiting the internal flow choking. The fact is that at the choked flow condition the critical-BPR is a unique function of BHCR. Briefly, the LCHI can be predicted (Eq. (4)) using the lowest value of the BHCR among the dominant gases present in the CVS of each subject (human being or animal). The upper critical hemorrhage index (UCHI) can be predicted (Eq. (5)) from the specific heat of blood at constant pressure (C_p) and the specific heat of blood at constant volume (C_v) using the differential scanning calorimeter [6].

4. In vitro methodology

In vitro data [6] shows that nitrogen (N_2), oxygen (O_2), and carbon dioxide (CO_2) gases are predominant in fresh blood samples of the human being/*Guinea-pig* at a temperature range of 37–40 °C (98.6–104 °F), which increases the risk of internal flow choking leading to the asymptomatic cardiovascular risk. It is evident from the reported results (**Figure 4**), exceeding the thermal tolerance level, that the possibilities of internal flow choking in the human being is higher than the animal (*Guinea pig*) under the same thermal loading condition as the BHCR of the dominant gas evolved in the animal is found consistently higher than the human being. As a result, the LCHI is higher for the healthy male *Guinea pig* as dictated by the Eq. (4). The mass spectrum of N_2 is reported higher in animal whereas in human being CO_2 is found higher [1, 6]. The BHCR of N_2 is 1.4 and that of CO_2 is 1.289 at a temperature of 300 K (80.33 F). At this thermal loading condition, an early internal flow choking occurs in the human artery at a BPR of 1.82 compared to an animal (*Guinea pig*) artery at a BPR of 1.89. It proves that the thermal tolerance level of the healthy *Guinea pig* is higher and the cardiovascular risk is lower than the human being under identical conditions. Therefore, increasing the thermal tolerance level in terms of BHCR of the human being is an important factor for reducing the risk of asymptomatic cardiovascular diseases caused by the shock waves as a result of internal flow choking. **Figure 5** is demonstrating the percentage variations of evolved gases (viz., N_2 -m/z = 28, O_2 -m/z = 32, CO_2 -m/z = 44, Ar -m/z = 40, an unknown composite gas -m/z = 28.5), from blood samples of four different healthy human beings and one healthy male *Guinea pig* of four weeks old, during the hyphenated technique at a blood temperature of 40 °C (104° F). The estimated UCHI of healthy human being of age 23–56 with different blood group is presented in **Table 1**.

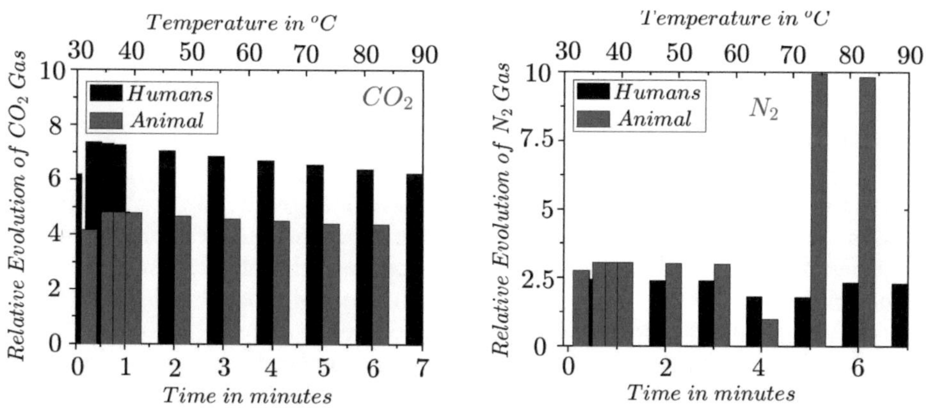

Figure 4.
The mass spectrum of CO_2 and N_2 evolved as a function of both time and temperature in the blood samples of healthy subjects [1].

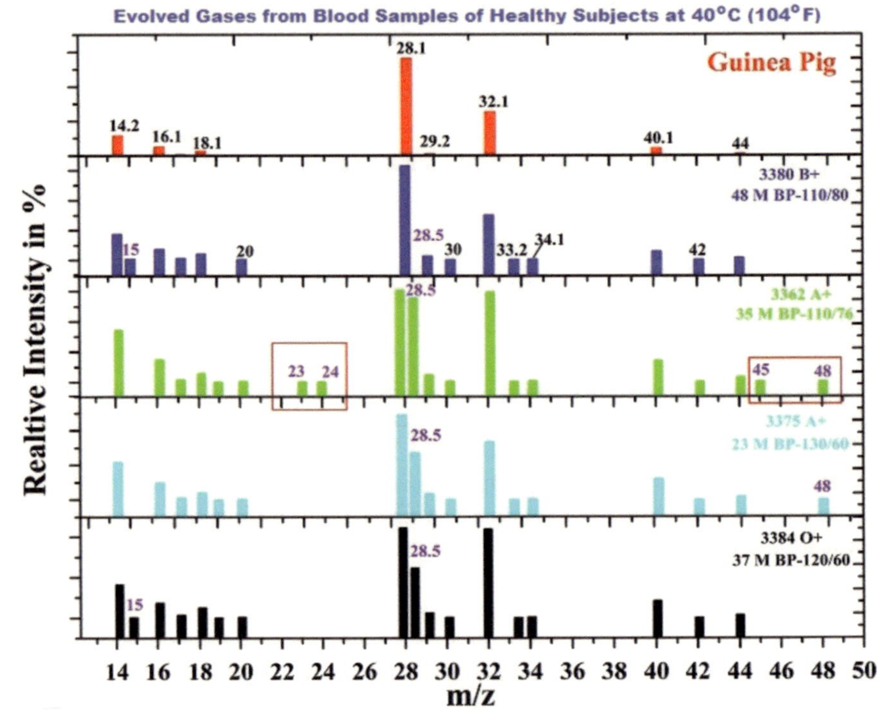

Figure 5.
Demonstrating the percentage variations of evolved gases (viz., N_2-m/z = 28, O_2 m/z = 32, CO_2-m/z = 44, Ar-m/z = 40, an unknown composite gas - m/z = 28.5) from the blood samples of four different healthy human beings and one Guinea pig during the hyphenated technique at a blood temperature of 40 °C (104° F) [2].

Batch No.	Blood Group	SBP/DBP	BPR	BHCR	UCHI @ 37.5° C
3073	O+	150/90	1.666	3.500	3.110
3074	A+	120/70	1.714	2.760	2.691
3078	B-	150/90	1.666	2.7292	2.709
3080	O+	150/90	1.666	2.9935	2.824
3082	A+	140/96	1.458	2.6759	2.640

Table 1.
Prediction of the UCHI from the heat capacity ratio of fresh blood samples of healthy human being of age 23–56 [2].

5. In silico methodology

Over the decades, bio-medical researchers have been relying on *in silico* simulation to model and cognize the natural mechanisms behind the creation and evolution of hemodynamic disorders. It has been recognized that the *wall-shear-stress* exerted on the walls of the blood vessel due to the flow of blood/biofluid is one of the main pathogenic factors leading to the occurrence of such disorders. The magnitude and distribution of the *wall shear stress* in a blood vessel can provide an insight into the locations of possible aneurysm growth. Furthermore, blockages that build up over time can be predicted by having a qualitative understanding of the flow profile. *In silico* methods can be used for modeling and understanding such vital internal flows. Obviously, the insights gained from the three-dimensional (3D) multi-phase *in silico* simulation can help design patient-specific treatments and forecast asymptomatic cardiovascular risk. In this book chapter, as a proof of the concept of fluid-throat persuaded shock waves, we are highlighting the single phase *in silico* results (**Figure 6**) demonstrating the Sanal flow choking phenomenon followed by pressure-overshoot in an idealized physical model of a blood vessel with divergent region (see **Figure 3**) with working fluid as gas. The modeling of non-Newtonian behavior of blood flow is an important task in any *in silico* simulation with fluid-structural interaction for forecasting asymptomatic cardiovascular diseases. Additionally, a realistic time-varying boundary condition need to be implemented in order to mimic the pulsatile nature of diabatic flow (flow involves transfer of heat) of blood in a thermo-viscoelastic vessel.

The in silico result presented in **Figure 6** is clearly demonstrating the phenomenon of the Sanal-flow-choking and the shock-waves generation at the subsonic inflow condition (creeping flow) leading to the transient pressure-overshoots (stroke) in the downstream region of an artery with divergent port. **Figure 6** provides the proof of the concept of fluid-throat persuaded flow choking in the CVS. The closed-form analytical prediction of the 3D blockage factor [1] at the sonic-fluid-throat location is a useful tool for the *in vitro* and *in silico* experiments in both the continuum and non-continuum flows with due consideration of heat transfer effects (real-world fluid flow effect). Note that the phenomenon of Sanal flow choking is a paradigm shift in the diagnostic sciences of asymptomatic CVD. Therefore, development of a multi-phase, multispecies, viscoelastic fluid-structural interactive *in silico* model capturing the memory effect (stroke history) is a meaningful objective for predicting *a priori* asymptomatic cardiovascular diseases with credibility [2]. Such an effort will be helpful for the diagnosis, prognosis, treatment and prevention of the hemorrhagic stroke and the acute heart failure of each and every subject with confidence.

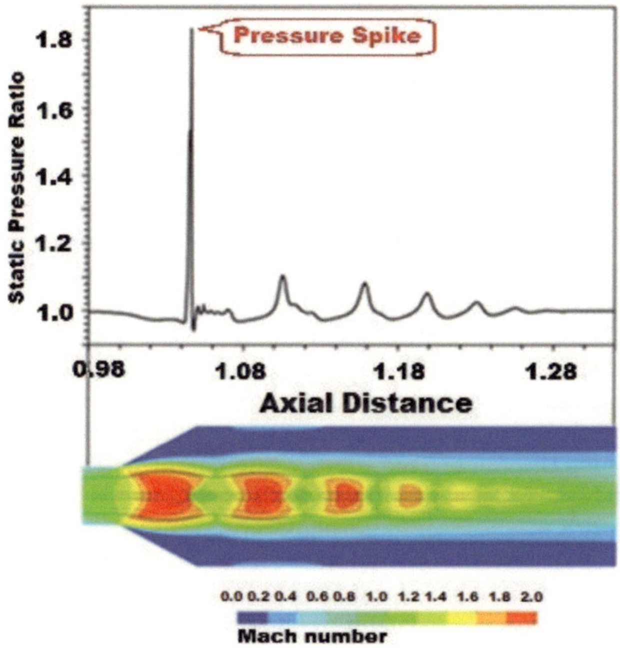

Figure 6.
Single phase in silico *result is demonstrating the transient pressure-overshoot (stroke) at 12 milli-second from Sanal flow choking time, after reaching the lower critical hemorrhage index (LCHI), in a simulated artery with the boundary layer blockage (a case of an internal flow choking and shock wave generation due to gas embolism and without any plaque [5]).*

6. Summary and conclusions

Although the diagnostic sciences have been advanced significantly during the last eight decades [32–40], until the theoretical discovery of the Sanal flow choking, the real occurrence of acute-heart-failure was poorly understood, largely for the reason that it was an under diagnosis condition [2]. Now the real cause of an acute-heart-failure comes to the foreground [1, 2]. All the findings reported in this chapter are complementing with the clinical data causing asymptomatic cardiovascular diseases. Analytical models, *in vitro* and *in silico* results presented herein corroborated that a vaccination or a single drug could reduce the risk of hemorrhagic stroke and acute heart failure [1, 2]. It could be achieved by increasing the BHCR and/or decreasing the BPR. We recognized through this comprehensive review that the internal flow choking, leading to the shock-wave generation and the transient pressure spike in a blood vessel, is the fundamental cause of asymptomatic cardiovascular diseases including hemorrhagic stroke and acute heart failure. Now the precipitating factor for the plaque rupture has come to the foreground. We concluded that the boundary-layer-blockage persuaded Sanal flow choking could occur anywhere in the circulatory circuit with gas embolism when BPR reaches LCHI. The boundary-layer-blockage-factor depends on the BHCR, flow Mach number, biofluid viscosity and turbulence, which could alter due to seasonal changes, variations in lipoprotein and other contributing factors. The greater the reduction in low-density lipoprotein (LDL) cholesterol, the lower the risk of stroke. The shock wave due to the Sanal flow choking could disrupt an atherosclerotic plaque or coronary artery wall. In a nutshell, the discovery of the biofluid/Sanal flow choking is a paradigm shift in the diagnostic sciences of coronary artery disease (CAD) and peripheral artery disease (PAD).

In vitro study shows that nitrogen (N2), oxygen (O2), carbon dioxide (CO2), and argon (Ar) gases are predominant in fresh blood samples of healthy subjects at a temperature range of 37 – 40 °C (98.6 – 104 °F), which enhances the chances of internal flow choking (with or without any coronary artery stent) leading to pressure-overshoot and acute heart failure. This physical situation is more dangerous in Covid-19 patients, which could lead to cardiac epidemic. We observed through *in vitro* study that (**Figure 4**), CO_2, the gas with the lowest heat capacity ratio (HCR), is relatively and consistently higher in the healthy males than the healthy male *Guinea pig* of four weeks old. It reveals that as a preventive measure for all subjects with a low BHCR, including patients who are taking blood-thinning medication must maintain their BPR always less than 1.82, as dictated by Eq. (4), for reducing the risk of asymptomatic CVD.

We concluded that a single anticoagulant drug capable to suppress the turbulence level and enhance the BHCR or a companion medicine along with the traditional blood-thinning medications is predestined for meeting the conflicting requirements (i.e., decrease viscosity and turbulence simultaneously) of all the subjects for reducing the risk of asymptomatic hemorrhage (AH) and acute heart failure (AHF). In high risk subjects, (i.e., BPR is very close to the LCHI), a slight oscillation in the BPR predisposes to the choking and the unchoking phenomena, which could lead to arrhythmia and memory effect. Briefly, this study sheds light for exploring new avenues in biological science for discovering new blood-thinning drugs for reducing the risk of internal flow choking causing asymptomatic cardiovascular diseases [1, 2]. The cardiovascular treatment should be targeted based on blood pressure ratio (BPR), instead of blood pressure levels alone, in chronic heart failure patients. We concluded that the risk of internal flow choking heading to asymptomatic cardiovascular diseases could be decreased by concurrently reducing blood viscosity and turbulence by enhancing the BHCR and/or reducing the BPR.

The discovery of the Sanal flow choking phenomena calls for continuous ambulatory blood pressure (BP) and thermal level monitoring in high risk patients in the diagnosis and preventive management of asymptomatic cardiovascular diseases. The continuous blood pressure and thermal level measurement could be done in a more pragmatic way by using a wearable BP monitor with the temperature sensor in the modern form of a wristwatch. Analytical methods such as machine learning could definitely enhance the accuracy and advance daily wearable device-based diagnoses [41–49]. Recent studies on heart failure management in gravity and microgravity environment (during the long human spaceflight) corroborate that the physical situation of the Sanal flow choking phenomena calls for continuous ambulatory BP and thermal-level monitoring in astronauts'/cosmonauts [6, 41–50]. Note that the Sanal flow choking is more susceptible at microgravity condition due to altered variations of blood viscosity, turbulence and the BPR. Microgravity environment decreases plasma volume and increases the hematocrit compared with the situation on the earth surface, which increases the relative viscosity of blood. We concluded that for a healthy-life all subjects (human being/animals) in the earth and in the outer space with high BPR necessarily have high BHCR. We also concluded that for reducing the cardiovascular risk, all the astronauts/cosmonauts should maintain the BPR lower than the lower critical hemorrhage index (LCHI) as dictated by the lowest heat capacity ratio (HCR) of the gas generating from the biofluid/blood for prohibiting the internal flow choking during the space travel. We recommend all astronauts/cosmonauts should wear ambulatory blood pressure and thermal level monitoring devices similar to a wristwatch throughout the space travel for the diagnosis, prognosis and prevention of internal flow choking leading to asymptomatic cardiovascular diseases. The scientific objective of this study and review was to discover the correlation between the thermal tolerance level in terms of BHCR, the BPR, blood viscosity, ejection fraction (EF) and the cardiovascular risk leading to AH and AHF, which we could achieve herein. We concluded that designing the precise blood thinning regimen is vital for attaining the desired therapeutic efficacy and negating undesirable flow choking leading to acute-heart failure. For a healthy-life all subjects with high-BPR inevitably have high-BHCR for reducing the risk of the internal flow choking (biofluid/Sanal flow choking) triggering the AHF due to the shock wave generation. We corroborated that, the acute-heart-failure (AHF) is a transient episode and not an illness. In a nutshell, a single drug capable to increase BHCR and/or decrease the BPR could reduce the risk of asymptomatic cardiovascular diseases without any prejudice.

Author details

Valsalayam Raghavapanicker Sanal Kumar[1,2,3*], Shiv Kumar Choudhary[4], Pradeep Kumar Radhakrishnan[5], Rajaghatta Sundararam Bharath[2], Nichith Chandrasekaran[2,3], Vigneshwaran Sankar[2,3], Ajith Sukumaran[3] and Charlie Oommen[2]

1 Indian Space Research Organisation, India

2 Indian Institute of Science, India

3 Kumaraguru College of Technology, India

4 Cardiothoracic and Vascular Surgery, All India Institute of Medical Sciences, New Delhi, India

5 Chief Division of Cardiothoracic and Vascular Surgery, GITAM University, India

*Address all correspondence to: vr_sanalkumar@yahoo.co.in

References

[1] V.R.Sanal Kumar, Vigneshwaran Sankar, Nichith Chandrasekaran, Ajith Sukumaran, Sulthan Ariff Rahman M, Bharath R.S, Charlie Oommen, Pradeep Kumar Rakrishnan, Shiv Kumar Choudhary, "Sanal Flow Choking: A Paradigm Shift in Computational Fluid Dynamics Code Verification and Diagnosing Detonation and Hemorrhage in Real-World Fluid-Flow Systems," *Global Challenges*, Wiley Publications, 2020 May 27; 4(9): 2000012, PMCID: PMC7267099

[2] V.R.Sanal Kumar, Shiv Kumar Choudhary, Pradeep Kumar Radhakrishnan, Rajaghatta Sundararam Bharath, Nichith Chandrasekaran, Vigneshwaran Sankar, Ajith Sukumaran, Charlie Oommen, "Lopsided Blood-thinning Drug Increases the Risk of Internal Flow Choking Leading to Shock Wave Generation Causing Asymptomatic Cardiovascular Disease," *Global Challenges*, Wiley Publication, 2021 January 29, 2000076

[3] M.Packer, JACC: Heart Failure, 2018, 6(1), 73-75.

[4] A.Mebazaa, JACC: Heart Failure, 2018, 6(1),76-79.

[5] V. R. S. Kumar, V. Sankar, N. Chandrasekaran, V. Saravanan, V. Natarajan, S. Padmanabhan, A. Sukumaran, S. Mani, T. Rameshkumar, H. S. N. Doddi, K. Vysaprasad, S. Sharan, P. Murugesh, S. G. Shankar, M. N. Nejaamtheen, R. V. Baskaran, S. A. R. M. Rafic, U. Harisrinivasan, V. Srinivasan, C. J. Rajshree, A. Krishnan, A. Pal, G. V. Panicker, A, Rajesh, AIAA-2018-3962, 2018.

[6] V.R.Sanal Kumar, Shiv Kumar Choudhary, Pradeep Kumar Radhakrishnan, Bharath, R.S, Nichith C, Charlie Oommen, Vigneshwaran Sankar, Ajith S, Amrith M, Thianesh U.K, Deviparameswari K, Nanoscale Flow Choking and Spaceflight Effects on Cardiovascular Risk of Astronauts – A New Perspective, AIAA SciTech 2021, 11-15 Jan 2021.

[7] Satoshi Iwase, Naoki Nishimura, Kunihiko Tanaka and Tadaaki Mano Satoshi Iwase, Naoki Nishimura, Kunihiko Tanaka and Tadaaki Mano, Effects of Microgravity on Human Physiology, Book chapter, Intechopen, 2020.

[8] Diedrich A, Paranjape SY, Robertson D. Plasma and blood volume in space. The American Journal of the Medical Sciences. 2007;334 (1):80-85.

[9] Antonutto G, di Prampero PE. Cardiovascular deconditioning in microgravity: Some possible countermeasures. European Journal of Applied Physiology. 2003;90:283-291, Epub 2003 Jul 8.

[10] Ertl AC, Diedrich A, Biaggioni I, Levine BD, Robertson RM, Cox JF, et al. Human muscle sympathetic nerve activity and plasma noradrenaline kinetics in space. The Journal of Physiology. 2002;538:321-329

[11] Grigoriev AI, Morukov BV, Vorobiev DV. Water and electrolyte studies during long-term missions onboard the space stations SALYUT and MIR. The Clinical Investigator. 1994;72:169-189.

[12] W. Caleb Rutledge, Nerissa U. Ko, Michael T. Lawton, and Helen Kim, Hemorrhage Rates and Risk Factors in the Natural History Course of Brain Arteriovenous Malformations, Transl Stroke Res. 2014 Oct; 5(5): 538-542.

[13] Hao, Y., Liu, W., Wang, H., Zi, W., Yang, D., Wang, W., ... Xu, G.

(2018). Prognosis of asymptomatic intracranial hemorrhage after endovascular treatment. Journal of Neuro Interventional Surgery, neurintsurg–2018-013848.

[14] M. Brust, C. Schaefer, R. Doerr, L. Pan, M. Garcia, P. E. Arratia, C. Wagner, "Rheology of Human Blood Plasma: Viscoelastic Versus Newtonian Behavior," Phys. Rev. Lett. 2013, 110, 078305.

[15] A.S. Varchanisa, Y. Dimakopoulosa, Christian Wagnerb, J. Tsamopoulosa, How viscoelastic is human blood plasma?, Soft Matter, 2018.

[16] J. D. Anderson, Jr., Modern Compressible Flow, with Historical Perspective, Fourth Edition, McGraw-Hill Publishing Company (2007).

[17] V.R.S.Kumar, V. Sankar, N. Chandrasekaran, V. Saravanan, V. Natarajan, S. Padmanabhan, A. Sukumaran, S. Mani, T. Rameshkumar, H. S. N. Doddi, K. Vysaprasad, S. Sharan, P. Murugesh, S. G. Shankar, M. N. Nejaamtheen, R. V. Baskaran, S. A. R. M. Rafic, U. Harisrinivasan, V. Srinivasan, AIP Advances, 2018, 8, 025315.

[18] S.Stewart, A.Keates, A.Redfern, J.V.M.John, Seasonal variations in cardiovascular disease, Nat Rev Cardiol, 2017, 14, 654-664.

[19] Luscher TF. Heart failure: the cardiovascular epidemic of the 21st century. Eur Heart J 2015; 36:395-397.

[20] Alexandra N. Nowbar , Mauro Gitto, James P. Howard, Darrel P. Francis, Rasha Al-Lamee, Mortality From Ischemic Heart Disease, Circulation: Cardiovascular Quality and Outcome, Vol.12, No.6, 2019.

[21] Elena Bartoloni, Alessia Alunno and Roberto Gerli, Hypertension as a cardiovascular risk factor in autoimmune rheumatic diseases, Nature Reviews Cardiology, (2017).

[22] Efremov, L., Jacobs, L., Thijs, L. et al. Risk factors for predicting heart failure: a subject-level meta-analysis from the HOMAGE database. Arch Public Health 73, P9 (2015).

[23] Helena Marti-Soler et al., Seasonal Variation of Overall and Cardiovascular Mortality: A Study in 19 Countries from Different Geographic Locations. PLoS ONE 9(11): e113500.

[24] Craig T. January, et al. 2019 AHA/ACC/HRS Focused Update of the 2014 AHA/ACC/HRS Guideline for the Management of Patients With Atrial Fibrillation. Circulation, 2019.

[25] Shikdar, S, Bhattacharya, PT. International normalized ratio (INR). StatPearls. https://www.ncbi.nlm.nih.gov/books/NBK507707/. Updated October 27, 2018.

[26] Rongjia Tao, Reducing blood viscosity and suppressing turbulence with magnetic field to prevent heart attack and stroke, Proceedings Volume 10926, Quantum Sensing and Nano Electronics and Photonics XVI; 1092605 (2019), 8 March 2019.

[27] R. Tao and K. Huang, "Reducing blood viscosity with magnetic fields," Phys. Rev. E 84, 011905 – Published 12 July 2011.

[28] Hans-Christoph Diener et al., Dabigatran for Prevention of Stroke after Embolic Stroke of Undetermined Source, N Engl J Med (2019).

[29] Amanda Fernandes, "Doctor, Should I Keep Taking an Aspirin a Day?" N Engl J Med (2019).

[30] Sharonne N. Hayes et al., Spontaneous Coronary Artery Dissection: Current State of the Science: A Scientific Statement From

the American Heart Association, Circulation. (2018).

[31] Deepanjali Pant, Krishan Kumar Narani, and Jayashree Sood, Significant air embolism: A possibility even with collapsible intravenous fluid containers when used with rapid infuser system, Indian J Anaesth. 2010 Jan-Feb; 54(1).

[32] Firas F.Mussa et al., Acute Aortic Dissection and Intramural Hematoma, A Systematic Review, JAMA, (2016).

[33] Lindsay, M. E., & Dietz, H. C. (2011). Lessons on the pathogenesis of aneurysm from heritable conditions. Nature, 473(7347), 308-316.

[34] Jesse F. Veenis, et al., Treatment Differences in Chronic Heart Failure Patients With Reduced Ejection Fraction According to Blood Pressure, Circulation: Heart FailureVol.13,No.5, May2020.

[35] ESC Guidance for the Diagnosis and Management of CV Disease during the COVID-19 Pandemic, https://www.escardio.org/Education/COVID-19-and-Cardiology/ESC-COVID-19-Guidance.

[36] Gheorghiade, M. Acute heart failure syndromes. BMC Pharmacol 9, S13 (2009).

[37] Tirfe, M., et al. Treatment outcome and its predictors among patients of acute heart failure at a tertiary care hospital in Ethiopia: a prospective observational study. BMC Cardiovasc Disord 20, 16 (2020).

[38] Ferreira, J.P., et al. Alogliptin after acute coronary syndrome in patients with type 2 diabetes: a renal function stratified analysis of the EXAMINE trial. BMC Med 18, 165 (2020).

[39] Baumgartner, J., Brauer, M. & Ezzati, M. The role of cities in reducing the cardiovascular impacts of environmental pollution in low- and middle-income countries. BMC Med 18, 39 (2020).

[40] Krittanawong, C., Rogers, A.J., Johnson, K.W. et al. Integration of novel monitoring devices with machine learning technology for scalable cardiovascular management.Nat Rev Cardiol (2020).

[41] Gaba, P., Gersh, B.J., Ali, Z.A. et al. Complete versus incomplete coronary revascularization: definitions, assessment and outcomes. Nat Rev Cardiol (2020).

[42] Heusch, G. Myocardial ischaemia–reperfusion injury and cardioprotection in perspective. Nat Rev Cardiol (2020).

[43] Adamo, L., et al. (2020). Reappraising the role of inflammation in heart failure. Nature Reviews Cardiology.

[44] Rosenbaum, A.N., Agre, K.E. & Pereira, N.L. Genetics of dilated cardiomyopathy: practical implications for heart failure management. Nat Rev Cardiol 17, 286-297 (2020).

[45] Ferrari, R., Fox, K. Heart rate reduction in coronary artery disease and heart failure. Nat Rev Cardiol 13, 493-501 (2016).

[46] Turk-Adawi, et al. Cardiovascular disease in the Eastern Mediterranean region: epidemiology and risk factor burden. Nat Rev Cardiol 15, 106-119 (2018).

[47] V.R.Sanal Kumar, Shiv Kumar Choudhary, Pradeep Kumar Radhakrishnan, Bharath R.S, Nichith C, C.Oommen, Vigneshwaran Sankar, Ajith Sukumaran, Amrith M, Thianesh U.K, Deviparameswari K, "Nanofluid Flow Choking and Spaceflight Effects on Cardiovascular Risk of Astronauts – A New Perspective," the 2021 AIAA SciTech Forum, 11-15 Jan 2021.

[48] Michael D. Delp, Apollo Lunar Astronauts Show Higher Cardiovascular Disease Mortality: Possible Deep Space Radiation Effects on the Vascular Endothelium, Scientific Reports, **2016**, 6:29901.

[49] K. Marshall-Goebel, et al. Assessment of Jugular Venous Blood Flow Stasis and Thrombosis During Spaceflight, JAMA Network Open, 2(11), 2019.

[50] V R S. Kumar, S.K.Choudhary, P.K.Radhakrishnan, Suresh Menon, Vrishank Raghav, K.K.N Namboodiri, Sapna E.Sreedharan, Bharath R.S, Nichith C, C.Oommen, V.Sankar, A.Sukumaran, Arun K, A.Pal, Tharikaa R.K, Abhirami R., “Lopsided Blood-thinning Drug Increases The Risk Of Internal Flow Choking And Shock Wave Generation Causing Asymptomatic Stroke,” International Stroke Conference, 17-19 March, 2021, American Stroke Association.